THE BIOLOGY AND TREATMENT OF CANCER

Understanding Cancer

Arthur B. Pardee

Department of Biological Chemistry
Harvard University
Dana-Farber Cancer Institute

Gary S. Stein

Department of Cell Biology
University of Massachusetts Medical School
and UMASS Memorial Cancer Center

⟨JW⟩WILEY-BLACKWELL

A JOHN WILEY & SONS, INC., PUBLICATION

Published by John Wiley & Sons, Inc., Hoboken, New Jersey
Published simultaneously in Canada

Wiley-Blackwell is an imprint of John Wiley & Sons, formed by the merger of Wiley's global Scientific, Technical, and Medical business with Blackwell Publishing.

For general information on our other products and services or for technical support, please contact our Customer Care Department within the United States at 877-762-2974, outside the United States at 317-572-3993 or fax 317-572-4002.

Wiley also publishes its books in a variety of electronic formats. Some content that appears in print may not be available in electronic formats. For more information about Wiley products, visit our web site at www.wiley.com.

Library of Congress Cataloging-in-Publication Data:

Pardee, Arthur B. (Arthur Beck), 1921–
     The biology and treatment of cancer : understanding cancer / Arthur B.
Pardee, Gary S. Stein.
       p. cm.
     ISBN 978-0-470-00958-1 (pbk.)
   1. Cancer – Popular works.   2. Cancer – Treatment – Popular works.   I.
Stein, Gary S. II. Title.
     RC263.P276 2006
     616.99′4 /dc22
                                                        2008001368

Printed in the United States of America

10 9 8 7 6 5 4 3 2 1

THE BIOLOGY AND TREATMENT OF CANCER

CONTENTS

CONTRIBUTORS

Rami I. Aqeilan, Department of Molecular Virology, Immunology, and Medical Genetics, Division of Human Cancer Genetics and Comprehensive Cancer Care, Ohio State University, Columbus, Ohio

Elizabeth A. Bronstein, UMASS Memorial Cancer Center, University of Massachusetts Medical School, Worcester, Massachusetts

Carlo M. Croce, Department of Molecular Virology, Immunology, and Medical Genetics, Division of Human Cancer Genetics and Comprehensive Cancer Care, Ohio State University, Columbus, Ohio

Michael W. Deininger, Oregon Health & Science University, Center for Hematologic Malignancies, Portland, Oregon

Konstantin H. Dragnev, Norris Cotton Cancer Center, Darthmouth-Hitchcock Medical Center, Lebanon, New Hampshire

Eleni Efstathiou, Department of Genitourinary Medical Oncology, M.D. Anderson Cancer Center, University of Texas, Houston, Texas

Christopher A. Eide, Howard Hughes Medical Institute, Oregon Health & Science University, Cancer Institute, Portland, Oregon

Otto S. Gildemeister, Department of Biochemistry and Molecular Parmacology, University of Massachusetts Medical School, Worcester, Massachusetts

James R. Hebert, Department of Epidemiology and Biostatistics, Arnold School of Public Health, South Carolina Statewide Cancer Prevention and Control Program, University of South Carolina, Columbia, South Carolina

Mark A. Israel, Norris Cotton Cancer Center, Darthmouth–Hitchcock Medical Center, Lebanon, New Hampshere

Khandan Keyomarsi, Department of Experimental Radiation Oncology, M.D. Anderson Cancer Center, University of Texas, Houston, Texas

Kendall L. Knight, Department of Biochemistry and Molecular Pharmacology, University of Massachusetts Medical School, Worcester, Massachusetts

Barry S. Komm, Wyeth Research, Collegeville, Pennsylvania

Donald H. Lambert, Department of Anesthesia, Boston University Medical School, Boston Medical Center, Boston, Massachusetts

Laura A. Lambert, Department of Surgical Oncology, M.D. Anderson Cancer Center, University of Texas, Houston, Texas.

Peng Liang, Vanderbilt–Ingram Cancer Center, Vanderbilt University, Nashville, Tennessee

Christopher J. Logothetis, Department of Genitourinary Medical Oncology, M.D. Anderson Cancer Center, University of Texas, Houston, Texas

Christopher P. Miller, Radius Health, Cambridge, Massachusetts

Catherine N. Norton, MBLWHO1 Library, Marine Biological Laboratory, Woods Hole, Massachusetts

Thomas O'Hare, Howard Hughes Medical Institute, Oregon Health & Science University Cancer Institute, Portland, Oregon

Arthur B. Pardee, Harvard Medical School, Dana–Farber Cancer Institute, 44 Binney Street, Boston, Massachusetts

Kenneth J. Pienta, Internal Medicine and Urology Departments, University of Michigan Comprehensive Cancer Center, Ann Arbor, Michigan

Alan Rosmarin, Division of Hematology/Oncology and UMASS Memorial Cancer Center, University of Massachusetts Medical School, Worcester, Massachusetts

Jay M. Sage, Department of Biochemistry and Molecular Pharmacology, University of Massachusetts Medical School, Worcester, Massachusetts

David Shepro, Biology Department, Boston University, Boston, Massachusetts and Marine Biological Laboratory, Woods Hole, Massachusetts

Gary S. Stein, UMASS Memorial Cancer Center, University of Massachusetts Medical School, Worcester, Massachusetts

F. Marc Stewart, Seattle Cancer Care Alliance, Fred Hutchinson Cancer Research Center, University of Washington, Seattle, Washington

Jessica A. Stewart, Seattle Cancer Care Alliance, Fred Hutchinson Cancer Research Center, University of Washington, Seattle, Washington

Nicola Zanesi, Department of Molecular Virology, Immunology, and Medical Genetics, Division of Human Caner Genetics and Comprehensive Cancer Care, Ohio State University, Columbus, Ohio

PREFACE

We and our families and friends, like too many others, have experienced cancers of various kinds. Some patients recovered, but sadly, many died. From these trying events and from our professional studies as cancer researchers, we decided that a source which briefly summarizes our current knowledge about cancer and its treatment in nontechnical language would be useful. We hope to provide explanations of cancer treatment and biology that are meaningful to cancer patients and their families. It is intended for an informed audience who are interested in learning about cancer and who are not specialists. We acknowledge a forerunner with this theme, John Cairns' *Cancer Science and Society*, published in 1978 by W.H. Freeman and Company, San Francisco.

This book is developed to explain the nature of the disease, current options for treatment, and emerging strategies for cancer detection and therapy, as provided from clinical experience and by spectacular advances in our understanding of cells, genes, and molecular biology. Insights have been gained into fundamental regulatory mechanisms that are faulty in cancers and that reveal prospects for new treatments.

The presentations are not encyclopedic. We cannot do better than to paraphrase the preface of *The Evolution of Physics* (1938) by Albert Einstein and Leopold Infeld, a book on an even more difficult subject. "We have not a written a textbook of physics. Our intention was rather to sketch in broad outline the attempts of the human mind to find connections. But our presentation had to be simple. Through the maze of facts and concepts we had to choose some highways. Some essential lines of thought have been left out because they do not lie along the road we have chosen."

Arthur B. Pardee

Gary S. Stein

I

INTRODUCTION

1

WHAT GOES WRONG IN CANCER

Arthur B. Pardee

Harvard Medical School, Dana-Farber Cancer Institute,
Boston, Massachusetts

Gary S. Stein and Elizabeth A. Bronstein

UMASS Memorial Cancer Center, University of Massachusetts
Medical School, Worcester, Massachusetts

INTRODUCTION

In this chapter we give a brief overview of current ideas about the biology of cancer. We paint with a broad brush and illustrate what goes wrong, using as examples some of the disease's more dramatic and central processes. We then summarize newer genetic and biochemical information and how it is being used in treatment. These ideas are discussed in more detail in later chapters.

THE DISEASE

About a third of humans develop cancer in a lifetime. Cancer starts as an abnormal cell which grows with time into a mass of cells, some of which can spread to other

The Biology and Treatment of Cancer: Understanding Cancer
Edited by Arthur B. Pardee and Gary S. Stein   Copyright © 2009 John Wiley & Sons, Inc.

locations in the body (*metastasize*), where they grow and upset normal bodily functions. It is one of the most frequent causes of human death. The rate of death varies greatly for different types of cancer. Lung and pancreatic cancer are the worst, usually fatal within a year. But not all cancers are fatal: Only one-fifth of breast cases result in death. Successful treatments utilize surgery, radiation, drugs, and immunology.

Cancer is a complicated set of diseases. About 200 varieties have been described, whose properties and treatments are different. There are three main types. *Carcinomas* (90%) are solid cancers (e.g., solid tumors) that arise from the epithelial cells that cover our inner and outer surfaces. *Sarcomas* are solid cancers developed from the connective tissue cells that form body structures such as muscle and bone. *Leukemias* and *lymphomas* are cancers of white blood cells. Leukemias of early childhood differ from adult leukemias in their properties and treatments. Cancers are named according to the organ from which they came. Retinoblastoma is mainly a cancer of the eye, osteosarcoma of bone, and melanoma of skin pigment cells. Lung, colon, prostate, and breast cancers are the most common.

Frequencies of various cancers vary greatly between countries. These differences are not inherited but are environmental; second-generation Japanese in California have a tenfold higher death rate from prostate cancer than do Japanese in Japan. Studies of population environments reveal carcinogenic agents: for example, particular diets high in calories, fat, and meat are bad, and diets high in fibers and fruits are good. Colon cancer is tenfold higher in women from countries in which high quantities of meat ($\frac{1}{2}$ pound per day) are eaten. Japanese have a high level of stomach cancer, related to the fern fronds that they eat. Lung cancer correlates with increased smoking; it is five times higher in Britain than in Norway, where only one-fourth as many cigarettes are smoked per person. It increased in men about 15-fold since 1930, when smoking became prevalent, but increased much later in women. Skin cancer develops based on excessive exposure to sunlight, especially for races with light skin pigmentation. The probability of getting cancer can be decreased by avoiding smoking, a high-meat diet, and excessive sun exposure. Leukemias are frequently developed following exposure to radiation.

GENES, MUTATIONS, AND CANCER

These connections with environmental factors suggest that some cancers could originate from agents that change a cell's genetic material (mutation). Each of the more than 100 trillion cells in a human body carries its genetic information in *deoxyribonucleic acid* (DNA), composed of long double-helical strands (see Figure 2) made of sequences of four building blocks (bases) linked in pairs. It is packaged in 23 pairs of chromosomes which can be seen with a microscope. The DNA in each cell carries information equal to the letters in 600 encyclopedia volumes. *Genes* are sequences of DNA that code for individual proteins.

Mutations are errors in DNA structure that alter this genetic information. Most mutations arise spontaneously, possibly from mistakes that arise while DNA duplicates during cell growth. Experiments have shown that foods contain many chemicals that cause carcinogenic damage to DNA. Errors can also be produced by damage from toxic chemicals (*carcinogens*) or radiation. Cell growth is stopped when molecular mechanisms termed *checkpoints* sense the damage, recruit the molecules to rectify the problem, and give time for corrections to be made. Then enzymes for repair are activated, and the cell may recover if the damage was not too severe. Genes designated *BRCA1* and *BRCA2* are involved in DNA repair and are mutated in some breast and ovarian cancers. The inability to repair damaged DNA may result in cancer.

Visible changes in the structure of chromosomes in cancer cells provide direct evidence for the genetic basis of cancer. Rearrangements at many definite positions have been observed repeatedly in many types of cancers (Figure 1). At the molecular level are found miscoding changes, including substitutions, deletions, duplications, and rearrangements of DNA building blocks. For example, in a recent study of breast and colon cancers, 189 genes (average 11 per tumor) were frequently found to be mutated. In several cancers, mutations change the functioning of genes located at their positions. DNA is often altered in human chromosome 6 at position p21, where the cancer-related K-*ras oncogene*, a gene that may modify cell growth aberrantly and lead to cancer, is located. Additional copies of a particular gene make a cell resistant to the anticancer drug methotrexate. Rare cancers are produced by virus infection; for example, introduction of genetic material by the human papilloma virus causes cervical cancers. This provides further evidence for the genetic basis of cancer.

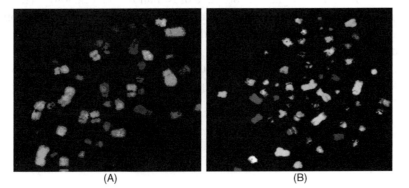

(A)   (B)

Figure 1. Cancer-related chromosomal aberrations. In early stages of cancer, chromosomes break and join with segments of other chromosomes that are not adjacent in normal cells (chromosomal translocations). As a consequence, genes that control cell growth and specialized properties of cells are frequently rearranged. Other cancer-related alterations that result from reorganization are in cell adhesion and motility as well as in capacity to invade and grow in tissues at distant sites from the initial tumor (metastasis). (A) normal chromosomes (note that each chromosome is a single color); (B) chromosomes in cancer cells that contain fused segments of multiple chromosomes (note multicolored chromosomes). (See insert for color representation.)

Some people who are related genetically carry a DNA defect that might cause a relatively rare inherited cancer, of which there are about 30 types. Seven percent of breast and ovarian cancers are hereditary; mutations of breast cancer–associated genes (BRCAs) are a common cause (50%). The hereditary autosomal polyposis gene (APC) causes growths (polyps) in the colon that develop into cancers. Spontaneous mutations of APCs are also found in nonhereditary cancers. Prostate cancer is more frequent in persons descended from Africans, whose sequence of a gene that involves the male hormone differs from that of Europeans.

A *tumor* is an excessive localized growth of cells which is usually not fatal if detected early and immediately treated. But many of its properties progress from bad to worse with time, from a series of mutations followed by selection of those multimutated cells that grow faster; hence, it develops into a mass of differently mutated cells. This multiple-step process must alter perhaps a half-dozen genes to produce a clinical cancer. Furthermore, mutational "hits" on both of a pair of genes are usually necessary for a biological effect, because one mutation can be masked by functioning of the nonmutated partner. In cases of such multiple hits, cells can lose control of their growth and their ability to develop into specialized cells (to *differentiate*). The consequences of mutations that set the stage for metastasis are particularly devastating. Tumors become lethal (*malignant*) cancers that spread to other locations in the body (metastasis), where their cells interfere with normal body functions. They can also release molecules that modify other cells. Metastasis causes 90% of cancer deaths.

After a tumor is initiated, it can take 20 to 30 years to become clinically apparent. Accumulation of all the mutations takes time, so human cancers can develop over decades. Cancer deaths increase dramatically (exponentially) with age; they are five times higher for 80-year-olds than for 50-year-olds. The normal mutation rate is not high enough to produce the several required mutations in a lifetime in even one of a person's 100 trillion cells. Some mutations can speed up the mutational process 25-fold or so. This accelerated mutation rate creates genetic instability, due to inactivation of DNA repair genes or changes at the ends (*telomeres*) of chromosomes that prevent their proper separation between cells at division.

CANCER CELL BIOLOGY

Cells are the units of life. Normal cells act on each other to control their growth and other properties in balance with the entire organism. They are closely regulated by a variety of genetic and biochemical processes. For example, biological feedbacks act in much the same way that a thermostat controls heat production by a furnace. Cancer is a disease of "outlaw" cells, cells that have lost their normal relationship to the whole organism. A tumor originates when single normal cells mutate and develop into cancer cells, termed *transformed cells*. Mutations produce defects in their cellular regulatory mechanisms, changing their biochemistry and biology so that they differ from normal cells in structure and functioning and grow at the wrong times and in the wrong places (Figure 2).

Briefly, each cell is surrounded by a membrane that separates it from its surroundings, which include other cells, nutrients, and molecules that regulate growth and other functions. Within the cell is a fluid, *cytoplasm*, containing proteins and structures, including mitochondria (the source of energy for a cell), that produce chemical energy and the machinery (ribosomes) that synthesizes proteins. The nucleus, which contains the genetic material, sits in the middle of the cell. Location within a cell can determine a molecule's possible biochemical interactions and effects. Cells of cancers develop into disorganized arrangements, and their nuclear shapes are abnormal, properties that are scrutinized carefully during diagnosis and are used to classify the *stage* of a cancer.

Regulatory machinery in the cells is organized architecturally within the nucleus and cytoplasm as well as in the plasma membrane that surrounds the cell and in the nuclear membrane that separates the nucleus from the cytoplasm (Figure 2). Solid tumors, leukemias, and lymphomas exhibit striking changes in cell and tissue structure that are linked to the onset and progression of cancer. Modifications occur in the cell size and shape; in the compartmentalization (packaging/location) of factors that control gene expression, replication, repair, protein synthesis, and exchange of regulatory signals; and in the representation and organization of cells within tumors.

General and tumor-type specific modifications in nuclear organization are long-standing indications of cancer. Many cancers have alterations in the number and composition of *nucleoli* (see the small orange spheres in the cell nucleus in Figure 2), the focal sites within the cell nucleus for ribosomal gene expression that supports protein synthesis. Chromosomal rearrangements are prevalent in cancer. Modifications in plasma membrane–associated receptors modify responses of the tumor cell to growth factors. Changes in *integrins*, molecules that mediate communication between the extracellular environment and the cytoplasm within a cancer cell, influence the transmission of information (Figure 3). Cancer-related alterations occur in the exchange of signals between the cell nucleus and cytoplasm, which are critical for control of cell regulatory machinery. These changes provide insight into cellular and molecular parameters of cancer that facilitate tumor diagnosis and are targets for therapy. Effects of mutation that are found in most cancer cells are failures of molecular mechanisms that limit growth and differentiation into specialized cells, causing their death (apoptosis), their movement out of the tumor (metastasis), and the activation of a blood supply, which is required to feed the tumor (angiogenesis).

Normal cells of an adult animal usually are not growing. They can be stimulated to increase in number (proliferate) upon changes in external conditions such as increased concentration of growth factor proteins or hormones, or elimination of contacting cells through death or by wounding. A single cell must double all its parts and divide to produce two daughter cells. This is a sequence of events termed

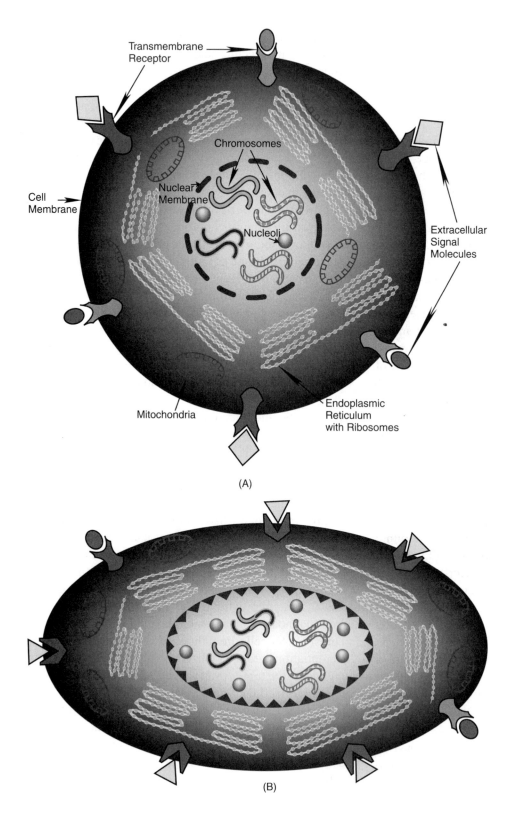

the *cell cycle* (Figure 4). It is similar in content and timing for normal and cancer cells. This process is repeated many times to produce the many cells of an organism. Cancers grow because they can initiate their cell cycles independent of external growth factors and inhibitions by contacting cells, or they are stimulated by their mutated internal machinery. Elimination by mutation or inactivation of inhibitory tumor suppressors (such as the retinoblastoma protein) releases constraints on proliferation, and control of cell division is lost (see below). Dozens of these genes are misregulated in cancers.

Stem cells are *multipotential* in nature. They can develop into *any* type of tissue (differentiate) and thereby create various tissues and eventually "build" organs such as muscle, liver, or blood. The differentiated cells function in specialized ways, and most of them stop growing. Stem cells fail to stop dividing. Tumors contain immature cells that exhibit differentiation failures. Such a rare defectively differentiated subset of stem cells in tissues has been proposed as the origin of tumor cells. An example is acute promyelocytic leukemia, where stem cells have been blocked from achieving differentiation.

Normal cells can stop growing permanently, a process of arrest that is designated cell *senescence*. Cells survive for varying lengths of times. At one extreme, brain cells might last a lifetime, but white cells in blood survive for only about two months. Cancer cells, in contrast, are immortalized and have an unlimited potential to proliferate. This indefinite proliferation requires activity of *telomerase*, an enzyme that at each cycle of the cell adds back DNA sequences of telomeres to the ends of chromosomes. Telomerase is active in malignant cancer cells but not in normal cells.

Cells sense defects in their functioning, which causes them to commit suicide, called programmed cell death or *apoptosis*, thereby removing defective cells. In fact, many cells of a tumor die spontaneously; the tumor's size increases because proliferation exceeds death. Cancer cells very often become mutated to decrease apoptosis. The p53 tumor suppressor gene is the most often altered growth regulatory gene in cancers. Because the p53 gene is central to activating apoptosis, it has been called the guardian of the genome. Again, in this struggle for survival the cancer cells that resist apoptosis are selected; they have an advantage for

---

Figure 2. Structure and organization of regulatory machinery in (A) normal and (B) cancer cells. The organization and location of machinery that controls genes is modified during the onset and progression of cancer. The transition from a round or cuboidal to an elongated cell is characteristic of early-stage tumors. Changes that are frequently observed in tumor cells are in the cell membrane, receptors for transduction of signals from the outside to the inside of the cell (the cell's communication system), exchange of chromosome segments, and an increased number of nucleoli which support synthesis of proteins. Often, the nuclear membrane that controls exchange of information between the cell nucleus and cytoplasm is modified (see the purple dashed-line circle surrounding the center of the "normal cell"). These changes in cell structure and location of genes and regulatory molecules result in the development and spread of cancer. The altered organization of the cell's regulatory machinery is important for cancer diagnosis and provides targets for treatment. (See insert for color representation.)

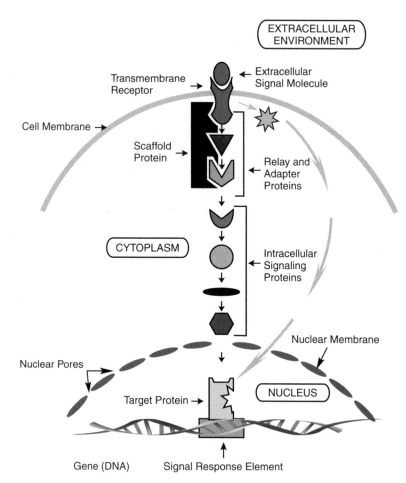

Figure 3. Cell signaling. Cells communicate and respond to the extracellular environment through a process designated *signal transduction*. Signal molecules bind to transmembrane receptors that span the cell membrane. The interaction of signal molecules with components of receptors located outside the cell modifies the intracellular components of the receptors. An environmental signal is thereby transduced into a cascade of regulatory steps that control genes which control cell proliferation and specialized properties of cells.

   In some signaling pathways, scaffold proteins assemble signaling molecules into complexes for the initial passage of information from the transmembrane receptor to relay and adaptor proteins. Subsequent steps in the signaling process amplify and integrate signals. A chain of intracellular signaling proteins processes regulatory information through the cytoplasm and into the cell nucleus to activate or suppress genes. In other signaling pathways the regulatory cascades are abbreviated. The transduction of regulatory information from the intracellular component of the transmembrane receptor is more direct, circumventing intermediary steps in information transfer. At an early stage in the signaling process a signaling protein enters the nucleus and interacts directly with genes to modify expression.

   Many cancer cells exhibit defects in one or more steps of signaling cascades that alter control of cell growth, specialized cell properties, cell–cell communication, cell motility, and cell adhesion. The components of signaling pathways that are modified in tumor cells are targets for treatments that are effective and specific. (See insert for color representation.)

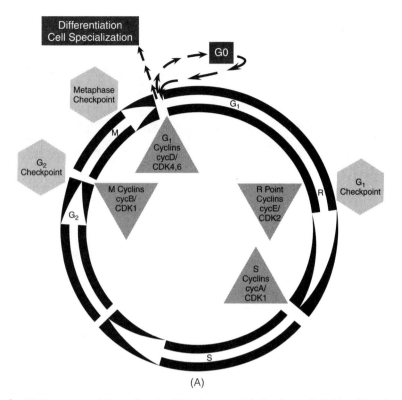

(A)

Figure 4. (A) The stages of the cell cycle. G1 is the period following cell division (M; mitosis) and precedes the S phase, the period when genes (DNA) are duplicated to provide an identical set of genes for progeny cells. Following gene duplication, the G2 period provides the cell time to prepare for cell division. The cell is regulated by cyclins (cys) and cyclin-dependent kinases (cdk) that regulate genes during each period. Early G1 is controlled by cyclin D, cdk4, and cdk6. At the restriction point (R point) late in G1, competency for gene replication and cell cycle progression is established. Control is by cyclin E and cdk2. During the S phase and into mitosis, control is by cyclin A and cdk1. During mitosis, control is by cyclin B and cdk1.

Checkpoints at three strategic locations during the cell cycle provide surveillance for effectiveness of the process. Progression of the cell cycle occurs only if fidelity of control is confirmed. The cell cycle is delayed or terminates if problems are encountered that cannot be corrected. The G1 checkpoint assesses DNA damage by chemicals or radiation and monitors adequacy of conditions to support DNA synthesis (gene duplication) and permits entry into the S phase. The G2 checkpoint determines that DNA replication has occurred after DNA is damaged and permits entry into mitosis. The metaphase checkpoint assures that chromosomes are attached to the mitotic spindle, the apparatus for distribution of genes to progeny cells during mitotic division.

(B) The stages of mitosis, the process of cell division. During prophase, the initial stage of mitosis, DNA in the nucleus (2 yards of DNA in each nucleus) is organized into chromosomes (two sets of 23 chromosomes in every human cell). The chromosomes attach to the spindle and at the completion of prophase, the membrane surrounding the nucleus disassembles. During metaphase the chromosomes attach to the mitotic spindle and align in the center of the cell. During anaphase the chromosomes move along the spindle fibers to the opposite poles of the cell. Identical sets of chromosomes (genes) are distributed to progeny cells that will be formed at the completion of cell division. Telophase, the last phase of mitosis (cell division), is initiated when the chromosomes reach the poles. The compact chromosomes now begin to disassemble. A cleavage furrow forms and deepens, culminating in the formation of two cells, each genetically, structurally, and functionally equivalent to the parent cell. (See insert for color representation.)

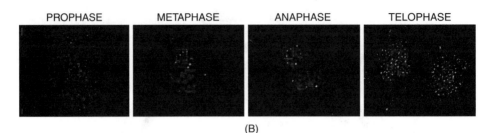

(B)

Figure 4. (*Continued*)

survival in the tumor environment. As an example, prostate cells undergo apoptosis if androgen (male sex hormone) is lowered. Prostate cancers that lose androgen dependence develop resistance to apoptosis.

Metastasis, which causes 90% of cancer deaths, makes surgery and radiation far less effective, because these treatments are local. Advanced cancers whose cells have undergone many different mutations develop metastases. A cell loses control of proliferation and multiplies into a primary tumor mass. Then additional mutations produce cells that escape and move through the blood or lymphatic system to other places in the body. The biology of metastasis is complex and is incompletely understood. Its several steps include increased cell migration, motility, escape into the blood, settling into a new site, and proliferation. Genes and proteins responsible for events of metastasis are being discovered; for example, cell–cell adhesion molecules that facilitate cell–cell interactions have antimetastatic activities. These adhesion molecules are dissolved by enzymes termed *proteases*, which increase in cancers, and their inhibitors are removed. Tumor cells are thereby released and enabled to populate sites that may be considerably distant from the primary tumor. A protein (maspin) that inhibits these proteases is eliminated as breast cancers progress. Metastatic cells may spread only to a specific organ in which normal cells and conditions permit attachment and growth into secondary tumors. For example, prostate cancer cells frequently metastasize to bone. This is the "seed and soil" hypothesis of metastasis, a framework for understanding relationships between the tumor and the tissues at the metastatic site.

Until traveling cancer cells are able to get the food and other molecules needed for growth into large cancers, they remain micrometastases. Once a critical mass of aggregate tumor cells develops in one location, a solid tumor is formed that requires sustenance to survive. *Angiogenesis* is the production by a tumor of a new blood vessel system for the purpose of providing nutrients to the tumor. Therapies for inhibiting angiogenesis are being investigated.

BASIC CANCER RESEARCH

Spectacular advances are being made in understanding mechanisms that self-regulate normal cells and defects in cancer cells. This helps us to understand the initiation and progression of the disease and can provide targets for its treatment. In cancer, there are numerous altered structures, and amounts and degrees of cell functioning of DNA, ribonucleic acid (RNA), and proteins. Mutations can alter a gene's expression of a protein by changing controls, both genetic and biochemical. There may be cancer-related alterations that modify structure and affect the rate of a protein's (or its messenger RNA's) synthesis and degradation, and its characteristics.

Studies with humans have taught us a great deal about cancer. But this research is limited by ethics and by the requirement for immediate surgical removal of the tumor, or chemotherapy or radiation treatment, to optimize survival and quality of life. Therefore, most fundamental research is performed with animals. Among the many living creatures used for cancer research are yeasts, flies, nematode worms, sea urchins, frogs, zebrafish, mice, and rats. Mice are the animals most frequently used for basic studies, including tumor growth, metastasis, and effects of gene modifications and drugs. In these animals, injected cancer cells respond based on interactions with adjacent normal cells. An animal provides comparisons of treatment outcomes as they relate to toxicity and growth within the context of cancer cells and normal cells. Many of the insights into growth control that have come from animal studies translate directly to elucidation of control of proliferation in human cells. Human and animal cancers are similar but of course not identical, so applications to humans have to be tested in human clinical trials. Yeasts have regulatory mechanisms similar to those of human cells and are much easier to investigate genetically. Yeast studies have provided important basic information about cell proliferation.

Much fundamental research is done with cells in culture dishes, in which they can be studied conveniently. In this setting, it is easy to provide or remove molecules, including nutrients, vitamins, inhibitors, and growth factor proteins such as insulin. By comparison, difficulties are encountered with cells in animals because of their internal environment. Normal cell growth and survival require adhesion to a surface (anchorage). Cells increase in number until they cover the surface of the culture dish. When cells come into close contact with neighboring cells, they stop proliferating. This arrest is called *density-dependent growth* or *contact inhibition of growth*. A protein coating can be applied to the culture dish to provide a more natural surface than plastic, to which a set of regulatory proteins located on the cell's surface binds. Three-dimensional culture in protein gels is even more physiological (i.e., more closely represents the three-dimensional environment in the body). In contrast, tumor cells can grow in suspension, without any of the supportive mechanisms required by normal cells.

CANCER MOLECULAR BIOLOGY AND BIOCHEMISTRY

An understanding of functioning at genetic and molecular levels is very important for comprehending the workings of cancer cells and for finding therapeutic *targets*.

Most genes are inactive most of the time. Molecules that enter the cell nucleus can activate specific genes to be copied into messenger RNAs (mRNAs), which act as the working blueprints that determine sequences of the amino acids in proteins. Proteins of many types are the cell's working machinery. These proteins have many functions, including forming structures, transfering nutrients and external signals into cells, activating gene expression, acting as enzymes that speed up biochemical reactions, and performing as regulators of these reactions.

Biochemistry is organized into many sequences of enzyme-catalyzed reactions, which can produce and degrade molecules and provide energy. These reactions are tightly regulated, primarily through molecules that bind to enzymes. For example, inhibitors are small molecules that can attach loosely to enzymes and decrease their activities. A very important component of regulation is the chemical attachment of a phosphate group to a protein; this can increase or decrease an enzyme's activity, affecting its location and even its degradation. These reactions are catalyzed by a set of enzymes called *kinases*, hundreds of which target different proteins. Kinases are balanced by *phosphatases*, enzymes that remove phosphates from proteins. For example, PI3K kinase is countered by PTEN phosphatase, a tumor suppressor which when lost frequently causes cancer and activates tumor progression.

Cell proliferation usually starts with binding of external molecules to receptors of the cell. For example, estrogen binding turns on expression of genes that release normal breast and ovarian cells from the nondividing "quiescent" state. Excessive estrogen receptors overactivate proliferation in 70% of breast cancers. Chemicals such as tamoxifen, used for breast cancer therapy, compete with estrogen for this binding. Cell proliferation can also be initiated by proteins called growth factors that bind to their receptors on the cell surface. Epidermal growth factor proteins activate excessive receptors on many breast cancers. These are more aggressive and more difficult to treat than are those activated by estrogen. Drugs and antibodies that block this interaction are being used clinically. An example is the antibody herceptin (Trastuzumab), which decreases by half the risk of reappearance of hormone-independent breast cancer.

Activating signals must pass through the cell's cytoplasm and into the nucleus within the cell, where genes are located. Molecular signals convey regulatory information into and out of cells as well as between cells. There are three major signaling pathways, each composed of a cascade of kinase reactions that move and amplify signals (Figure 3). Various mutant genes in cancers turn on these processes. Changes in the multiple steps in signaling cascades often occur during the onset and progression of cancer, providing options for cancer detection and are also targets for treatment.

Of primary interest to cancer research is the cycle of events during a cell's duplication (Figure 4). A growing cell can pass though the cell cycle in a day or so to produce two daughter cells. At different times during this cycle all components of the cell must be duplicated. DNA is duplicated near midcycle, which divides the cycle into four biochemically different phases (G1, S, G2, and M), followed by division.

In the initial phase (G1) of the cell cycle, molecular machinery for DNA synthesis is produced and activated. The regulating circuitry is complicated; details are discussed in later chapters. Briefly, *cyclins*, a series of short-lived proteins that increase and then decrease at definite times in the cell cycle, are central to regulating all stages of cell proliferation. Their defects are important in cancer. Cyclin D1, which appears early in the G1 phase of the cell cycle, activates a cyclin-dependent kinase (Cdk) that adds phosphate molecules to proteins that control progression through the cell cycle. It is overexpressed in many types of human tumors (e.g., 50% of human breast cancers). This causes contact-independent growth by the cells and thereby increases the risk of early metastasis. Breast cancers that have progressed to overproduce altered cyclin E are no longer responsive to drug treatment. Cyclin A1 activity is a variant form of cyclin A that is elevated in cancer cells but is normally produced only in embryos. Other proteins, such as INK4, inhibit Cdks, are negative regulators of proliferation, and are frequently mutated to be inactive or are lost in cancers.

The *restriction point* is a most critical event for control of the cell cycle. Normal cells in the G1 phase select between continuing to proliferate or returning to quiescence, which depends on whether external conditions are suitable for growth. The cell must accumulate enough of a protein to activate a Cdk that phosphorylates retinoblastoma protein (pRb), a regulatory factor that suppresses cell growth. Thereby, pRb releases the gene-activating protein that is designated E2F-1. Enzymes are then produced that catalyze DNA synthesis. Restriction point control is diminished in cancers, and tumor cells therefore proliferate under conditions that would stop normal cells from dividing. pRb, a principal regulator of growth control, is mutated in the majority of human cancers. Loss of growth regulatory proteins makes the cells insensitive to antigrowth factors and to the requirement for Cdk-cyclins. Under these conditions, the ability of a cell to control proliferation is out of reach.

The second cell cycle phase is S, named for the synthesis of DNA. During this period of the cell cycle, proteins designated *histones* are synthesized to package newly replicated DNA into chromosomes. Then follows the short G2 phase, which is preparatory for the cell to enter mitosis (M phase). In mitosis the duplicated chromosomes are distributed equally to the two progeny cells produced by cell division. Errors of chromosome separation take place in a cancer cell during mitosis and cell division, especially if their DNA has been damaged, which creates further mutations and advances the cancer.

As a summary of self-regulation, a mutation alters the structure of a gene, which can change a regulatory protein and in turn cause the loss of control of cellular processes such as proliferation, leading to cancer. The mutations that cause cancer alter structures and positions of genes controlling biochemical balances in cells. These, in turn, change the amounts and properties of critical regulatory proteins. These proteins are specifically designed to modify the function of an enzyme or another protein involved in cell regulation. Proteins do this by binding to a location of the target protein other than the normal site for activity, thereby changing its structure. Regulation mechanisms are even more complex. The structure and function of an active protein or its regulatory partner are often modified by strong bonding of a small molecule, such as phosphate or acetate, as mentioned above, or by weaker binding of other molecules. Among the most frequently mutated proteins are the cyclins, which activate cyclin-dependent kinases; the retinoblastoma protein, which inactivates protein E2F-1 and thereby disrupts the copying of many genes into their mRNAs; and the p53 protein, which activates the programmed death mechanism, which can eliminate cancer cells.

CHEMOTHERAPY

Surgery is the primary method of treating cancer. For example, the standard for patients with early breast cancer is surgical removal with a wide local margin, followed by x-radiation. Why are they not cured? Surgery can be effective only if the cancer has not already metastasized. A cancer that does not get early treatment is likely to reappear. These procedures are therefore often followed by chemotherapy (often referred to as *adjuvent chemotherapy*). Chemotherapy poses many difficult problems. Anticancer drugs are poisons that must kill most of the cancer cells but also must not kill too many normal cells and thereby the patient. Selection is difficult because the cells are similar. Cells can develop resistance to drugs, so a carefully tested small set of drugs is applied to the tumor, chosen from the several dozen currently available. These drugs must be applied with proper dosage and schedule and be supervised carefully. Illnesses can develop from treatment. Also, not all drugs can help all patients, since each person and each tumor is genetically different. Some cells treated by chemotherapy can survive and grow into drug-resistant cancers. Treatment-related diseases can develop later. Many of the drugs that kill tumors can cause mutations that transform normal cells to cancer. Quality of life for the cancer survivor after completion of treatment is an important consideration. Cancer prevention and reduction in the risk of recurrence can significantly influence the life-threatening consequences of cancer. Ongoing research is determining methods of cancer prevention (e.g., intake of substances such as antioxidants that can prevent cancer or tumor recurrences, management of diet, and use of natural products or synthetic compounds that can decrease the risk of mutations).

Research on drug treatments is a continuous competition of human inventiveness against the constantly changing defenses of cancer cells. Discovery of differences between normal and tumor cells is necessary to provide a selective drug target. A cell is in a dynamic "steady-state" balance between positive and negative control systems, similar to the motor and brakes that control movement of an automobile. These regulatory balances operate at many levels: genetic, biochemical, structural, and cellular. Examples are cell proliferation versus death, oncogenes and tumor suppressor genes, syntheses versus removal of proteins and mRNAs, and kinases versus phosphatases. These complex components of cellular control are different in normal and cancer cells.

The molecular changes that create cancers have been found to provide targets for therapy. This is the Achilles' heel principle: an advantage can create a weakness. A major difference in cancer cells from normal cells is that cancer cells frequently make DNA to support the rapid rate of proliferation. This has provided a therapeutic target for drugs that attack the DNA replication process. These include the DNA building block analogs that disrupt DNA replication (e.g., 5-fluorodeoxyuridine, cytarabine) and inhibitors of DNA synthesis (e.g., methotrexate). Cells in the S phase are more sensitive to therapeutic agents that damage DNA (e.g., radiation, cyclophosphamide, *cis*-platinum). A therapeutic challenge here is that normal blood-forming and intestinal cells also divide frequently, so they too are killed. Destruction of these healthy cells results in side effects from chemotherapy that can cause considerable discomfort for cancer patients undergoing treatment. Another difference between normal and tumor cells may be the inability of tumor cells to repair DNA damage correctly. In this way, cancer cells become mutated. Cancer cells also frequently enter mitosis, and compounds that block mitosis (e.g., taxol, vincristine) preferentially kill them. Hormone-dependent cancer can be treated by decreasing the hormone's level or its activity with a competing compound. But cancer cells can become independent of hormones and resistant to such hormone-based therapies. Another treatment is the application of an antibody that targets a growth factor's receptor on the cell surface, blocking the passage of signals for proliferation, as mentioned above.

New ways to treat cancers are being investigated. Twenty-six drugs were approved by the U.S. Food and Drug Administration in the past decade. Some are based on new knowledge about targets, often discovered in academic centers and in biotechnology companies. Newly developed therapeutic inhibitors are being applied, such as Gleevec, which inhibits the oncogenic growth regulatory factor Abl kinase, which is overexpressed in some cancers. A problem frequently encountered in cancer therapy is low specificity (i.e., the drug targets normal as well as cancer cells). Toxicity to vital organs can result from treatment with such drugs. Other therapeutic targeted drugs are modifications of established compounds. Many are marginally effective, extending life only for months. They might be most effective in combination with a classic generally toxic drug.

Novel targets are being investigated. Several mechanisms are responsible for resistance of cancer cells to apoptosis. Certain drugs can reactivate apoptosis of cancer cells and thereby make them die. For example, proteasomes are large enzymes that degrade proteins, including the p53 tumor suppressor. As a consequence, a reaction is blocked, which prevents the killing of cancer cells. Velcade inhibits proteasomes, which increases p53 tumor suppressor levels and reactivates apoptosis. Velcade is used effectively to treat various cancers, including multiple myeloma.

Expression of genes provides new therapeutic targets. The structure and function of chromatin are altered by attaching acetyl groups to the histone proteins that package genes (DNA) within the nucleus of the cell. For example, the compound SAHA inhibits removal of these acetyl groups, restores differentiation (cell specialization), and inhibits cancers. SAHA has been approved for clinical use. A major development (rewarded by the Nobel Prize in Physiology for 2006) is the discovery of naturally existing small RNA molecules that inhibit expression of specific genes. An exciting possibility is the use of these inhibitory small RNA molecules or related synthetic molecules clinically to block expressions of oncogenes.

Cancer prevention is an active area of investigation to which clinical trials are being applied, especially with persons who are at high risk, those with a premalignant condition, or those who have been treated for an initial cancer. For example, the antiestrogen drug tamoxifen has decreased the incidence of hormone-dependent breast cancer by about 50%. It has not been used widely as a preventive agent for women who are not at high risk because of problematic side effects. Compounds found in plant foods such as green tea are being tested for chemoprevention. Such plant compounds can affect cells by removing or blocking carcinogens. It is important to develop molecular tests to determine the effectiveness of chemoprevention compounds on tumors.

EARLIER DETECTION

There is no substitute for early detection. This is the patient's best opportunity for a competitive advantage against a tumor. Cancers are often detected when the disease has progressed beyond an early stage. Tumors of 100 million cells can be detected clinically, are palpable at 1 billion cells (pea size), and lethal at 1 trillion cells. Physical detection methods include x-rays and computerized tomography (CT) scan. Tumors are more likely to be treated successfully in early stages. This is demonstrated by the Papanicolaou tissue test (Pap smear), which detects early cervical cancer and has saved many lives. Other examples are mammographic breast examination and prostate-specific antigen protein tests (PSA is a protein that appears in the blood of men with prostate cancer, the level of which changes during treatment and recurrence). Methods for earlier detection of most cancers are being developed. These methods are based on detecting molecular markers such as changed DNA, mRNAs, or proteins and identifying them in tissues, blood, and other body fluids. An example is the detection of excess or structurally altered cyclin E protein, which controls cell growth during breast cancer progression and correlates with unsuccessful treatment. Simultaneous assessment of dozens or even hundreds of frequently altered biomarkers that provide a "signature" for a tumor will be needed. The sensitivity of these tests must be sufficient to reveal the few cancer cells among many normal cells.

SUMMARY

Cell growth and death are closely regulated by special mechanisms. The controlling molecules are specialized and are additional to a cell's functional molecules. A variety of these molecules act at multiple molecular levels to keep normal cells in balance metabolically. Cancer arises from mutations that damage these mechanisms and thereby allow cells to multiply when and where they should not. Solid cancers, leukemias, lymphomas, and myelomas exhibit changes in cell size and shape, ability to grow, compartmentalization of regulatory machinery, and competency for motility. Metastatic cancer cells result, which can be lethal. Intense scrutiny of the differences between normal and cancer cells provides targets for therapy.

Acknowledgment

The authors are appreciative of the artistic assistance of Priscilla Vazquez for her creation of Figures 2, 3, and 4.

DETAILED REVIEWS OF MATERIAL IN THIS CHAPTER

Bertino J, ed. 2002. *Encyclopedia of Cancer*, 2nd ed. Amsterdam: Academic Press.
Stein GS, Pardee AB, eds. 2004. *Cell Cycle and Growth Control*, 2nd ed. Hoboken, NJ: Wiley-Liss.
Weinberg RA. 2006. *The Biology of Cancer.* New York: Garland Sciences.

SOURCES OF FURTHER INFORMATION

National Institutes of Health website
PubMed (http://www.ncbi.nlm.nih.gov/entrez), especially for searches on reviews and key word combinations
Local libraries
Yellow Pages under "Social Services and Health Agencies"
Cancer Information Service Hotline, 1-800-4-CANCER. National Cancer Institute, Building 31, Bethesda MD 20892
American Cancer Society, 1-800-ACS-2345. 1599 Clifton Rd. N.E., Atlanta, GA 30329.

II

CLINICAL PERSPECTIVE

2

CANCER AS A DISEASE: TYPES OF TUMORS, THEIR FREQUENCIES, AND THEIR PROGRESSION

Kenneth J. Pienta

Internal Medicine and Urology Departments, University of Michigan Comprehensive Cancer Center, Ann Arbor, Michigan

HOW CANCERS FORM

The disease *cancer* refers to the process by which genetic mutations accumulate in normal cells such that they exhibit uncontrolled growth. Virtually every cell type in the body has the capacity to accumulate mutations and become a tumor. The process by which a normal cell becomes a tumor is referred to as *carcinogenesis* or *tumorigenesis*. If the tumor has the ability to spread (metastasize) from its site of origin (the primary), it is considered to be malignant.

In the simplest terms, cancer is the result of deoxyribonucleic acid (DNA) damage that occurs in a normal cell and leads toward a growth and survival advantage [1–3] (Figure 1). A mutation to the DNA must occur in a place where it (1) does not lead to the death of the cell, (2) does not occur in a sequence of DNA that does not change behavior, and (3) occurs in a place that conveys a growth or survival advantage. Meaningful DNA damage is the result of gene–environment interactions on multiple levels. First, cells may inherit "susceptibility" for damage from parental genes. This can be at a very recognizable and measurable level: for example, a damaged DNA repair enzyme in Li–Fraumeni syndrome, a

The Biology and Treatment of Cancer: Understanding Cancer
Edited by Arthur B. Pardee and Gary S. Stein   Copyright © 2009 John Wiley & Sons, Inc.

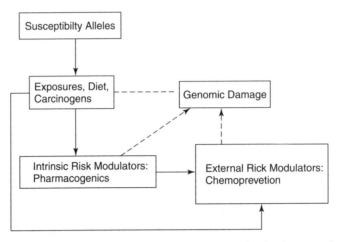

Figure 1. Cancer is a result of gene–environment interactions that lead to genetic mutations in pieces of DNA that lead to survival advantage. Every person inherits a different set of genes from their parents. Some of these genes carry with them an inherent risk or susceptibility to cancer. On this genetic background, we are exposed to multiple different carcinogens in the form of diet, infections, chemicals, radiation, and so on. These exposures are processed by the body to varying extents. The carcinogen can cause DNA damage directly, or its risk may be modulated by intrinsic modulators. For example, each person processes the chemicals in tobacco smoke differently based on the genetic doses of modifying enzymes. In addition, the relative risk of exposures can be altered by extrinsic modulators, such as the antioxidants found in chemoprevention agents. Finally, the damaging factor must mutate a relevant part of the DNA. Many mutations occur in sequences of DNA that do not provide a survival advantage, but rather, in survival-neutral or deleterious genome sequences.

syndrome that makes people more susceptible to developing multiple cancers, or the inheritance of the gene *BRCA1*, which makes women more susceptible to developing breast and ovarian cancers [4,5]. On this inherited genetic background, the cells are assaulted by a variety of gene-damaging exposures, including radiation, viruses, microbes, carcinogens, chemicals, and hormones, as well as the free radicals that are by-products of normal cellular processes that accumulate with age. These DNA-damaging agents are modulated by both organ- and non-organ-specific risk modulators.

Intrinsic risk modulators are inherited traits that do not contribute directly to DNA damage, but modulate the environment to which the cells are exposed. Examples include how well metabolizing enzymes function to modulate drug and hormone activity as well as how well a hormone such as testosterone binds to its receptor, based on factors that change the avidity of the gene [6]. In addition, before the damaging agent can cause mutation, it must evade extrinsic risk modulators. Extrinsic risk modulators are best characterized by chemoprevention agents such as antioxidants. Dietary factors such as selenium and vitamin E have been demonstrated to remove damaging oxygen radicals from the intracellular environment by catalyzing their breakdown to water [7,8]. If the damaging agent escapes all of these potential protective mechanisms, it still must damage the DNA in a susceptible place that will allow a survival advantage [1,3]. Most mutations to the DNA are either deleterious or neutral—very few are adaptive [9]. In bacteria, for example, it is estimated that only 1 in 10,000 mutations provides an adaptive advantage [9,10]. It is estimated that in the much more complex human genome, this ratio would be much higher, on the order of 1 in 1 to 10 million mutations.

COMMON CHARACTERISTICS OF CANCERS

Although each cancer exhibits a unique set of behaviors and growth character-istics (its phenotype), cancers do share a group of common characteristics or *hallmarks* [3,11,12]. A tumor is the result of a collection of cancer cells that are actively dividing and acquiring mutations that allow the emergence of a success-ful group or clone of cells. This is a highly inefficient process, and tumors are filled with cells that will not survive and are undergoing *apoptosis* (programmed cell death) as a result of harmful mutations, lack of oxygen (*hypoxia*) and other vital nutrients, and destruction by the immune system. Some cells, however, manage to acquire enough mutations and acquire the hallmarks of a successful cancer cell [3] (Table 1 and Figure 2). These hallmarks are discussed in detail below.

Unlimited Replicative Potential

Cancer and cancer cells are immortal. This does not mean that each cell itself lives forever, but rather, that the cell population doubles without limit and creates uncontrolled clonal expansion. In noncancerous cells, a cell can double

TABLE 1. Traits That a Tumor Needs to Grow and Spread Successfully

Trait to Allow Growth and Dissemination	Cancer Cell: Clonal Expansion
Unlimited replicative potential	Asexual reproduction, activation of telomerase
Adaptation	Genetic instability, natural selection
Protection from death	Loss of apoptotic pathway activation
No growth inhibition	Anchorage-independent growth
Nutrient supply	Stimulate new blood vessel growth
Population expansion	Activation of proteases to break down surrounding tissue
Evasion of enemies	Evasion of the immune surveillance system (e.g., as cells circulate prior to establishing themselves in a new organ)
Successful colonization	Adaptation to the use of growth factors in the new environment and applying all of the traits above in a new environment

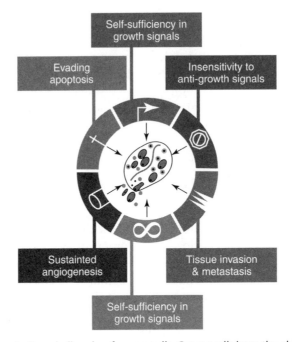

Figure 2. Common traits or hallmarks of cancer cells. Cancer cells have the ability to continually divide, avoid cell death, attract new blood vessels, and metastasize. (From ref. 3.)

approximately 50 times before the population undergoes senescence and dies [13]. Termed the *Hayflick number*, this is the result of an internal cell-doubling clock a *telomere* built onto the end of each chromosome [14]. Telomeres are specific strands of DNA that shorten with each cell division. At a critical shortened length, the cells undergo apoptosis. Cancer cells reactivate an enzyme, telomerase, which maintains the length of telomeres with each cell division by adding base pairs back onto the telomeres, thereby maintaining length integrity.

Adaptation, Mutation, and Natural Selection

A fundamental property of cancer is the generation of tumor cell heterogeneity, that is, cells with multiple mutated characteristics or *phenotypes*, through a mechanism of DNA or genetic instability [15–20]. When a normal cell divides, it makes an exact copy of its DNA. When a cancer cells divides, the DNA of the daughter cells is not copied exactly, resulting in new mutations that may or may not help the cells have a survival advantage. This genetic instability, caused by a wide variety of mechanisms, is a fundamental hallmark of cancer cells. It is likely that the initial mutations within a cell destined to become cancer happen as a result of a low mutation rate within a large population of cells. These mutations occur as a result of the interplay between susceptibility alleles and the environment as outlined above. Within the expanding clone, a mutation even-tually occurs that induces a "mutator phenotype" with coincident high mutation rates and the generation of tumor cell populations with a heterogeneous set of properties over a relatively short period of time. Although this mutator phenotype may occur as a result of chance, it may also be facilitated by the exposure of the cells to stresses such as hypoxia as the size of the tumor increases [21–23]. The emergence of the genetic instability rapidly selects cells with the most robust survival advantages.

Protection from Death

There are multiple redundant pathways in place to maintain the fidelity of normal cells to prevent mutation and damage. More often than not, deleterious mutations lead to the initiation of apoptosis. This may kill a particular cell, but protects the rest of the cell population. There are multiple apoptotic pathways within cells in response to different types of cellular damage [24–26]. Cancer cells have acquired mutations that allow damage to occur and accumulate without activating apoptotic pathways.

Loss of Growth Inhibition

For an organism or organ such as the liver to function in a coordinated fashion, it must control the individual cells that comprise it. In normal cells, this growth inhibition is controlled by anchorage-dependent growth and maintenance. If a normal cell becomes disconnected from its neighbors or the basement membrane on which it resides, apoptosis is triggered and the cell dies. Thus, a liver cell is not usually found in other places in the body. Cancer cells have acquired mutations that allow them to grow independent of attachment to a basement membrane or to other cells [27–29]. This anchorage independence releases the cell from com-municating with its neighbors and breaks down the fundamental fidelity of tissue, organs, and ultimately, the body. Several cell attachment proteins have been identified that have been demonstrated to be altered in cancer cells. These mutations also allow the cancer cell the freedom to leave the primary tumor environment and start down the path of metastasis [30].

Ability to Ensure a Nutrient Supply

A group of cancer cells undergoing clonal expansion can become only approxi-mately a cubic millimeter in size (20 population doublings, 1 million cells, i.e., the size of a pen tip) without a blood supply to oxygenate the cells and bring them other nutrients [31]. A critical step in successful cancer development is the release of factors such as vascular endothelial growth factor (VEGF) from the cancer cells to attract new blood vessel growth (neovascularity of angiogenesis) [32,33]. The growth of new blood vessels to the tumor also gives the cancer cells an additional avenue to metastasize.

Population Expansion and Growth Beyond Natural Boundaries

Cancer rarely kills its host because of its growth in a single organ. The majority of these cancers can be treated successfully by surgery and/or radiation, resulting in cure of the patient. Even untreated, a solitary cancer can grow in the primary organ for years before becoming clinically evident. Cancer kills because it spreads to other organs (*metastasizes*). This requires mutations that allow uncontrolled growth, anchorage-independent growth, apoptosis evasion, and new blood vessel growth, but also requires the acquisition of several other adaptation properties. For the cancer cell population to grow, it must break down its surrounding tissue environment using proteases that breakdown the confining extracellular matrix of surrounding tissue [34]. Cancer has been likened to a wound that does not heal. A cut to skin causes the skin cells to secrete proteases actively to allow tissue remodeling and VEGF to supply new blood vessels to the area. The difference is that when the wound closes, these cell programs turn off—in cancer they stay activated, allowing continued growth of the cancer.

Evasion of the Immune System

At every level in its life, a cancer cell, and its daughter clones, must evade the immune system. The immune system is a remarkably adaptable system that seeks out and destroys foreign and harmful agents within an organism. Cancer cells have developed several ways to evade the surveillance of the immune system [35]. Many cancer cells have lost proteins (antigens) on their cell surface that let the body recognize them as foreign. Other cancer cells secrete cytokines such as transforming growth factor beta (TGFβ), which inhibits the function of the immune system cells [36].

Successful Colonization or Metastasis

All of the acquired mutations, whether they were acquired through selective pressure via adaptation to continued hostile environmental hurdles or by chance accumulation, result in a cancer cell population that metastasizes successfully and grows in multiple new organ sites [4,30,37]. These cells have all of the traits that are needed to leave the primary site, survive in the circulation, and invade and flourish in new environments [38] (Figure 3).

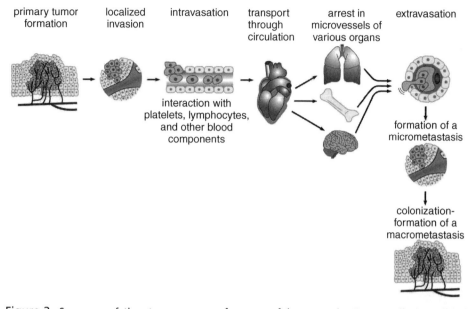

primary tumor | localized | intravasation | transport | arrest in | extravasation
formation | invasion | | through | microvessels of |
| | | circulation | various organs |

interaction with
platelets, lymphocytes,
and other blood
components

formation of a
micrometastasis

colonization-
formation of a
macrometastasis

Figure 3. Summary of the steps necessary for successful metastasis. Cancer cells must break down the tissue surrounding them, invade their environment, and attract a blood supply. They must then enter the blood stream or lymphatics and survive the circulation to arrest in a distant organ, extravasate into it, and grow. (From ref. 39. Copyright @ Garland Science 2007.) (See insert for color representation.)

TYPES OF CANCER

The human body is made up of billions of cells. The different types of cells can be grouped together or classified according to the job they do or the type of body tissue they make up. For example, there are epithelial tissue cells, connective tissue cells, and cells of the blood and lymphatic systems. Eighty-five percent of all cancers are cancers of the epithelial cells and are termed *carcinomas* or *adenocarcinomas*. Cancers arising from cells in the blood are termed *leukemias*; if they arise in the lymph nodes they are termed *lymphomas*; those that arise in the connective tissue are sarcomas (Table 2).

TABLE 2. Types of Cancer

Type of Cancer	Area of Origination
Adenocarcinoma	Glandular tissue
Blastoma	Embryonic tissue of organs
Carcinoma	Epithelial tissue (i.e., tissue that lines organs and tubes)
Leukemia	Tissues that form blood cells
Lymphoma	Lymphatic tissue
Myeloma	Bone marrow
Sarcoma	Connective or supportive tissue (e.g., bone, cartilage, muscle)

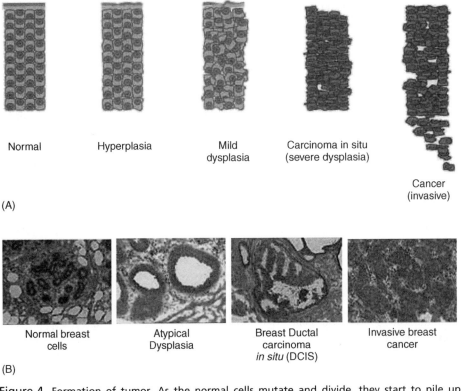

Normal   Hyperplasia   Mild   Carcinoma in situ
                                     dysplasia   (severe dysplasia)

                                                                          Cancer
                                                                          (invasive)
(A)

Normal breast	Atypical	Breast Ductal	Invasive breast
cells	Dysplasia	carcinoma	cancer
		in situ (DCIS)	

(B)

Figure 4. Formation of tumor. As the normal cells mutate and divide, they start to pile up (hyperplasia): (A) artists drawing; (B) actual pictures of this occurring in the breast. Over time, these cells develop added mutations and begin to look abnormal (atypical dysplasia). If this process occurs in an organ with ducts, such as the breast, they fill in the normal breast ducts before they come invasive (ductal carcinoma in situ). Overall, this process is thought to take years to occur. [(A) From ref. 40.] (See insert for color representation.)

Generally, no matter what organ a cancer arises in, it follows a general pattern of growth (Figure 4). As the cells become abnormal and start to grow, they start to look abnormal (dysplasia). If they are in an organ that has ducts, such as the breast and prostate, these cells pile up and fill in the duct (carcinoma in situ) before they start to invade the surrounding tissue (invasive cancer).

The most common cancers in adults in the United States are skin, lung, colorectal, breast, endometrial, ovarian, and prostate (Figure 5). According to the American Cancer Society (Table 3), the most common type of cancer is nonmelanoma skin cancer, with more than 1 million new cases expected in the United States in 2008, representing about half of all cancers diagnosed in this country. This type of cancer rarely causes death to the patient and is often not included in cancer statistics. Cancer has surpassed heart disease as the leading cause of death for those younger than age 85 (Figure 6). The death rate from all cancers combined has decreased by 1.5% per year since 1993 among men and by

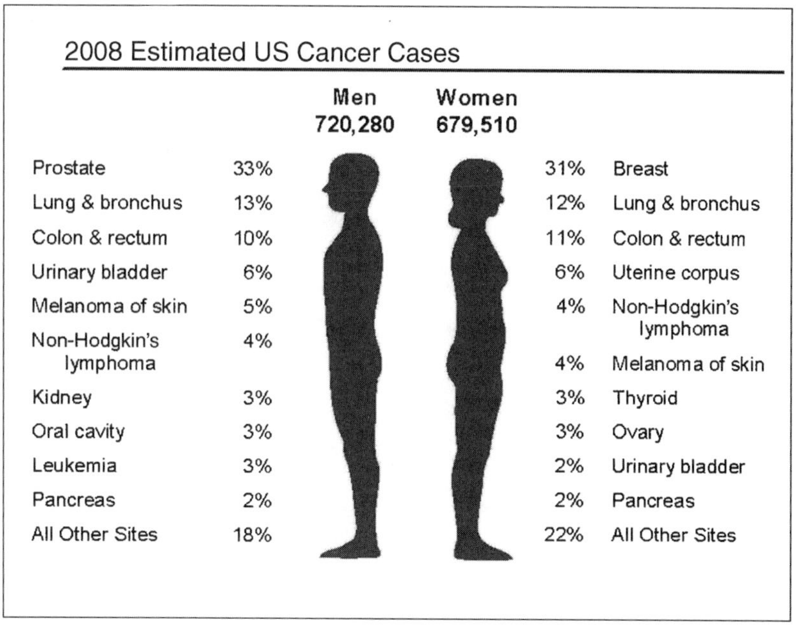

2008 Estimated US Cancer Cases

	Men 720,280		Women 679,510	
Prostate	33%		31%	Breast
Lung & bronchus	13%		12%	Lung & bronchus
Colon & rectum	10%		11%	Colon & rectum
Urinary bladder	6%		6%	Uterine corpus
Melanoma of skin	5%		4%	Non-Hodgkin's lymphoma
Non-Hodgkin's lymphoma	4%		4%	Melanoma of skin
Kidney	3%		3%	Thyroid
Oral cavity	3%		3%	Ovary
Leukemia	3%		2%	Urinary bladder
Pancreas	2%		2%	Pancreas
All Other Sites	18%		22%	All Other Sites

Figure 5. American Cancer Society 2008 cancer incidence statistics. (From ref. 41.)

0.8% per year since 1992 among women. The mortality rate has also continued to decrease for the three most common cancer sites in men (lung, colorectal, and prostate) and for breast and colorectal cancers in women. These decreases are the result of better screening programs as well as treatments.

Over 2000 years ago the Greek physician Hippocrates observed a disease that spread out and grabbed on to another part of the body like "the arms of a crab"

TABLE 3. Estimated Number of New Cases, Prevalence, and Death Attributable to Cancer in 2008

Cancer Type	Estimated New Cases	Estimated Deaths	Prevalence (2002)
Bladder	68,810	14,100	499,000
Breast	184,450	40,930	2,290,000
Colon and rectal (combined)	148,810	49,960	223,000
Endometrial	40,100	7,470	572,000
Leukemia (all)	44,270	21,710	189,000
Lung (including bronchus)	215,020	161,840	351,000
Melanoma	62,480	8,420	630,000
Non-Hodgkin's Lymphoma	66,120	19,160	347,000
Pancreatic	37,680	34,290	26,000
Prostate	186,320	28,660	1,832,000
Skin (non-melanoma)	>1,000,000	Not available	Not available
Thyroid	37,340	1,590	327,000

Source: Ref. 41.

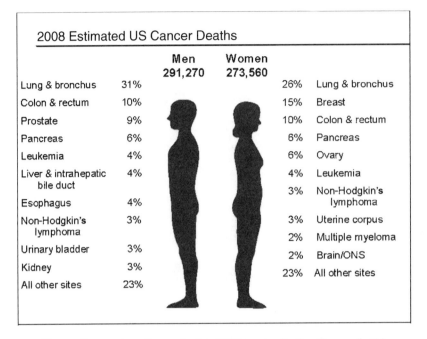

<figure>

2008 Estimated US Cancer Deaths

	Men **291,270**	**Women** **273,560**	
Lung & bronchus	31%	26%	Lung & bronchus
Colon & rectum	10%	15%	Breast
Prostate	9%	10%	Colon & rectum
Pancreas	6%	6%	Pancreas
Leukemia	4%	6%	Ovary
Liver & intrahepatic bile duct	4%	4%	Leukemia
Esophagus	4%	3%	Non-Hodgkin's lymphoma
Non-Hodgkin's lymphoma	3%	3%	Uterine corpus
Urinary bladder	3%	2%	Multiple myeloma
Kidney	3%	2%	Brain/ONS
All other sites	23%	23%	All other sites

</figure>

Figure 6. American Cancer Society 2008 cancer deaths. (From ref. 41.)

and named it cancer. Although we have made in-roads into describing the steps involved in tumorigenesis and metastasis, this observation remains unchanged. It can be appreciated, more than ever, that cancer is a complicated disease that will probably not be cured by a single discovery or drug. Much of the progress in cancer research and treatment is now focusing on the development of inter-disciplinary teams to understand and fully explore the interplay among environ-mental, lifestyle, genetic, and molecular variables contributing to cancer and take advantage of the technological resources available to help them do this.

REFERENCES

1. Greaves M. 2002. Cancer causation: the Darwinian downside of past success? *Lancet Oncol* 3: 244–251.
2. Nowell PC. 1976. The clonal evolution of tumor cell populations. *Science* 194:23–28.
3. Hanahan D, Weinberg RA. 2000. The hallmarks of cancer. *Cell* 100:57–70.
4. Iwakuma T, Lozano G, Flores ER. 2005. Li–Fraumeni syndrome: a p53 family affair. *Cell Cycle* 4(7):865–867.
5. Sogaard M, Kjaer SK, Gayther S. 2006. Ovarian cancer and genetic susceptibility in relation to the *BRCA1* and *BRCA2* genes: occurrence, clinical importance and intervention. *Acta Obstet Gynecol Scand* 85(1):93–105.
6. Coffey DS. 2001. Similarities of prostate and breast cancer: evolution, diet, and estrogens. *Urology* 57:31–38.

7. Pathak SK, Sharma RA, Mellon JK. 2003. Chemoprevention of prostate cancer by diet-derived antioxidant agents and hormonal manipulation [review]. *Int J Oncol* 22:5–13.

8. Farinati F, Cardin R, Della Libera G, Herszenyi L, Marafin C, Molari A, Plebani M, Rugge M, Naccarato R. 1994. The role of anti-oxidants in the chemoprevention of gastric cancer. *Eur J Cancer Prev* 3(Suppl 2):93–97.

9. Radman M, Matic I, Taddei F. 1999. Evolution of evolvability. *Ann NY Acad Sci* 870:146–155.

10. Taddei F, Radman M, Maynard-Smith J, Toupance B, Gouyon PH, Godelle, B. 1997. Role of mutators in adaptive evolution. *Nature* 387:700–702.

11. Marusic M. 1991. Evolutionary and biological foundations of malignant tumors. *Med Hypotheses* 34:282–287.

12. Pienta KJ, Partin AW, Coffey DS. 1989. Cancer as a disease of DNA organization and dynamic cell structure. *Cancer Res* 49:2525–2532.

13. Neumann AA, Reddel RR. 2002. Telomere maintenance and cancer—look, no telomerase. *Nat Rev Cancer* 2:879–884.

14. Rubin H. 2002. The disparity between human cell senescence in vitro and lifelong replication in vivo. *Nat Biotechnol* 20:675–681.

15. Pienta KJ, Ward WS. 1994. An unstable nuclear matrix may contribute to genetic instability. *Med Hypotheses* 42:45–52.

16. Nowak MA, Komarova NL, Sengupta A, Jallepalli PV, Shih Ie, M, Vogelstein B, Lengauer C. 2002. The role of chromosomal instability in tumor initiation. *Proc Natl Acad Sci USA* 99: 16226–16231.

17. Anderson GR, Stoler DL, Brenner BM. 2001. Cancer: the evolved consequence of a destabilized genome. *Bioessays* 23:1037–1046.

18. Hoglund M, Gisselsson D, Sall T, Mitelman F. 2002. Coping with complexity: multivariate analysis of tumor karyotypes. *Cancer Genet Cytogenet* 135:103–109.

19. Kerbel RS, Cornil I, Korczak B. 1989. New insights into the evolutionary growth of tumors revealed by Southern gel analysis of tumors genetically tagged with plasmid or proviral DNA insertions. *J Cell Sci* 94:381–387.

20. MacPhee DG. 1991. The significance of deletions in spontaneous and induced mutations associated with movement of transposable DNA elements: possible implications for evolution and cancer. *Mutat Res* 250:35–47.

21. Yuan J, Narayanan L, Rockwell S, Glazer PM. 2000. Diminished DNA repair and elevated mutagenesis in mammalian cells exposed to hypoxia and low pH. *Cancer Res* 60:4372–4376.

22. Reynolds TY, Rockwell S, Glazer PM. 1996. Genetic instability induced by the tumor microenvironment. *Cancer Res* 56:5754–5757.

23. Coffey DS, Isaacs JT. 1981. Prostate tumor biology and cell kinetics: theory. *Urology* 17 (Suppl):40–53.

24. Hussein MR, Haemel AK, Wood GS. 2003. Apoptosis and melanoma: molecular mechanisms. *J Pathol* 199:275–288.

25. Bowen AR, Hanks AN, Allen SM, Alexander A, Diedrich MJ, Grossman D. 2003. Apoptosis regulators and responses in human melanocytic and keratinocytic cells. *J. Invest Dermatol* 120:48–55.

26. Hoglund M, Gisselsson D, Hansen GB, Sall T, Mitelman F. 2002. Multivariate analysis of chromosomal imbalances in breast cancer delineates cytogenetic pathways and reveals complex relationships among imbalances. *Cancer Res* 62:2675–2680.

27. Abraham S, Zhang W, Greenberg N, Zhang M. 2003. Maspin functions as tumor suppressor by increasing cell adhesion to extracellular matrix in prostate tumor cells. *J Urol* 169:1157–1161.

28. Su ZZ, Gopalkrishnan RV, Narayan G, Dent P, Fisher PB. 2002. Progression elevated gene-3, PEG-3, induces genomic instability in rodent and human tumor cells. *J Cell Physiol* 192:34–44.

29. Kondoh N, Shuda M, Arai M, Oikawa T, Yamamoto M. 1998. Activation of anchorage-independent growth of HT1080 human fibroblasts. *Mutat Res* 199:273–291.

30. Cooper CR, Chay CH, Gendernalik JD, Lee HL, Bhatia J, Taichman RS, McCauley LK, Keller ET, Pienta KJ. 2003. Stromal factors involved in prostate carcinoma metastasis to bone. *Cancer* 97:739–747.

31. Folkman J. 2002. Role of angiogenesis in tumor growth and metastasis. *Semin Oncol* 29:15–18.

32. van Nieuw Amerongen GP, Koolwijk P, Versteilen A, van Hinsbergh VW. 2003. Involvement of RhoA/Rho kinase signaling in VEGF-induced endothelial cell migration and angiogenesis in vitro. *Arterioscler Thromb Vasc Biol* 23:211–217.

33. Chang L, Kaipainen A, Folkman J. 2002. Lymphangiogenesis new mechanisms. *Ann NY Acad Sci* 979:111–119.

34. Chung AS, Yoon SO, Park SJ, Yun CH. 2003. Roles of matrix metalloproteinases in tumor metastasis and angiogenesis. *J Biochem Mol Biol* 36(1): 128–137.

35. Nambu Y, Beer DG. 2003. Altered surface markers in lung cancer: lack of cell-surface Fas/APO-1 expression in pulmonary adenocarcinoma may allow escape from immune surveillance. *Methods Mol Med* 74:259–266.

36. Ivanovic VV, Todorovic-Rakovic N, Demajo M, Neskovic-Konstantinovic Z, Subota V, Ivanisevic-Milovanovic O, Nikolic-Vukosavljevic, D. 2002. Elevated plasma levels of transforming growth factor-beta(1) [TGF-beta(1)] in patients with advanced breast cancer: association with disease progression. *Eur J Cancer* 39:454–461.

37. Keller ET, Zhang J, Cooper CR, Smith PC, McCauley LK, Pienta KJ, Taichman RS. 2001. Prostate carcinoma skeletal metastases: cross-talk between tumor and bone. *Cancer Metastasis Rev* 20:333–349.

38. Pienta KJ, Loberg RD. 2005. The emigration, migration, and immigration of prostate cancer. *Clin Pros Cancer* 4(1):24–30.

39. Weinberg RA. 2007. *The Biology of Cancer*. New York: Garland Science, p. 591.

40. http://www.arctur.com/consumer_portal/images/breast_cancer_progression.gif.

41. Jemul A, Siegel R, Ward E, Hao Y, Xu J, Murray T, Thun MJ. 2008. Cancer Statistics, 2008. *CA Cancer J Clin,* 58:71–96.

3

ENVIRONMENTAL, GENETIC, AND VIRAL CAUSES OF CANCER

Rami I. Aqeilan, Nicola Zanesi, and Carlo M. Croce

Department of Molecular Virology, Immunology, and Medical Genetics, Division of Human Cancer Genetics and Comprehensive Cancer Care, Ohio State University, Columbus

OVERVIEW

Cancer is a genetic disease that consists of different combinations of genetic alterations. Several types of genetic alterations contribute to malignant transformation. The genome of an early-transforming cell acquires activated alleles of oncogenes, mutated or lost tumor suppressor genes, and alterations of other genes responsible for genome stability. Recently, genetic alterations in a new group of noncoding genes called microRNA genes have also been described in several types of human cancer. These combinations of genetic abnormalities generate cells that divide more rapidly or evade cell death, thus liberating it from growth control and cell cycle checkpoints. Mammalian cells have multiple safeguards to protect them against these genetic changes, and only when several genes are defective, does a cancer develop. It has been widely accepted that cancer is caused by both external factors, such as mutagens, radiation, tobacco, and infectious agents, and internal factors, such as inherited mutations (genetic and epigenetic) and immune conditions. These causal factors may act together or in sequence to initiate carcinogenesis or assist it to progress. Although all neoplastic

The Biology and Treatment of Cancer: Understanding Cancer
Edited by Arthur B. Pardee and Gary S. Stein   Copyright © 2009 John Wiley & Sons, Inc.

transformation involves genetic alterations, most cancers are sporadic and a minority of cases are hereditary. In hereditary cases, there is clear evidence that the initiating events occurred within a person's germ cell. Despite that, these inherited genetic abnormalities are not sufficient for development of cancer, indicating that other sporadic changes are required. Alterations in a single cancer gene increase the risk of cancer, but a single genetic change is rarely sufficient for the development of a malignant tumor. Thus, cancer is the result of a multistep process involving sequential genetic alterations. The initiating genetic alterations are extremely important to uncover since development of malignancy depends on that specific genetic alteration. Targeting the initiating event should be the first priority in the development of rational therapy. Other genetic alterations take place during tumor progression which probably result in heterogeneity of tumors. Tumor heterogeneity has a great clinical impact, due to the differences in clinical behavior and responses to treatment of tumors of the same diagnostic type. In summary, identifying early genetic and epigenetic alterations and changes during tumor progression has a great impact on cancer treatment.

GENETIC BASIS OF CANCER

Sporadic and Hereditary Cancers

Cancer that is not due to an obvious inherited pattern is called *sporadic*. It is believed that perhaps 90 to 95% of all cancers are sporadic. People who have sporadic cancer did not inherit cancer-causing mutations from their parents. Instead, certain cells in their body (somatic cells) developed mutations that led to cancer. *Mutation* is defined as any change in the sequence of the genome. Those changes can affect single deoxyribonucleic acid (DNA) bases or can be a result of small or large deletions or insertions, amplification, or translocations (see below). If a mutation occurred in somatic cells, it results in sporadic tumors. These mutations can be caused by environmental factors such as exposure to sun (which can lead to skin cancer), to radiation, or to carcinogenic or mutagenic chemicals, such as those present in tobacco smoke. To date, scientists know about several genes that are commonly mutated in sporadic cancers and use them as markers or parameters in diagnosis and prognosis or for therapy.

The other type of cancer is called *hereditary*. Hereditary cancers occur when a person is born with a change or mutation in a single copy of a gene that she or he inherited from parents. In other words, if a mutation occurred in the germline cell (reproductive cells: oocytes and sperm), it results in hereditary cancer transformation. Most common mutations in the germline are subtle (point mutations or small deletions or insertions). Because people with an inherited mutation have only one working copy of a protective gene, damage to that remaining gene may occur over a shorter period of time. Inheriting a gene mutation does not necessarily mean that a person will develop cancer, but it increases the risk. Nevertheless, these changes do not increase the risk for every type of cancer and not everyone who is born with a gene change will develop cancer; risks vary according to the exact mutation that was inherited. For instance, the main hereditary breast cancer syndromes—caused by mutations in the *BRCA1* or *BRCA2* gene—are also associated with an increased risk for ovarian cancer. The main hereditary colon cancer syndrome, called hereditary nonpolyposis colorectal cancer (HNPCC), can also be associated with an increased risk for ovarian cancer or uterine cancer.

Sporadic cancer and hereditary cancer differ in several ways that may affect health care decisions. Whereas hereditary cancer tends to occur at an early age, the sporadic form of the same cancer occurs at later ages. Hereditary gene changes can be passed on to children, whereas changes in somatic cells cannot. Individuals who have inherited a gene change may be at a higher risk for more than one type of cancer. In people who have already been diagnosed with a cancer, this may affect their cancer treatment or follow-up care. In hereditary cancers, the germline mutation is the "head start" of the neoplastic process; however, for a lesion to take place, additional mutations have to accumulate in the body. That is, germline mutations by themselves are not enough to cause cancer. Specific screening or risk-lowering options exist for people who know that they are at high risk for certain types of hereditary cancer.

Protein-Coding Cancer Genes

Three classes of protein-coding genes are involved in cancer formation when they are altered: oncogenes, which show a dominant gain of function; tumor suppressors, which show a recessive loss of function; and stability genes, which maintain the integrity and stability of the human genome. Oncogenes are activated in cancer (Figure 1) when genetic alterations give rise to a gain of function at the gene level. Oncogenes encode proteins that are involved in the control of cell proliferation, apoptosis (programmed cell death), or both. They can become activated by translocation to a highly active promoter by change of a single amino acid (building block of proteins), by producing a truncated protein product that is hyperactive, or by genetic amplification. All of these types of mutations are almost dominant with respect to the unaltered copy (allele) of the oncogene and can contribute to transformation in the heterozygous condition. The fact that oncogenes are turned on in cancer makes them rational targets for gene-specific cancer treatment. The role of oncogenes in the pathogenesis of cancer has been validated in transgenic mice (see the section "Model Organism of Human Cancer" below) that carry in the germline genetic alteration present in a human tumor. Such mice, after variable periods of time, develop malignancies similar to the human tumor.

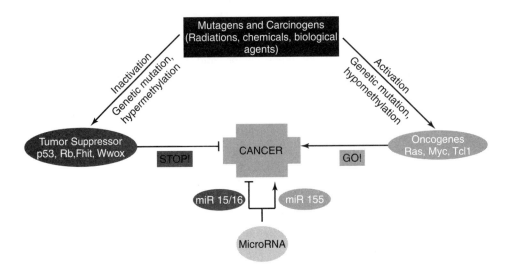

Figure 1. Schematic representation showing the complex relationships among genetics, epigenetics, and environmental factors (radiations, chemicals, and microorganisms) in causing cancer. Oncogenes and tumor suppressors are protein-coding genes, whereas microRNA genes are noncoding genes (see the text). (See insert for color representation.)

In addition to the presence of dominantly acting oncogenes, the functional loss of proteins encoded by tumor suppressor genes also contributes to the neoplastic phenotype (Figure 1). A tumor suppressor gene is a gene that reduces the probability that a cell will turn into a tumor cell. In many cases, inactivation of tumor suppressor genes occurs through mutation or deletion of a large portion of their DNA sequence. Usually, both copies (alleles) of a given tumor suppressor gene are mutated or lost. By contrast to oncogene activation, which normally is sporadic, tumor suppressor inactivation occurs in both sporadic and inherited cancer predisposition syndromes. Tumor suppressor genes or, more precisely, the proteins for which they code, have either a dampening or a repressive effect on regulation of the cell cycle or promote cell death, and sometimes do both. The functions of tumor suppressor proteins fall into several categories:

1. Repression of genes that are essential for continuation of the cell cycle. If these genes are not expressed, the cell cycle will not continue, effectively inhibiting cell division.
2. Coupling the cell cycle to DNA damage. As long as there is damaged DNA in the cell, it should not divide. If the damage can be repaired, the cell cycle can continue. If the damage cannot be repaired, the cell should initiate apoptosis to remove the threat it poses for the greater good of the organism.

Unlike oncogenes, tumor suppressor genes generally follow the *two-hit hypothesis*, which implies that both alleles that code for a particular gene must be affected before a damaging effect is manifested. If only one allele for the gene is damaged, the second can still produce the correct protein. However, there are cases where mutations in only one allele will cause an effect, a condition that is called *haploinsufficiency*. A notable example for this is the gene that codes for p53.

A third class of protein-coding cancer genes, the stability genes, serve as caretakers of DNA replication. Some stability genes are responsible for repairing subtle mistakes made during DNA replication or induced following exposure to environmental carcinogens. Other stability genes control processes involving large portions of chromosomes, such as mitosis. The main function of these types of genes is to keep genetic alterations to a minimum. If the first mutation occurs in a gene that repairs or prevents other mutations, additional changes can quickly accumulate and eventually lead to cancer development. Therefore, when stability genes are inactivated, mutations in other genes, such as oncogenes and tumor suppressor genes, take place.

MicroRNA Genes in Cancer

Until recently, it was thought that only alterations in protein-coding genes, such as oncogenes and tumor suppressor genes, were responsible for tumor development. Recently, however, a new class of genes that are noncoding genes, the micro-ribonucleic acid (miRNA) genes, have been shown to be implicated in the development of human cancer. miRNAs are encoded by genes that are transcribed from DNA but not translated into protein. The function of miRNAs appears to be in gene regulation through degradation of target RNA transcripts or a block of target protein translation. Mapping of all miRNAs genes to their chromosome locations indicated that many miRNAs genes occur in chromosomal regions that undergo rearrangements, deletions, and amplifications in cancer cells. Indeed, miRNAs can be up-regulated (such as oncogenes) or down-regulated (such as tumor suppressor genes) in cancer (Figure 1). For example, miRNA 155 is found up-regulated in diffuse large B-cell lymphoma (DLBCL) and in an aggressive form of chronic lymphocytic leukemia (CLL). Overexpression of miRNA 155 in the B- cell lymphocytes of mice led to increased B-cell proliferation and development of lymphoma, indicating that deregulation of a single miRNA can lead to cancer. Another example of miRNA genes that are implicated in human cancer are miRNA 15a and miRNA 16-1. Both of these miRNAs are deleted or underexpressed in CLL. Recent studies have shown that miRNA 15a and miRNA 16-1 target the expression of BCL2, an oncogene that inhibits cells to undergo apoptosis miRNA 15a and miRNA 16-1 down-regulate expression of *BCL2* and thus lead to cell death. In other cancers, alteration of miRNA 15a and miRNA 16-1 results in overexpression of the *BCL2* oncogene and thus cells continue to grow. Therefore, restoration of deleted miRNAs or silencing of overexpressed miRNAs can be of therapeutic potential in the war against cancer.

Genetic Instability in Human Cancer

As stated above, stability genes maintain the integrity and structure of DNA. If stability genes get mutated, numerous genetic alterations take place, contributing to genetic instability. There is now evidence that most cancers may indeed be genetically unstable. In other words, tumor-cell genomes usually reveal higher instability than do normal-cell genomes. This observation supports the notion that an increased mutation rate is required for the development of many types of cancer in humans. In normal cells that contain unstable DNA, cellular mechanisms (such as apoptosis) are responsible for eliminating such cells; this mechanism is often compromised in tumor cells, resulting in the survival of a mutated cell which possibly grows to a large population of its similarly mutated descendants.

Types of Genetic Alterations in Tumors

Genetic changes that lead to oncogene activation and genetic instability can be divided into four major categories:

1. *DNA sequence changes.* These changes involve small deletions, insertions, or substitutions of a few nucleotides. These instabilities are uncommon in human cancers, but when present, cause dramatic phenotypes. If these changes happened to a gene that maintains genome integrity or repairs damage caused by environmental carcinogens, other mutations will accumulate. If these mutations hit important cancer genes that control cell cycle or apoptosis, they may well contribute to tumor development. Examples of genes that are frequently mutated or deleted in human cancer are the *RAS* gene (involved in carcinomas of the lung, colon, and pancreas); and the *FHIT* and *WWOX* genes (involved in most common types of human carcinomas and lymphomas).

2. *Chromosome number changes.* Alterations in chromosome number involve losses or gains of entire chromosomes, a phenomenon called *aneuploidy* (Figure 2). The mechanism underlying aneuploidy is not well known. Nevertheless, study of chromosome gain or loss (karypotyping) has indicated that the majority of human cancers exhibit chromosome instability. Since many cancer genes can be affected by aneuploidy, this may result in activation or inactivation of these genes, which can eventually contribute to tumor development.

3. *Chromosome translocations.* These alterations result in fusion of different chromosomes or segments of a single chromosome (Figure 2). Initially, chromosomal translocations were thought to be a result of the cancer phenotype; however, we know today that chromosomal translocation causes cancer. If a portion of a chromosome that harbors the regulatory element of a highly active gene is moved to drive an oncogene, the result

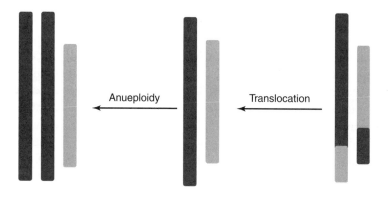

Figure 2. Examples of chromosome alterations in tumors. The two central chromosomes represent the normal situation. On the left, gain of a whole chromosome is one of the possible cases of aneuploidy (see the text). On the right, a case of balanced chromosomal translocation is shown, where an even exchange of genetic material occurs with no extra or missing information.

will be an increased expression of this oncogene and thus activation of an entire pathway that may be indispensable for tumor development. This is exactly what happens in some hematopoietic malignancies, such as Burkitt's lymphoma and follicular lymphoma. In Burkitt's lymphoma, the *MYC* gene, which is an oncogene, is activated due to the translocation of a portion of chromosome 8 to chromosome 14, chromosome 22, or chromosome 2. In the case of follicular lymphoma, a portion of chromosome 18 is translocated to chromosome 14, leading to high expression of the *BCL2* gene. Both *MYC* and *BCL2* have oncogenic potential and are well implicated in liquid and solid tumors. To date, there are catalogs and atlases that tabulate these translocations in each specific type of cancer.

4. *Gene amplification.* Gene amplification is a multiplication of a small region of a chromosome and is usually observed in advanced stages of cancer. Amplification usually affects one gene and usually occurs during tumor progression, whereas chromosomal gain affects more than one gene and usually takes place early in tumorigenesis. One example is the amplification of the *HER2* gene in breast cancer.

Epigenetics

In previous sections we focused on genetic changes that occur in DNA sequences and contribute to development of cancer. The cellular information, other than the DNA sequence itself, that is heritable during cell division is referred to as *epigenetics*. The main mechanism of epigenetic inheritance is methylation. DNA methylation is a chemical modification of DNA that can be inherited without changing the DNA sequence. DNA methylation involves the addition of a methyl group to DNA. In humans, approximately 1% of DNA bases undergo DNA methylation. In adult somatic tissues, DNA methylation typically occurs in a CpG dinucleotide context. The functional relevance of DNA methylation is the silencing of the gene, resulting in loss of gene function. In cancer, CpG methylation usually occurs in an unregulated fashion, and hence the expression of various genes, such as tumor suppressor genes, may be silenced. In many cases indeed, inactivation of tumor suppressor genes occurs through methylation of nucleotides in the promoter sequences that control the expression of these genes. The first link between hypermethylation and the tumor suppressor gene (Figure 1) was made on the retinoblastoma gene *RB*. The *RB* promoter is methylated in a significant subset of sporadic and even hereditary retinoblastomas, causing inactivation of pRb and thus impairing cell cycle regulation. On the other hand, hypomethylation of oncogenes (Figure 1), causing their activation and increased expression, has been demonstrated in cancer. Hypomethylation of the *RAS* oncogene and the *MLH1* DNA repair gene has been reported in an array of human tumors.

Methylation can also affect genomic imprinting. *Imprinting* is usually referred to as relative silencing of one parental allele compared with the other parental allele. It is maintained, at least in part, by methylation of the promoter regulatory regions of these imprinted genes. Loss of imprinting has been shown to contribute to malignancies such as Wilms' tumor. Finally, methylation can also affect histone modification, which has also been linked to cancer. Histones are the chief protein components that complex with DNA to make up chromatin and thus chromosomes. They act as spools around which DNA winds and they play a role in gene regulation. Histone chemical modification includes acetylation and phosphorylation; both are important in transcriptional regulation and cell division. Improper histone modification may lead to abnormal gene expression and hence pathological conditions. The contribution of epigenetics to the inactivation of key pathways that are involved in carcinogenesis has been well investigated. Drugs that target epigenetic modifications have been shown to have antitumor potential; some are already approved by the U.S. Food and Drug Administration for treating certain types of cancer.

Carcinogens and Mutagens

The term *carcinogen* refers to any substance or radiation that contributes directly to cancer or facilitates its propagation (Figure 1). This may be due to genomic instability or to the disruption of cellular metabolic processes. Common examples of carcinogens are inhaled asbestos, benzene, benzopyrene, tobacco-specific nitrosamines such as nitrosonornicotine, and reactive aldehydes such as formaldehyde. Carcinogens may increase the risk of getting cancer by altering cellular metabolism or damaging DNA directly, thus interfering with biological processes and leading to uncontrolled malignant division, leading ultimately to the formation of tumors. Usually, DNA damage, if too severe to repair, leads to apoptosis, but if the apoptosis pathway is damaged, the cell cannot prevent itself from becoming a cancer cell. Carcinogens can be classified as genotoxic or nongenotoxic. *Genotoxins* cause irreversible genetic damage or mutations by binding to DNA. Genotoxins include chemical agents such as *N*-nitroso-*N*-methylurea (MNU) or nonchemical agents such as ultraviolet (UV) light and ionizing radiation. Certain viruses can also act as carcinogens by interacting with DNA. *Nongenotoxins* do not affect DNA directly but act in other ways to promote growth. These include hormones and some organic compounds.

A *mutagen* is a physical or chemical compound that changes the DNA and thus increases the frequency of mutations above the natural background level. As many mutations cause cancer, mutagens are typically also carcinogens (Figure 1). The nature of mutagens varies; they are usually chemical compounds (e.g., ethidium bromide, sodium azide) or ionizing radiation (e.g., UV, gamma, alpha radiation). Mutagens can get inserted into the DNA strand during replication, react with DNA, and cause structural changes, or work indirectly by causing the cells to synthesize chemicals that have a direct mutagenic effect. By exerting their modification, carcinogens and mutagens have the potential to activate oncogenes or inactivate tumor suppressor genes, thus contributing to the neoplastic process (Figure 1).

Infectious Agents and Cancer

During the past decades it has become apparent that several infectious diseases also contribute to the development of certain types of cancer. The first evidence that infectious organisms such as viruses and bacteria (Figure 1) might be causative to cancer was provided early in the twentieth century by Peyton Rous. Rous demonstrated that tumors in chickens can be transmitted by transferring cell extract that later was found to be a virus and named Rous sarcoma virus (RSV). His observation gave a lot of hope since it was speculated at that time that infections are the causes of cancer, and if we were able to prevent infections, we could cure cancer. To date, we know that most people who have oncogenic viral or bacterial infections do not get cancer. They probably escape because cancer is multifactorial in origin. The same can be said of other exposure to carcinogenesis, such as tobacco smoke and mutagens; not all people are affected in the same way when exposed.

Infections are thought to cause cancer through one of two pathways: either by causing chronic inflammation or more directly, by causing cell transformation. In general, inflammation is usually associated with formation of reactive oxygen and nitrogen species, which can damage DNA, proteins, and cell membranes. DNA damage results in point mutations and other genetic alterations that if hitting an important cancer gene can result in cancer development. Chronic inflammation is also associated with increased cell division, increased proliferation, block-in differentiation, and enhanced necrotic cell death (accidental death, not apoptosis). All are factors that increase the rate of genetic alterations and hence the risk of development of cancer. In theory, increased cell division will increase the probability of genetic alterations. It is well accepted today that the cells that are most relevant to cancer are stem cells, which are the pluripotential cells that give rise to all different cell types. An increase in the rate of division of stem cells increases the mutation incidence and hence increases the cancer risk. This increase in the host cell division rate is often accompanied by block-in differentiation, causing immature cells to accumulate, a condition that also resembles the neoplastic process.

The inflammatory process is normally accompanied by three main responses: (1) The affected area is supplied by an increased volume of blood; (2) there is increased permeability of the endothelial cells, allowing inflammatory mediators to pass through; and (3) there is migration of white blood cells (leukocytes) to surrounding and inflamed tissues. Migration of the leukocytes will result in activation of the immune response that will cause recruitment of the phagocytes, which will recognize the foreign cells and subsequently kill the ingested organism through a battery of microbicidal agents such as activated proteases (enzymes) and potent oxidants.

Oxidative damage caused by the release of oxidants, such as reactive oxygen species and nitric oxides, can lead to DNA breaks, mutations, and chromosome abnormalities. The type of mutation depends on the severity of the inflammation, on the host cell type, and on the DNA repair machinery by the host cell. By the end, if these inflammation-mediated lesions took place, it increases the risk of developing cancer. Antioxidants were shown to be protective against certain forms of cancer, such as skin cancer; however, the mechanism is not known. One possible mechanism is that antioxidants scavenge oxidants that would otherwise damage DNA. Nevertheless, the evidence that oxidants contribute to cancer associated with inflammation suggests that antioxidant intervention could be protective. Therefore, epidemiological data based on studies of fruit and vegetable consumption, which contain a rich diversity of antioxidants, indicate a protective effect against cancer.

The other mechanism by which infectious agents contribute to malignancies is through their direct oncogenic potential. Some pathogens can alter the cell cycle of the host cells directly by inserting active oncogenes, inhibiting tumor suppressor genes, or mimicking growth factors. It is well accepted that cancer risk can be increased by an agent that either interacts with DNA directly, causing mutation, or that increases the number of replications of the DNA, or both. Certain infectious organisms have the ability to increase the host cell proliferation and to induce changes in cell cycle, thus contributing to the transformation process. Once again, the key to any infectious agent causing cancer is to affect the genetic structure of the host cell either directly or indirectly; once several mutations have accumulated or other genetic alterations have taken place, a cancer develops.

At present, an etiological relationship between virus infection and tumor development can be demonstrated in about 15% of the worldwide cancer burden. Approximately two-thirds, of these cancers are caused by papilloma virus infection, and the remaining third is dominated by hepatitis B. Although often necessary, neither of these infections is sufficient for the induction of the respective cancer. Additional modifications have to take place within the genome of the infected host cell, or secondary events have to paralyze the host's immune system.

The direct and indirect effects of these infectious agents on the carcinogenic process present an opportunity for prevention of cancer development by treatment of the infection or by vaccination against initial infection. For example, since bacterial infections can be cured with antibiotics, identification of bacterial causes of malignancy could have tremendous implications for cancer prevention. Another example is development of the Gardasil vaccine, which is the first vaccine developed to prevent cervical cancer, precancerous genital lesions, and genital warts caused by human papilloma virus (HPV).

The interaction of infectious agents with other environmental carcinogens and mutagens enhances the carcinogenic risk of the infection process. A very well studied example, is the relationship between specific chemicals, such as nitrosoamines, and *Helicobacter pylori* in the etiology of stomach cancer. Even in situations where an infectious organism is only one contributor to the carcinogenic process, removing it should greatly reduce the incidences of certain types of tumors worldwide.

Cancer Evolution

How does cancer evolve? Scientists believe that the first genetic alteration, due to spontaneous mutation, exposure to environmental carcinogens, or infectious agents, is the key initiating event for cancer development. The first somatic mutation in an oncogene or a tumor suppressor gene that causes a clonal expansion that initiates the neoplastic process. Accumulation of mutation in the three classes of protein-coding cancer genes and noncoding microRNA genes enhances cell proliferation and leads to tumor progression. Scientists gain a lot of knowledge about this issue through studying genetics of mice, yeast, flies, and worms (see the following section). Alterations in oncogenes and tumor suppressor genes drive cancer formation by increasing tumor cell numbers through enhancing cell proliferation or the inhibition of cell death. This increase can be caused by activating genes that drive cell cycle, inhibiting genes responsible for the apoptosis machinery or by facilitating the supply of nutrients to tumor cells, a process called *angiogenesis* (see below). Subsequent mutations usually result in tumor progression toward malignancy and metastasis.

Several cancer genes directly regulate cell cycle stages. For example, certain cancer genes control transitions from a resting stage to a replicating stage of the cell cycle. Many of those genes become inactivated by mutations during the neoplastic process. Importantly, mutations affecting individual cancer genes result in alterations of vital cellular pathways controlled by these genes. One example is the *TP53* tumor suppressor gene. *TP53* expression is either mutated or missing in more than 50% of human cancers. Following activation by DNA damaging agents, p53 can lead to cell growth arrest or to apoptosis, depending on the cell type and stimulus. p53-mediated growth arrest will allow enough time for the cell to correct the DNA damage. If unsuccessful, p53 will promote cells to undergo apoptosis. In cancer cells where p53 is mutated or deleted, cells will neither arrest nor apoptose and thus continue to grow. Another well-studied pathway is controlled by the retinoblastoma protein (pRb), which plays a central role in determining whether a cell will proceed through cell cycle phases. In several types of human cancer, such as retinoblastomas and small-cell lung carcinomas, the pRb protein is absent because of mutations that disable the *RB* gene, whereas in cervical carcinomas, the pRb protein is degraded very effectively by the E7 oncoprotein of the human papillomavirus. In other tumors, the inactivation of *RB* is mediated through inactivation of another gene, such as $p16^{INK4A}$.

If cells escape apoptosis, they continue to grow. The balance between cell proliferation and apoptosis will determine cell growth. The proliferation of normal cells depends on the presence of growth factors in their surrounding. Normal cells will not proliferate when they are deprived of growth factors. By contrast, cancer cells have a strongly reduced dependence on external proliferation stimulation. This acquired independence of cancer cells is derived from activated oncogenes that generate constitutive proliferation signals. For example, the *RAS* oncogene, which is mutated in 25% of all human tumors, encodes a mutated protein that sends constitutive proliferating signals to the tumor cell, enabling it to grow without a need for growth factors from its external environment. Another example is the alteration of growth factor receptors that transmit proliferating signals from the cell surface into the cell body. In different types of human tumors, these growth factor receptors are overexpressed or structurally altered.

Increasing tumor cell numbers can also be achieved by facilitating the supply of nutrients, an indispensable process for tumor growth: angiogenesis. This is a physiological process involving the growth of new blood vessels from preexisting vessels. Tumors beginning to develop cannot grow greater than 2 mm in diameter unless they are ensured access to the circularity system. They do so by releasing angiogenic factors that induce the formation of new blood vessels. Indeed, in all solid cancers there is enhanced angiogenesis, which provides the tumor cell with nutrients and oxygen and facilitates the evacuation of metabolic wastes. In the last two decades, several antiangiogenic drugs were developed to deprive tumor cells from oxygen and other nutrients.

In summary, cancer evolves when an array of genetic changes take place in cancer genes, leading to enhanced cell proliferation and escape from apoptosis.

MODEL ORGANISMS OF HUMAN CANCER: MICE AND BEYOND

There are two main reasons to model cancer in animals. The first is to determine the causal relationship between specific genetic alterations found in cancer, and the second is to engineer living organisms with defined tumor models for use in studies involving novel technologies and testing novel therapies. Although cell culture experiments certainly provide some information as to the mechanisms being studied, experiments in living animals are required to determine the complex interactions between tumor cells and the host environment. Legitimate concerns exist regarding the use of animals, particularly mammals, in biomedical research. However, most people can reconcile the use of animals if the goal is to combat a lethal human disease such as cancer.

Mice

Modeling human cancer in the mouse (*Mus musculus* and a few other species) has become an extremely important source of knowledge in biomedical research by deepening our understanding of human tumorigenesis and generating experimental systems for the evaluation of novel therapeutic approaches. Mice were originally used for such studies because of the ease with which they are genetically manipulated and because mammals with smaller brains pose fewer ethical problems than those with more intellectual complexity. Over time, the number of available genetic alterations in mice and the expanding number of technologies developed to produce them further reinforced the advantages of using this species. Thus, mice remain the primary mammalian species used in cancer studies and are the main focus of this review on model organisms. The mouse shares conspicuous physiologic, anatomic, and genetic similarities with humans. During the past quarter of a century, an impressive arsenal of genetic tools, along with the recent availability of the mouse genome sequence, have made the laboratory mouse the key organism for modeling human genetic diseases.

Historically, mouse strains that develop certain types of tumors either spontaneously or following treatment with carcinogenic agents were studied to understand aspects of disease causes. These earlier models were, nevertheless, characterized by long tumor latency and, more important, by the lack of a defined correlation between genes and disease. In the 1980s a new and revolutionary conceptual framework for the creation of faithful mouse models opened the way to study tumor biology through the manipulation of mouse germ cells (oocytes and sperm) with consequent genetic modifications of all the other body cells in the offspring. So far, a considerable number of genetically altered and engineered mice have been generated. These cancer-prone mouse strains have provided interesting insights into the role of individual genes and their mutated counterparts in tumorigenesis and of the cooperation of individual mutations in tumor development. However, cancer is a disease characterized by the progressive accumulation of genetic abnormalities (mutations) in regular body cells (somatic cells) more than in germ cells. Such sporadic lesions eventually lead to tumor growth inside a genetically normal environment, which often contributes actively to tumor progression. Therefore, the conventional technology that targets germ cells does not mimic sporadic multistep tumorigenesis because the initiating mutation is present throughout the body. Moreover, germ cell genetic abnormalities, also called *germline mutations*, of oncogenes or tumor suppressor genes sometimes lead to the death of the embryos (embryonic lethality), which makes it unfeasible to study the effects of mutations on tumor development in adult mice. Consequently, various strategies have been developed to allow the induction of somatic mutations in the mouse in a tissue-specific and time-controlled fashion. These advancements are currently making possible the creation of sophisticated models that better mimic tumor onset and progression. Such improved models allow, for instance, the generation of compound mutants carrying different copies of a single gene, called *alleles*, in which the contribution of individual mutations to the tumor can be evaluated accurately.

Tumorigenic mutations exert their effects through either oncogene activation or tumor suppressor inactivation (see the preceding section). To model the effects of deregulated oncogenes or tumor suppressor mutations in the mouse, various germline modification strategies have been developed based on two fundamental approaches: (1) the transgenic approach and (2) the gene-targeting approach. The former is based on the random transfer, into the mouse genome, of foreign DNA sequences coming, for instance, from a different organism and called *transgenic DNA*. The latter approach, on the contrary, introduces exogenous DNA into specific regions of the mouse genome with the purpose of targeting only the DNA of those regions, and for this reason, the procedure is called *genetargeting*. Both procedures have the purpose of mimicking in mice the pathological alterations found in human genes. The transgenic approach is usually adopted in the case of oncogenes. These genes cause cancer when overexpressed, which means that their proteins are more abundant than the physiological amounts required by the normal functioning of the cell. When a gene is overexpressed by a transgenic process (transgene) and is able to induce cancer in the host organism, its biological behavior corresponds to that of an oncogene (Figure 3A). Two examples of mouse models of oncogenes are *HER-2* transgenic mice, in which transfer and overexpression of the human *HER-2* gene induces breast cancer, and *TCL-1* transgenic mice, which develop different types of leukemias depending on the types of lymphocytes affected by the overexpression of human *TCL-1* gene.

The gene-targeting method is classically used to inactivate genes and is typically exploited with tumor suppressor genes. Many cancers are caused by inactivation of tumor suppressors, and a convincing way to prove that a gene actually has a tumor suppressor function is to produce a mouse model that develops cancer because of inactivation of that specific gene (knockout mouse).

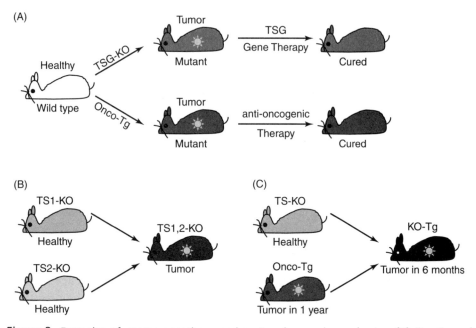

Figure 3. Examples of cancer genetics experiments using engineered mice. **(A)** Creation of knockout and transgenic mice and their use to test novel experimental therapies (see the text). **(B)** Two knockout mice, each inactivated with a single tumor suppressor, are healthy. When they are crossed together, their offspring, lacking both genes, develop tumors (see the text). **(C)** A transgenic mouse develops cancer in one year, but when crossed with a knockout mouse, their progeny develop the disease in six months, showing that the two cancer genes are involved in the same pathological process. (See insert for color representation.)

Thus, through gene targeting, a gene that in physiological conditions makes a regular amount of a protein protective against cancer, stops to do so, and the host organism will start to develop some kind of tumor (Figure 3A). Recently described examples of tumor suppressor mouse models are the Fhit and Wwox knockout mice. The first one tends to develop more lymphomas and benign tumors, while the second is prone to juvenile osteosarcomas and adult lung carcinomas. Contrary to the transgenic mice that have additional copies of a gene, the knockout mice exist in two forms, the heterozygous form, in which only one copy of the gene is inactivated, and the homozygous form, where neither copy is functioning.

The number of copies inactivated in a tumor suppressor gene may be of great relevance for the development of cancer. Indeed, a major focus in the study of knockout mice is based on the relationship between genotype and phenotype, where genotype expresses the number of inactivated copies of a gene (wild type, heterozygote, and homozygote) and phenotype expresses the sum of all clinical manifestations induced by a specific genotype. In the relatively long history of knockout models of cancer, many different situations occurred. For instance, both heterozygous and homozygous Fhit knockout mice display the same phenotype (lymphomas and benign tumors) at approximately the same time (less than two years of age). On the other hand, the knockout model of the *TP53* gene, the first tumor suppressor to be investigated, shows in the heterozygote an intermediate phenotype between the healthy wild type and the homozygote that dies of cancer before 10 months of age and starts developing malignancies around one year and a half. These two different situations reveal that in the case of the Fhit mouse, the amount of Fhit protein produced by either genotype, hetero- or homozygote, is insufficient to protect the cells from cancer, while for the p53 mouse, a half-dosage of the p53 protein (haploinsufficiency) is able to delay the onset of the carcino-genic phenotype significantly compared to complete loss of the gene. A com-pletely different paradigm occurs when the tumor suppressor gene inactivated in a knockout mouse also has some indispensable function in the embryonic develop-ment of the animal. In this case the homozygote is lethal and the mouse dies as an embryo before birth or immediately after birth. Usually, such a situation does not allow studying the cancer phenotype in the homozygous animals, as their lifespan is too short to develop any malignancy. However, a fortunate exception is represented by the Wwox knockout mouse, where 100% of the homozygous mice die by 4 weeks of age, but some of them live long enough to develop osteosarcomas spontaneously. In all cases of early lethality of the homozygotes, interest for cancer studies shifts to the heterozygotes, which in the case of Wwox, for example, develop lung cancer later as adult animals, thus demonstrating that the *WWOX* gene may be fully considered a tumor suppressor.

Sometimes, mice genetically engineered to simulate human cancers with mutations and alterations in specific cancer genes, are not able to recapitulate the disease, and they do not have any clear clinical phenotype. However, in many cases these animals are still useful models of the human condition, as they bear an intrinsic and hidden susceptibility to certain tumors. These models reveal only a more complex pattern in which the predisposition to tumors of their genotypes is not enough to make a cancer phenotype occur. In such situations one way to overcome the problem is to expose wild-type and mutant mice to carcinogens and see whether the mutants are more sensitive than wild type to the malignancies induced by these agents. The rationale behind the experiments with carcinogens is the following: As cancer is a multistep disease where most times an array of mutations or genetic alterations is needed to reach the final clinical outcome, a single gene inactivated or overexpressed may be necessary but not sufficient to drive the entire cancer process. At this point the use of carcinogenic agents would complete the work, disrupting other genes and cellular processes until the amount of damage is sufficient for the development of cancer. For instance, Fhit knockout mice do not develop spontaneous gastric cancer, but when administered with *N*-nitrosomethyl benzylamine (NMBA) by mouth, they are much more susceptible to stomach cancer than are their wild-type siblings. Also Wwox heterozygous mice, although they present a spontaneous phenotype of their own (lung tumors), develop more lung tumors and lymphomas in than do their wild-type littermates when treated with the chemical carcinogen ethyl nitosourea (ENU), which alters the chemical structure of the DNA of other genes. Another approach to bypassing the problem of lack of phenotype is to breed two different silent strains and see whether the combination of the two mutations is able to give an effect that neither of them alone can (Figure 3B). An interesting example of this situation is shown with two strains of animals, the homozygous Fhit and the heterozygous Vhl knockout mice. Neither mouse is affected by lung cancer, but this malignancy occurs frequently when a double-mutant mouse is generated. This experiment showed not only that the two genotypes involved are cryptically critical to lung cancer development but also that Fhit and Vhl cooperate in protecting lungs from cancer.

Mouse models of human cancer are important in biomedical research not only to study the function of cancer genes and how they interact with each other, but also to test new therapies based on knowledge provided by the models themselves (Figure 3A). A typical approach, for instance, is represented by the gene delivery applied to the cancers developed in knockout mice. These animals develop malignancies associated with the loss of tumor suppressor genes, as described above; therefore, a logical way to overcome this problem is to replace a disrupted gene with an intact and functioning gene. As an example, NMBA-induced gastric cancer in Fhit knockout mice represents an attractive model for gene delivery experiments since all these animals develop tumors reasonably fast after carcinogen exposure and the anatomical location of neoplastic lesions is easily accessible for a topical treatment. Gene delivery is often based on the administration of harmless viruses engineered such that they carry a specific gene and are able to transmit the gene to the cells they infect. When Fhit knockout mice are treated with NMBA, two situations are possible: one is waiting for the tumors to develop and then administering the Fhit viruses to attempt to cure the tumors (gene therapy) and the other is administering the Fhit viruses immediately after the carcinogen and trying to prevent the development of tumors (prevention). In the Fhit experiment, either approach, gene therapy and prevention, worked properly to reduce the size and number of tumors significantly compared to mice treated only with carcinogen. These experiments showed that the administration of a tumor suppressor gene strongly reduces the burden of tumors occurring with loss or reduction of that gene.

Other Model Organisms

Modern technologies of genetic engineering made mice the primary animal models in cancer research. However, by no means should they be considered the only ones. One of the simplest unicellular organisms to have a cell containing its genetic material in a nucleus separated from the other cellular components is the budding yeast *Saccharomyces cerevisiae*. This primitive fungus is being used widely to investigate fundamental processes common to all living organisms. Alterations in many of these processes, such as cell cycle, DNA replication, chromosome segregation, maintenance of genomic integrity, and stress responses, are involved in cancer. Therefore, yeast has emerged as an attractive model for cancer research. The genetic tractability of budding yeast represented by a vast number of mutant strains, its ease of manipulation, and the wealth of functional tools available make this organism ideal for analysis of biological functions related to cancer and antitumor drug discovery.

In the last 25 years, genetic studies in a worm, the nematode *Caenorhabditis elegans*, have made important contributions to the understanding of gene function, and some areas of cancer research have particularly benefited from the use of this model organism. First, genes very similar to human oncogenes and tumor suppressors have been found to control well-defined biological processes in *C. elegans*, and the interactions among these genes appear widespread in the animal kingdom, including humans. Thus, significant insights have been obtained into the function of human cancer genes by studying their counterparts in the worm. Second, although tumorigenesis per se is rarely studied in *C. elegans*, growth and differentiation processes, whose abnormalities are often involved in cancer, have been investigated extensively. Such studies have identified novel mechanisms and novel genes that have proven or predicted human counterparts and potential relevance in cancer formation. Third, *C. elegans* is being used in screens for therapeutic agents. Such investigations have enormous potential since oncogenic mutations can be incorporated in specific strains of worms, allowing the selection of drugs that affect mutant but not wild-type animals.

As it happens for *C. elegans*, many fundamental questions of cancer biology might find answers in other experimental systems that use simple organisms. For example, the fruit fly *Drosophila* has been important to an understanding of the mechanisms of complex signaling networks evolved to mediate both local cell interactions and communication across tissues and organs. Recently, issues addressing cancer more directly have become the focus of novel research projects. For instance, an area relevant to cancer is the genetics of tissue size, a complex coordination of cell proliferation and cell death that is mediated by a network of tumor suppressors. The evolutionary conservation of these tumor suppressors extends beyond the similarity of DNA sequence: The human counterparts can often functionally replace the *Drosophila* genes, suggesting that they have a similar function in regulating tissue growth. In addition to proliferation and apoptosis, cancer is characterized by the misregulation of cell adhesion to the tissues and cell movement across tissues. The importance of this aspect of cancer has become more and more appreciated in recent years, and several models in *Drosophila* have proven ideal for exploring its details. In conclusion, *Drosophila* is being used for what it does best: identifying novel oncogenes and tumor suppressors, and linking cancer-related genes together into complex networks of communication.

Another invertebrate, the sea urchin, was among the first animal models to explore cancer theories about a century ago. Centrosomes are cellular organelles that play a crucial role in the union of sperm and egg during fertilization and in the equal separation of chromosomes during cell division (mitosis). Every cell usually has a pair of centrosomes, and before mitosis starts, these organelles duplicate and migrate to the opposite poles of the cell, contributing to the successive migration of chromosomes when the cell divides. Classic studies by the German zoologist Theodor Boveri in the sea urchin egg model had shown that fertilization of an egg with two sperm results in abnormal cell division because of multiple centrosomes contributed by sperm. Since then, abnormal cell division has also been induced by chemical alterations of centrosomes. Abnormalities of centrosome structure are studied with chemicals such as formamide that induce the production of mono- or multipolar abnormal mitosis instead of regular bipolar division and unequal distribution of chromosomes. The patterns of abnormal centrosomes resemble those seen in cancer cells, where structural defects of centrosomes are frequently accompanied by abnormal mitosis and multipolar cells. In summary, the sea urchin model has been most useful to gain information on the role of centrosomes during cell division as well as on centrosome dysfunctions important for cancer.

Although invertebrates such as worms, flies, and sea urchins can develop abnormalities in cell proliferation and division, what is recognized clinically and pathologically as cancer is present almost exclusively in vertebrates, from fish to humans. Thus, to understand the formation, growth, and spread of malignant tumors, vertebrate models are necessary and invaluable.

Despite the more than 300 million years separating the last common ancestor of fish and humans, the biology of cancer is very much the same in these two organisms. Cancer is commonly seen in fish in the wild, and straightforward assays involving waterborne carcinogen exposure have demonstrated that teleosts, the bony fish, develop a wide variety of benign and malignant tumors in virtually all organs, with a histology closely resembling that of human tumors. As in humans, cancer in fish is a genetic disease. A comparison of the human and the zebrafish (*Danio rerio*) genome sequences demonstrates conservation of cell cycle genes, tumor suppressors, and oncogenes. There are also other advantages to modeling cancer in the zebrafish system. Collections of genetic mutant strains in yeast, *Drosophila*, and *C. elegans* (see above) have already revealed key genes regulating the cell cycle, cell proliferation, and cell death. Similar collections in the zebrafish examine the conservation of gene function in these biological pathways, establishing any vertebrate-specific event that leads to cancer. Most important, via the carcinogenesis assay, the zebrafish system provides a direct way to test if a mutation causes cancer predisposition in this animal. Once a cancer-related mutation is found, it is possible to identify interacting genes. Imagine using a zebrafish strain with a tumor suppressor gene mutation to find a second gene which, when inactivated, prevents cancer formation. This modifier would become an excellent target for an antineoplastic drug. In addition to traditional genetic screens, the zebrafish system is amenable to chemical genetic screens. Large numbers of embryos can be arrayed into multiwell plates containing water and aliquots of chemicals. Chemical screens using embryos select for drugs active in a multicellular organism, an advantage over traditional screens using transformed cell lines. Embryos exhibit many features of cancer, including rapidly dividing cells, extensive cell death (apoptosis), and vigorous neovascularization (angiogenesis). Screens for compounds that affect these embryonic properties could identify compounds that are useful for the treatment of cancer or are tools to study cancer pathways. Therefore, the zebrafish cancer system can be viewed as a combination of vertebrate tumor biology, classical and chemical genetics, and genomics.

The African clawed toad (*Xenopus laevis*) is another vertebrate that can be exploited for tumorigenesis studies. The *Xenopus* embryo provides a very useful model system for the analysis of gene function in a living organism. One very useful aspect of this model is the rapidity with which experiments can be performed. *Xenopus* embryos are fertilized in a test tube and subsequently microinjected with artificially synthesized messenger RNA encoding the protein to be tested. Hundreds of *Xenopus* embryos can easily be injected in one afternoon, allowing several different proteins to be examined in parallel. These embryos live happily in a dish of simple saline and develop to swimming tadpoles in just 3 days. Furthermore, these tadpoles have fully developed nervous systems, eyes, kidneys, hearts, and muscles. After 3 hours from fertilization, the embryo is composed of 32 cells each of which develops into a different tissue. Thus, injection of RNA into different cells at this stage of embryonic development will target expression of a specific gene in different tissues. Moreover, injections made into one side of the embryo usually have no effect on the other side, providing effective internal control in each embryo. So, in a one-week set of experiments, the effects of several different proteins can be tested in different cell types in the living organism with internal controls. In this way, by expressing a variety of tumor suppressors and oncogenes, the *Xenopus* embryo becomes a powerful model system for studying tumor formation.

SUMMARY

Cancer is a genetic disease caused by alterations in protein-coding genes, oncogens, and tumor suppressor genes, and in noncoding genes such as microRNA genes. For the most part, these alterations occur as somatic genetic changes, although germline events have been described in several types of heritable cancer. Malignant tumors are usually caused by accumulation of genetic changes in oncogenes, tumor suppressor genes, and microRNA genes. Exposure to external factors such as carcinogens, mutagens, and infectious agents can result in sequential alterations in the various classes of cancer genes and thus contribute to cancer development. The identification of genetic alterations involved in the initiation and progression of human tumors is indispensable for treatment of cancer. Indeed, intensive advanced research during the last decades has generated targets for the development of new drugs for treatment of human malignancies. One important lesson to identify targets was to identify targets that are involved in cancer initiation and/or for which tumor dependency occur. Identifying causes of cancer have strongly affected the incidence of human cancer. Uncovering mechanisms of cancer development through in vitro (laboratory bench work) studies and in vivo (modeling cancer in mice) experiments have greatly aided us in solving many questions and providing clinicians with important answers.

RECOMMENDED READING

Amatruda JF, Shepard JL, Stern HM, Zon LI. 2002. Zebrafish as a cancer model system. *Cancer Cell* 1(3):229–231.

American Cancer Society 2007. *Cancer Facts and Figures 2007*. Atlanta, GA: American Cancer Society, pp. 1–56.

Ames BN, Christen S, Hagen. TM, Shigenaga MK. 1999. Infection, inflammation and mutation. In: Parsonnet J, ed. *Microbes and Malignancy: Infection as a Cause of Human Cancers*. New York: Oxford University Press.

Aqeilan RI, Croce CM. 2007. WWOX in biological control and tumorigenesis. *J Cell Physiol* 212 (2):307–310.

Croce CM. 1991. Genetic approaches to the study of the molecular basis of human cancer. *Cancer Res* 51(18 Suppl):5015s–5018s.

Feinberg AP, Tycko B. 2004. The history of cancer epigenetics. *Nat Rev Cancer* 4(2):143–153.

Grisendi S, Pandolfi PP. 2004. Germline modifications strategies. In: Holland EC, ed. *Mouse Models of Human Cancers*. Hoboken, NJ: Wiley-Liss, pp. 43–66.

Hanahan D, Weinberg RA. 2000. The hallmarks of cancer. *Cell* 100(1):57–70.

Holland EC. 2004. Preface. In: Holland EC, ed. *Mouse Models of Human Cancers*. Hoboken, NJ: Wiley-Liss, p. vii.

Jones PA, Baylin SB. 2002. The fundamental role of epigenetic events in cancer. *Nat Rev Genet* 3(6):415–428.

Lengauer C, Kinzler KW, Vogelstein B. 1998. Genetic instabilities in human cancers. *Nature* 396(6712):643–649.

Menacho-Marquez M, Murguia JR. 2007. Yeast on drugs: *Saccharomyces cerevisiae* as a tool for anticancer drug research. *Clin Transl Oncol* 9(4):221–228.

Parsonnet J. 1995. Bacterial infection as a cause of cancer. *Environ Health Perspect* 103 (Suppl 8):263–268.

Pekarsky Y, Zanesi N, Aqeilan RI, Croce CM. 2007. Animal models for chronic lymphocytic leukemia. *J Cell Biochem* 100(5):1109–1118.

Poirier MC. 2004. Chemical-induced DNA damage and human cancer risk. *Nat Rev Cancer* 4(8):630–637.

Saito RM, van den Heuvel S. 2002. Malignant worms: what cancer research can learn from *C. elegans*. *Cancer Invest* 20(2):264–275.

Schatten H, Hueser CN, Chakrabarti A. 2000. From fertilization to cancer: the role of centrosomes in the union and separation of genomic material. *Microsc Res Tech* 49(5):420–427.

Vidal M, Cagan RL. 2006. *Drosophila* models for cancer research. *Curr Opin Genet Dev* 16(1): 10–16.

Vogelstein B, Kinzler KW. 2004. Cancer genes and the pathways they control. *Nat Med* 10(8): 789–799.

Wallingford JB. 1999. Tumors in tadpoles: the *Xenopus* embryo as a model system for the study of tumorigenesis. *Trends Genet* 15(10):385–388.

Zanesi N, Pekarsky Y, Croce CM. 2005. A mouse model of the fragile gene FHIT: from carcinogenesis to gene therapy and cancer prevention. *Mutat Res* 591(1–2):103–109.

4

DIAGNOSIS AND TREATMENT OF MALIGNANT DISEASES

F. Marc Stewart and Jessica A. Stewart

Seattle Cancer Care Alliance, Fred Hutchinson Cancer Research Center,
University of Washington, Seattle, Washington

INTRODUCTION

Over the past three decades major progress has been made in the treatment of malignant diseases. In both men and women, from 1992 to 2003, cancer death rates have declined due largely to a decrease in the use of tobacco, improved screening techniques, and advances in treatment. Five major approaches are used to treat patients with cancer: (1) surgery, (2) radiation, (3) drug therapy, (4) integrative medicine, and (5) palliative care (Figure 1). The choice of treatment approaches depends on a number of factors: (1) the organ or tissue in which the cancer originated (e.g., lung, kidney, blood); (2) the type of cancer determined by the pathologist, who examines the tissue under the microscope (e.g., adenocarcinoma, germ cell cancer); (3) specific biological factors analyzed in the laboratory (estrogen receptor proteins detected on the surface of breast cancer cells, which predict that the tumor is likely to respond to hormonal therapy), chromosomal analyses, which identify particular types of leukemias or lymphomas and give prognostic information; (4) the stage of the cancer determined by the TNM system [T represents the size of the primary (originating) tumor, N, the extent of the lymph

The Biology and Treatment of Cancer: Understanding Cancer
Edited by Arthur B. Pardee and Gary S. Stein   Copyright © 2009 John Wiley & Sons, Inc.

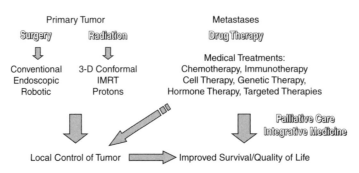

Figure 1. Cancer therapy involves five primary services (surgery, radiation, drug therapy (medical oncology), palliative care, and integrative medicine. Each service offers potential cutting-edge treatments discussed later in the text. Many important services not shown (pathology, radiology, social work, pastoral services, pain clinics, psychiatry, nutrition, etc.) play very important roles in the management of patients with cancer.

node metastases, and M the presence of metastatic disease to areas outside the primary tumor and immediate lymph node drainage].

Case 1

A 45-year-old woman with a newly discovered breast lump undergoes an excisional (tumor removed) biopsy. The pathologist examines the tissue, determines that the primary tumor measures 2×2 cm in diameter, and prepares tissue for examination under the microscope and for other special studies. The tumor is classified as an *infiltrating ductal carcinoma* [infiltrating = invading the normal breast (ductal) tissue] with a high number of *mitoses* (cell divisions) and clear margins (the tumor nodule has been removed completely, with no remaining cancer tissue left in the breast). Laboratory studies on the tissue identify a high concentration of estrogen receptors on the surface of the cells. A sampling of the lymph nodes under the arm (*axillary lymph nodes*) shows tumor involvement and the patient undergoes a *lymph node dissection.* Radiology studies show no evidence of spread to other parts of the body. Therefore, the breast cancer appears to be localized to the breast and lymph nodes. Unfortunately the patient still has a significant risk for recurrence at other sites in the body. Since the pathologist determined that the *surgical margins* were clear, no further surgery is required. However, because small undetectable numbers of cancer cells may have spread into the breast tissue surrounding the tumor mass, radiation is added to reduce the risk that the cancer might recur locally in the breast at some time in the future. Also, since there is a significant risk that small numbers of cells may have escaped from the primary tumor or lymph nodes into the bloodstream and onto other organs, hormonal therapy (a medication called *anastrazole*) is added. This drug reduces the level of estrogen in the body. Without estrogen, the estrogen receptor protein on the surface of the breast cancer cells fails to stimulate breast cancer cells causing the cells to die. Finally, chemotherapy treatments are given for four months to further reduce the risk of cancer recurrence. With these treatments it is hoped that the patient will be cured.

Discussion: This multimodality therapy is a typical treatment approach to localized cancers that respond to surgery, drug therapy, and radiation. The role of the pathologist is key for establishing a diagnosis and helping determine prognosis. In some diseases the very earliest stages of cancer can be treated with surgery alone or sometimes, radiation alone. When cancers have spread or metastasized to lymph nodes or other organs and tissues, drug therapy plays a primary role. In many cases of localized cancer and in some cases of metastatic cancer, cure is possible depending on the tumor type. When cure is not possible, treatments may improve symptoms by causing temporary shrinkage of the tumor. Palliative care services and integrative medicine approaches complement the other forms of treatment by focusing on symptom control and prompting a feeling of well-being for as long as possible. Research studies are a very important part of cancer treatment, and a clinical trial often represents the best available approach. Newer approaches called targeted therapies have been developed to treat very specifically the biological basis of the cancer and promise to improve outcomes with much less toxicity to normal tissues.

SURGERY

William Halstead, noted for many surgical and medical achievements, performed the first *radical mastectomy* for breast cancer in 1882. For the next three to four decades, surgery played the primary role in the treatment of breast cancer. With breast cancer as a model, cancer operations were developed for other tumors, which involved, for example, removal of large parts of the stomach in patients with gastric (stomach) cancer and segments of the colon and patients with colon cancer. In these early times it was felt but never proven that radical surgery was required to control or cure the cancer. As a result, many patients suffered disability and disfigurement since the tumor plus large amounts of extra tissue were removed. For example, the classic Halstead radical mastectomy removed the entire breast, surrounding muscle tissue, and lymph nodes draining the region. Women often had weakness and swelling in the associated arm and suffered due to removal of normal muscle tissue and the lymph nodes, which allow lymph to drain from the tissues in the arm. Over the past 30 years, clinical investigators in oncology have come to understand that removal of the tumor mass (lumpectomy or partial mastectomy) plus radiation to the breast provides the same survival and cure rate as the more radical approach described above. In addition, the use of techniques to inject the tumor with a mildly radioactive 'dye' that traverses the lymph node channels into the axillary lymph nodes allows surgeons to remove the first likely lymph node (referred to as the *sentinel lymph node*) that has the highest probability of containing tumor. If tumor cannot be found in the sentinel lymph node, lymph node dissection (removal) is not indicated and the patient is spared more surgery and the small risk of arm swelling; if tumor is present, a partial (first- or low-level) lymph node dissection is indicated. These approaches have improved the quality of life in women with breast cancer by minimizing disfigurement and reducing weakness and swelling in the associated arm.

The advances in surgery in the years that followed the Halstead era included improvement in sterile technique and wound control. More recently, technical advances have allowed surgeons to remove cancers using endoscopic approaches. *Endoscopes* are long, flexible tubes with a channel for video and mechanical devices that are used by the surgeon to biopsy or cut tissue. *Laparoscopy*, a technique that introduces an endoscope into the abdomen through very small incisions, has now been used to remove small colon cancers. This procedure is associated with a quicker recovery time than with a conventional partial colon resection (*partial colectomy*).

Robotic Surgery

Laparoscopic surgery can be assisted by the use of *robotics* (Figure 2). Robotic technology offers a number of advantages during surgery. Robotic arms filter the tiny tremors coming from the surgeon's hands to increase steadiness. Cameras controlled by the robot provide a three-dimensional stereoscopic image of the body's interior with sharp visualization of tiny structures such as nerves. This

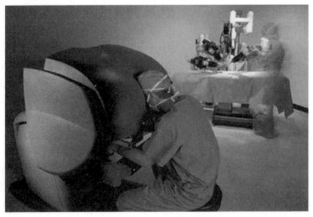

(A)

Figure 2. (A) Surgeon operates from a console located adjacent to the patient and the operative field. (B,C) Robotic arms are used to transect the tumor. Hand controls offer stability and precision in movement. (D) Simulated surgical approach to prostate cancer: robotic arms allow careful separation of nerves away from site of tumor/prostate resection, preserving urinary and sexual function. (Images © 2008 Intuitive Surgical, Inc.) (See insert for color representation.)

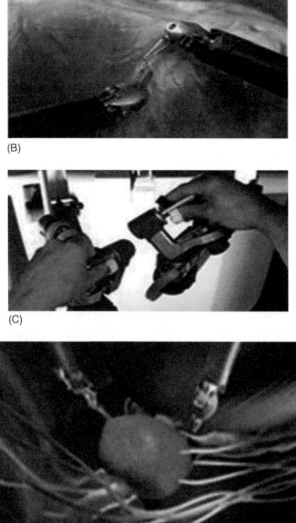

(B)

(C)

(D)

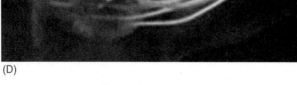

Figure 2. (*Continued*)

approach has been used, for example, in the treatment of localized prostate cancer. With conventional radical surgery (*radical prostatectomy*), complications such as *erectile dysfunction* (impotence) and *urinary incontinence* (inability to control urinary function) are common. The robot itself consists of four "arms" and "wrists" connected to hand and foot controls. Two arms hold video cameras and *retractors* (instruments that stabilize or hold tissue while the surgeon operates) and two arms replicate the hand movements initiated by the surgeon. The prostate tumor is removed very carefully and the tiny nerves important for sexual and urinary function are carefully preserved. Robotic surgery for prostate cancer often results in less pain, shorter hospital stay, less blood loss, and a quicker recovery time compared to standard surgery. Large tumors that extend outside the prostate gland may be more suitable for other approaches, such as radiation therapy. Computer stimulated operations allow surgeons to practice a complicated robotic procedure using 3-D images of the patient's tumor inside the body.

Case 2

A 55-year-old male noting a two-year history of frequent urination presents for evaluation. His father and uncle have a history of prostate cancer. A *digital rectal exam* reveals a firm, hard nodule in the left lobe of his prostate gland. PSA (*prostate-specific antigen*) reveals a slight elevation. He undergoes a biopsy, which reveals adenocarcinoma of the prostate, *Gleason grade* 4. Radiological studies show no spread to other body sites. A urologist experienced in robotic/cancer surgery removes his prostate gland by introducing the four robotic arms through four tiny incisions in his lower abdomen. Four months after his surgery he has slight, occasional urinary incontinence but begins to have normal sexual function again. His PSA is undetectable and he continues to be followed by his primary care physician.

Discussion: Prostate cancer is the second-leading cause of cancer-related deaths in males. The detection of PSA in the serum of men has led to earlier detection of prostate cancer. Although whether the detection of early prostate cancer by PSA improves survival from prostate cancer is controversial, it is used widely as a screening tool for men over the age of 50. The risk of prostate cancer is increased in families of men with prostate cancer. The patient's symptoms, and in particular the digital rectal exam in this case, led to the detection of prostate cancer. Robotic surgery is one approach that reduces the morbidity of prostatectomy since it is accomplished by laparoscopic techniques. Other options for patients with prostate cancer include radiation therapy (*IMRT, proton therapy, brachytherapy*—see below). To date in patients with *operable disease*, there are no definitive studies about whether radiation or surgical treatments are best. In the future the presence of specific gene mutations may serve as a biomarker to separate patients who might benefit from radical prostate cancer therapy from those who potentially need much less treatment.

Cryosurgery/High-Intensity-Focus Ultrasound Surgery/Laser Surgery

Researchers have developed technologies that may offer advantages over the traditional scalpel. The use of cold as a treatment for cancer is called *cryosurgery*.

Currently, it is used to treat precancerous lesions of the skin and uterine cervix. A *cryoprobe* introduced into the tumor or precancerous area delivers *liquid nitrogen or argon*, which destroys abnormal tissue by freezing it. High-intensity-focus ultrasound therapy, pioneered in China and Europe, uses inaudible sound waves to destroy, for example, prostate cancer tissue. *Laser surgery* applies *high-intensity light* to superficial tumors on the skin, vagina/cervix, or anus. Laser light is more precise than a scalpel and patients have less pain and a faster recovery. All of these approaches are being tested in other tumors, sometimes in conjunction with radiation or drug therapy.

RADIATION THERAPY

One of the most effective treatments for controlling cancer localized to a specific area of the body is radiation therapy. Radiation energy comes in the form of *photons* (a unit of electromagnetic radiation showing properties of both *particles and waves*), *electrons, carbon ions*, or *protons* (Figure 3).

There are several ways in which radiation is generated or delivered: (1) by an *external beam* (radiation generated by a machine such as a *linear accelerator*), (2) by *brachytherapy,* which uses *radioisotopes* (*atoms* with an *unstable nucleus* that gives off *gamma rays* and other atomic particles) in the physical form of seeds or rods which are implanted and/or then removed after a time interval, and (3) radioisotopes that are ingested or injected. Radiation interacts with water to cause the formation of *free radicals*, molecules that become very chemically reactive and cause breaks in the cells' deoxyribonucleic acid (DNA) strands, impairing cell division. Fortunately, cancer cells have a slower ability to repair these breaks than do normal tissue. However, radiation often requires oxygen to

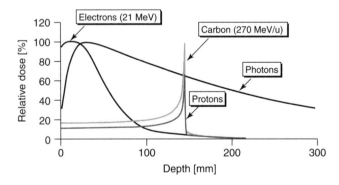

Figure 3. Various types of radiation, showing the amount of radiation released at a particular depth of treatment. Most treatment is delivered as photons from a linear accelerator. Electrons release energy early and are ideal for treating superficial tumors (e.g., skin tumors). Carbon ion and protons release energy completely at a specified depth and therefore have the potential to deliver more radiation to the tumor and less to surrounding normal tissues.

ensure that the damage to DNA is permanent without the ability to repair. Some malignant tumors that outgrow their blood supply have areas with very little oxygen, and the effectiveness of radiation is diminished. Efforts to increase oxygen to tumors during therapy or to use drugs that increase cancer sensitivity to radiation are active areas of research.

The dose of radiation is calculated in grays, abbreviated Gy. Many tumors have a much slower ability to recover from the effects of radiation than that of normal tissue exposed at the same dose. With increasing doses, tumor control is greater, but so are the risks for complications (Figure 4). For many tumors, radiation is more effective when given in fractions rather than in a single large dose. *Fractionation of radiation* allows the normal tissues exposed to radiation to recover. Hence, fractionated radiation treatments are more effective against tumor cells and less likely to damage normal cells permanently.

Radiation therapy is usually delivered by a *linear accelerator*, which generates a beam of radiation (*gamma rays* or *electron particles*) directed to the site of the cancer. In a patient with a localized lung cancer, the radiation beam is aimed at the tumor from several different directions. The tumor is treated to a specific dose based on overlap of beams in the area of the tumor internally. To treat the tumor in the lung, radiation must pass through the chest wall, through the normal lung tissue, through the tumor, continuing out through the opposite side of the body and through more normal tissues. Thus, the tumor and, to a lesser extent, the normal body tissue receive large amounts of radiation. With newer techniques such as three-dimensional conformal radiation and an even more sophisticated approach called *intensity-modulated radiation therapy* (IMRT), radiation may be concentrated very precisely in the region of the tumor, with greater sparing of normal tissues. These techniques use multiple beams often generated through a

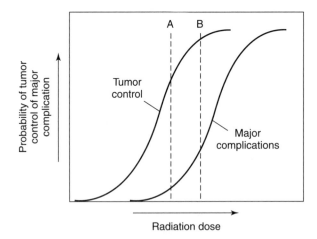

Figure 4. Relationship between radiation dose, tumor control, and complications related to treatment. Radiation dose A gives acceptable tumor control with minimal complications; Radiation dose B gives optimal tumor control with higher risk of major complications.

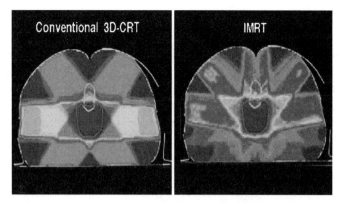

Figure 5. Comparison of three-dimensional conformal radiation therapy with intensity-modulated radiation therapy for prostate cancer (red). IMRT utilizes greater number of beams (yellow) tailored with various shapes and intensities to deliver more radiation to the tumor and less to the normal tissues. (See insert for color representation.)

series of opening and closing lead slats (a *multileaf collimator*). Both the shape of the beam and the intensity of the beam can be regulated rather than relying simply on overlap of beams, described above. In IMRT special software is required to calculate the number of beams and, for each beam, its intensity and angle of delivery (Figure 5). Image-guided radiation treatments link three-dimensional computerized tomography (CT) scans directly to radiation therapy units so that normal internal structures can be identified (and avoided) while the tumor can be targeted very precisely. Prior to this approach, skin tattoos have been employed to guide the beam direction, but the potential for slight changes in body position make this approach less accurate. Radiosurgery using a *cyberknife* is another technological advance that is similar to surgery in its precision. It is used to treat brain tumors, spinal tumors, and more recently, selected lung and other tumors. The Cyberknife integrates an image-guidance system as described above and a multijointed robotic arm with a number of degrees of freedom providing maneuverability in targeting tumors. A high-energy x-ray source mounted on the robotic arm locates the position of the tumor in the body and delivers pinpoint radiation from more than 1200 angles within a fraction of a millimeter accuracy. It is important to utilize these more precise and more costly methods appropriately since not every patient, particularly those undergoing palliative care, requires highly precise radiation therapy.

Electron beam therapy releases energy very superficially, an ideal for treatment of skin cancers or cancers that involve the body surfaces. *Brachytherapy* is a form of radiation generated by radioactive seeds or rods, which are implanted directly into such tumors as prostate, cervical, or uterine cancer. This approach has been used more recently in lung cancer and breast cancer. Radioactive plaques have been used to treat the rare patient with melanoma of the internal eye (uveal melanoma).

Case 3

A 35-year-old woman with a strong family history of breast cancer completes her first mammogram, which is reported as normal. On the *mammogram* her breast tissue is noted to be dense and a breast MRI (*magnetic resonance image*) is recommended (Figure 6). A right breast mass is detected and she is advised to undergo further evaluation. The breast mass is biopsied using stereotactic procedure (biopsy needle guided while the breast mass is being imaged). The pathology reveals cancerous cells and she undergoes removal of the 2.5-cm mass (*lumpectomy*). A sentinel lymph node biopsy is obtained which is normal. *Brachytherapy* is used to treat the tissue surrounding the breast tumor (Figure 7). The total radiation treatment time is 4 days, compared to the usual six weeks of treatment with conventional external beam radiation (radiation generated by linear accelerator and aimed at the breast) approaches. The pathology of the tumor showed an infiltrating ductal cancer and was completely removed. The tumor contains no estrogen receptors on its cell surfaces but a protein called *her-2-neu* is detected in abnormal amounts (Figure 8). Following radiation therapy, the patient is given chemotherapy to prevent the tumor from recurring. In addition, she is treated with *trastuzumab*, a special antibody which attacks or attaches to the her-2-neu surface protein on any microscopic numbers of remaining breast cancer cells. This *monoclonal antibody* is a manufactured product that kills tumor cells expressing the her-2-neu protein.

Discussion: Patients with strong family histories of breast cancer sometimes need to begin screening tests at an earlier age based on their higher risk of developing breast cancer. In this patient her breasts appeared very dense on mammograms limiting the ability to visualize any abnormalities. Breast MRIs create images based on the response of body tissues to strong magnets and

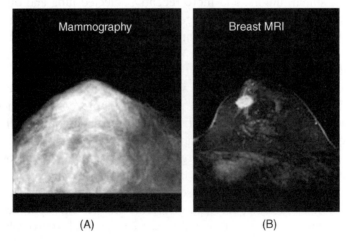

(A)   (B)

Figure 6. Mammogram of dense breast shows no abnormality (left). MRI shows an abnormality subsequently determined to be cancerous (right).

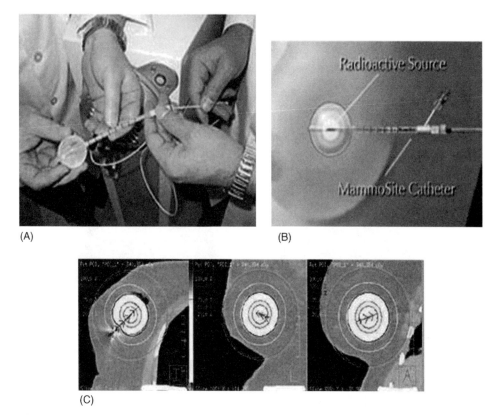

(A)

(B)

(C)

Figure 7. Brachytherapy for breast cancer. (A) Special balloon and catheter prior to insertion into tumor site following lumpectomy. (B,C) Radioactive seeds introduced into balloon through the catheter and removed after various time intervals. Extent of radiation effects show by concentric circles. (Image 7A used with permission of The University of Toledo Medical Center. Images 7B and 7C courtesy of Hologic.) (See insert for color representation.)

radio-wave pulses and can sometimes "see through" breast tissue that appears dense on conventional mammography. This patient therefore received surgery and radiation to treat the local cancer and chemotherapy and antibody therapy (or *immunotherapy*) to treat any tiny amounts of cells that have escaped from the tumor into the blood stream or lymph nodes. Hormone therapy is not indicated since estrogen receptors were not found on the surface of the breast cancer cells. Therapy is tailored to the biology of the tumor.

PROTON THERAPY

One of the newer forms of treatment uses protons to carry radiation energy to the tumor. Unlike other forms of radiation, a stream of protons releases radiation energy suddenly and completely to tumors deep in the body without passing through the opposite side of the body (Figure 9). This minimizes the radiation

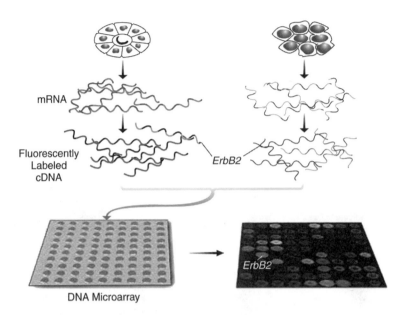

Figure 8. Microarray analysis used to detect abnormal expression of *ErbB2*. Flurorescent-labeled cDNA for the *ErbB2* gene combines specifically with a patient's mRNA containing *ErbB2*. If a patient with breast cancer (right) has a large amount of *ErbB2* in her cells, it will appear as a bright fluorescent spot on the array plate. (See insert for color representation.)

energy delivered to tissues on the opposite side of the beam (Figure 9). This form of radiation has great promise for cancers that are surrounded by fragile normal tissue structures. For example, proton therapy has been used to treat localized prostate cancer, sparing the bladder and rectum from significant amounts of

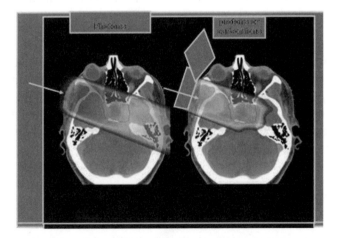

Figure 9. Comparison of photon delivery by linear accelerator and proton therapy by cyclotron to a brain tumor. (A) Photon radiation passes through normal tissue, tumor (center, circular structure), and more normal tissue. (B) Proton beam released in the tumor stops at the far edge if the tumor, sparing normal tissue. (See insert for color representation.)

radiation. Also, by sparing the nerves in the normal surrounding tissue that are important for sexual and urinary function, this form of treatment preserves quality of life while delivering large amounts of radiation to the tumor itself. Proton therapy is particularly useful for treating localized tumors in children. Spinal tumors, brain tumors, intraocular melanoma, and other forms of cancer require precision delivery of radiation in a way that spares sensitive nerve or brain tissue and preserves intellectual, motor, and sensory function.

DRUG THERAPY

Anticancer drugs commonly interfere with cell division by inhibiting the replication of DNA. Although these drugs often affect rapidly dividing cancer cells, most are relatively nonspecific and therefore may cause harm to normal body tissues (e.g., rapidly dividing normal cells such as hair cells and cells lining the intestines and mouth).

Ancient Egyptians were the first to use compounds from plants and animals to treat cancers of the uterus and stomach. Centuries later, during World War I, it was learned that soldiers exposed to *mustard gas* had lowered blood counts. Eventually, a related compound, *nitrogen mustard*, was used to treat *leukemia* and *lymphomas*. Since that time many chemicals have been studied and tested for their effects on cancer cells, and a large number now play a role in oncology treatment.

From studies conducted in the laboratory and in animals with cancer, promising drugs are tested in humans using a three- or four-phase series of clinical trials. In phase I studies a promising drug's safety/symptoms/side effect profile and the body's ability to metabolize the drug is determined while slowly increasing dose levels in groups of patients until the maximum tolerated level is achieved. In phase II studies the agent's effect on a particular kind of cancer (e.g., metastatic colon cancer) is evaluated. In phase III studies the new agent is compared directly to standard therapy, usually in a *randomized controlled trial* (patients consent to be randomly selected for standard treatment or the new treatment to be tested), to prove scientifically that the new treatment is indeed more effective than previous treatments. Phase IV studies further evaluate the long-term safety and effectiveness of a new treatment.

Tumor cells are heterogeneous and not infrequently develop resistance to the mechanism of action of a particular chemotherapeutic agent. Therefore, most chemotherapy is given using combinations of drugs, since each drug may be associated with a different biological mechanism of action. With this approach large numbers of heterogeneous tumor cells may be killed and resistance to treatment more effectively minimized.

Advances in understanding the genetic changes that transform a normal cell into a malignant cell have led to the creation of a new generation of targeted treatments. As the precise biological abnormality present in cancer cells is targeted, theoretically, larger numbers of normal cells are spared from toxicity.

Chemotherapy

Chemotherapy refers to a wide range of drugs used to treat cancer (Table 1). Some of the drugs are compounds extracted from various plants, while others are manufactured. Individual chemotherapy drugs act on cancer cells by different The most common routes of administration are by mouth, intravenously, and into a muscle. To increase the concentration of drug in a particular region of the body where the tumor resides, chemotherapy can be injected into a specific cavity, such as the abdomen (intraperitoneal), the brain and spinal column (intrathecal), the lung (intrapleural), or spread on the skin as topical therapy. Chemotherapy drugs each have their own unique toxicity profile. Side effects can be early, intermediate (within a few weeks), or late (occurring years after administration). Examples of early toxicities include nausea and vomiting. Lowering of blood counts [anemia (red cells), thrombocytopenia (platelets), leukopenia (white cells)], diarrhea, alopecia (hair loss), weakness and rarely kidney failure, lung scarring, and heart failure are examples of intermediate toxicities. Rare late toxicities include development of the leukemia, perhaps as the result of the DNA mutating effects of chemotherapy on normal blood stem cells.

Case 4

A 17-year-old male notes a painless swelling in his testis for the past eight months. He begins to notice that his breathing has become more difficult. A chest x-ray shows many tumor nodules in the lungs (Figure 10). Examination of his right testis shows a large, firm mass. An ultrasound study confirms the urologist's impression that this is a tumor and not a hernia or an infection. A blood sample is obtained which shows very high levels of β-HCG (the hormone used to detect pregnancy in women). His urologist removes the testis and the attached mass

TABLE 1. Chemotherapy Agents and Their Cellular Mechanisms of Action

Category	Mechanism	Example Drugs
DNA-altering drugs	May cause breaks or mutations in DNA	Cyclophosphamide, carboplatin, cisplatin
Antibiotics	Bind to DNA and prevent RNA synthesis leading to cell death	Doxorubicin, bleomycin, mitoxantrone
Antimetabolites	Block DNA synthesis	Cytarabine, fludarabine, gemcitabine
Microtubule inhibitors	Prevent microtubules in cells from supporting cell division	Vincristine, vinblastine
DNA repair enzyme inhibitors	Inhibits natural enzymes whose normal function is to repair DNA mutations	Etoposide
Steroids/hormones	Interact with receptors and cell membranes to kill cells	Prednisone, tamoxifen

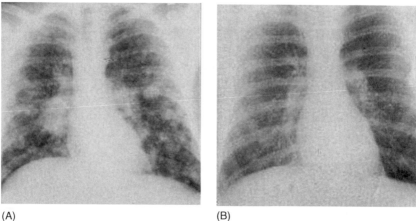

(A)   (B)

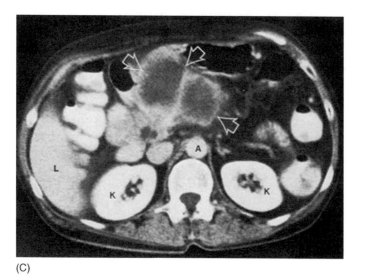

(C)

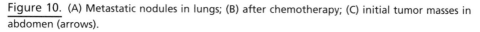

Figure 10. (A) Metastatic nodules in lungs; (B) after chemotherapy; (C) initial tumor masses in abdomen (arrows).

surgically. The mass is found to be an *embryonal carcinoma* of the testis. A CT scan of his abdomen shows massively enlarged lymph nodes. He undergoes four cycles of chemotherapy with cisplatin, etoposide, and bleomycin and his lung masses disappear completely and his β-HCG level becomes undetectable. A moderate-sized residual abdominal mass (Figure 10) is removed surgically and found to be scar tissue without any evidence of cancer. Ten years later he has no signs of cancer and is considered to be cured of his disease.

Discussion: Testicular cancer is the most common malignancy in young men. It is highly curable when detected early, However, even in very advanced cases, cure can be achieved with chemotherapy in over 70% of patients. Chemotherapy randomly attacks various parts of the cell structure, including DNA. Although it affects normal cells, rapidly dividing tumor cells are more sensitive to its effects. In this case the testis cancer cells (unlike some other types of cancer) are exquisitely sensitive to chemotherapy, and all cancer cells are destroyed. The malignant cells secrete β-HCG, a substance detected in the blood and indicative of active tumor when present, called a *tumor marker.* Since the chemotherapy has killed all of the tumor cells, this substance is no longer detected.

TARGETED THERAPY

The development of targeted agents is a natural evolution of major advances in the understanding of specific cellular mechanisms that cause cancer. Targeted agents block specific cellular pathways involving cell growth, proliferation, *angiogenesis*, and *metastasis* (Table 2). Although these treatments are highly specific for a particular tumor mechanism, cancers are hetergeneous, often composed of multiple clones of cells and prone to continued mutation. Thus, the challenge for targeted therapies will be the emergence of resistant clones of

T A B L E 2. Examples of Targeted Therapies for Malignant Disease

Drug	Major Target(s)	Disease
Small Molecule		
Sorafenib	BRAF, VEGFR; EGFR	Renal cell cancer; liver cancer
Sunitnib	VEGFR, c-kit, FLT3	Renal cell cancer; Gl stromal tumor
Erlotinib	EGFR	Non-small cell lung cancer; pancreatic cancer
Gefitinib	EGFR	Non-small cell lung cancer
Bortezomib	Proteosome	Myeloma
Lapatinib	Her-2/Neu	Breast cancer
Imatinib	Bcr-abl; c-kit	Chronic myelocytic leukemia; acute lymphoblastic leukemia; Gl stromal tumor; mastocytosis
Dasatinib	Bcr-abl; c-kit	Chronic myelocytic leukemia; acute lymphoblastic leukemia
Monoclonal Antibodies		
Bevacizumab	VEGF	Colorectal cancer; non-small cell lung cancer
Rituximab	CD20	B-cell lymphoma
Cetuximab	EGFR	Colorectal cancer; head and neck cancer
Gemtuzumab	CD33	Acute myelogenous leukemia
Alemtuzumab	CD52	Chronic lymphocytic leukemia
^{90}Y-ibritumomab	CD20	Non-Hodgkin's lymphoma

cells. Targeted therapies may be divided into two categories (1) *small-molecule inhibitors* and (2) *monoclonal antibodies*.

Small-Molecule Therapy

Protein tyrosine kinases have proven to be good targets for small-molecule inhibitors. Tyrosine kinases help other enzymes function in the cell. Defects or mutations in tyrosine kinases can lead to malignancy. Small-molecule inhibitors can pass through the cell membranes and inhibit tyrosine kinases inside the cell and thus can inhibit malignant cell growth. *Monoclonal antibodies* attack specific cell proteins or antigens on the surface of the malignant cell, either destroying the cell or blocking other factors in the blood from stimulating its growth.

Case 5

A 45-year-old man presents with weight loss. His appetite is good at the beginning of a meal, but he fills up quickly after a few bites of food. He notes abdominal fullness and a firm mass in the upper left portion of his abdomen. His physician palpates (feels) a very large spleen (i.e., the mass in his abdomen) and orders a complete blood count, which shows a very high white blood cell count, consistent with leukemia (Figure 11). The 52 chromosomes from a single leukemia cell are analyzed and show exchanged or translocated pieces of chromosomal material (a part of chromosome 9 has broken off and attached to chromosome 22) (Figure 12). This *chromosomal rearrangement* or *translocation*

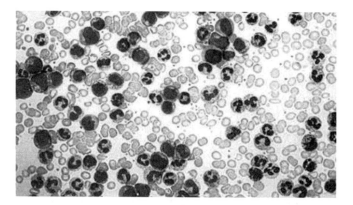

Figure 11. Blood smear showing a tremendously increased number of white blood cells (leukemia). White blood cells have the dark-staining nuclei; red cells (small cells with central pale area) lost their nucleus prior to leaving the bone marrow.

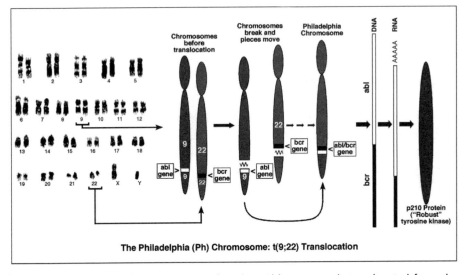

The Philadelphia (Ph) Chromosome: t(9;22) Translocation

Figure 12. Philadelphia chromosome translocation. Abl oncogene is translocated from chromosome 9 to chromosome 22 (left, photo of actual chromosome analysis). The region on chromosome 22 close to the breakpoint is called the breakpoint cluster region (bcr). The combination of bcr and abl forms a new hydrid gene, *bcr-abl* (right). This gene causes chronic myelocytic leukemia (CML). (See insert for color representation.)

creates a new *hybrid gene, bcr-abl*, adjacent to the new attachment area of chromosome 22. A diagnosis of chronic myelocytic leukemia is made. *Bcr-abl*, the new hybrid gene, transcribes a messenger ribonucleic acid (mRNA) molecule which translates a protein (tyrosine kinase) that causes the leukemia (Figure 12). The patient is treated with a drug manufactured specifically to inhibit the *bcr-abl protein*, imatinib (Figure 13). The effects of this drug are so specific that toxicities to normal cells are reduced. The patient achieves a complete remission (the white blood cell count decreases to normal and the bone marrow appears normal by microscopic exam). No cells containing the *bcr-abl* gene are detected using the very sensitive PCR (polymerase chain reaction) test. The patient continues the medication and the remission lasts for five years. At that time the patient develops a new, different chromosomal abnormality and progressive leukemia. *Dasatinib*, another designer drug that inhibits new mutations, is used for several months to control the more resistant leukemia. However, the leukemia progresses again and the patient is referred for high-dose chemotherapy and a stem cell transplant. Chemotherapy doses and whole-body irradiation are administered at very high levels to kill resistant leukemia cells. The infusion of matched stem cells from the patient's brother gives the patient new, normal bone marrow cells (Figure 14). This procedure is successful and the patient is cured of the disease.

Discussion: This patient has a chronic myelocytic leukemia (CML), a malignancy of blood stem cells leading to an overproduction of white blood

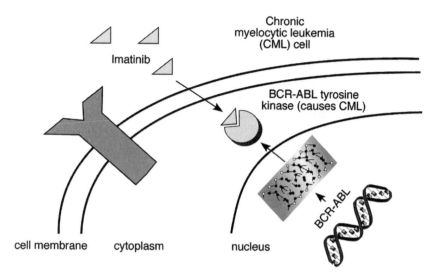

Figure 13. (A) Activation of bcr/abl by ATP; (B) inhibition of bcr/abl by Gleevec (imatinib).

cells. These cells circulate through the blood and bone marrow and also are sequestered by the spleen, which eventually becomes quite large. The enlarged spleen sometimes compresses the adjacent stomach, leading to the sensation of *early satiety*, a term used to describe the fullness that one feels after only a few bites of food. The *chromosomal rearrangement* in this case is very specific for

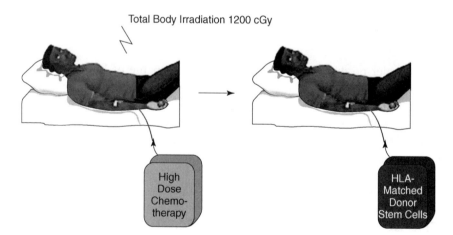

Figure 14. Treatment for relapsed CML. Patient is given high-dose chemotherapy and total body irradiation followed by infusion of tissue compatible stem cells. The very intense therapy is designed to destroy resistant leukemia cells. The infused cells from a normal donor provide new marrow to the patient and a new immune system that may help destroy leukemia cells that might have survived the intense chemoradiotherapy.

CML. When scientists use molecular techniques to cut the piece of DNA called bcr-abl and *transduce* (insert) it into the DNA of an animal's blood cells (e.g., a mouse), the animal will develop a leukemia similar to human CML. The treatment for this disease is revolutionary since *imatinib* is the first designer drug; that is, a drug that acts specifically on cells that have the *bcr-abl gene* abnormality (not randomly on all cells, normal and abnormal, like chemotherapy) (Figure 13). Although many people remain in remission with continued imatimib therapy, some patients' blood cells *mutate spontaneously* (develop new genetic abnormalities) and become resistant to imatimib therapy. Other designer drugs such as dasatinib have been developed for those patients, but the cure for the disease at that point would require high-dose therapy and stem cell transplant from a tissue-matched brother or sister or tissue-matched unrelated donor (Figure 14). The combination of high-dose chemotherapy and the immune reaction of the donor cells against any residual leukemia cells [called the graft versus leukemia effect (the graft comprises the donor cells infused into the patient)] both contribute to the potential cure of this disease. The procedure is risky since the donor cells sometimes attack the patient's normal tissues, a disease called *graft-versus-host disease*, which can be fatal if severe.

Small-molecule inhibitors may also affect tumors overexpressing the extra cellular growth factor receptor (EGFR) (Figure 15). Gefnitinib and erlotinib inhibit EGFR and have shown some effectiveness against EGFR-expressing tumors such as non-small-cell lung cancer and head and neck cancer. Cancer patients with mutations in EGFR are particularly susceptible to the effects of these drugs. Sorafenib, another small-molecule compound, inhibits multiple kinase enzymes, affecting both cell proliferation and angiogenesis.

Monoclonal Antibodies

In 1975, Kohler produced monoclonal antibodies capable of binding to specific tumor antigens. The fusion of mouse spleen cells with a human myeloma cell line (myeloma is a malignant disease of plasma cells in humans; these clones of cells produce a single antibody in large amounts) produced a "hybridoma" capable of producing large quantities of monoclonal antibodies. It is possible to produce antibodies to a specific cancer cell surface protein or antigen for therapeutic purposes. When monoclonal antibodies attach to a specific antigen on a tumor cell, the antibody may prevent other growth factors from stimulating the cancer cell. In colon cancer, too, many molecules of extracellular growth factor receptor (ECGFR) are produced on the surface of the cells. Cetuximab is a monoclonal antibody which blocks the ECGFR so that the normal growth factor, ECGF, cannot stimulate the cell to grow (Figure 16). Monoclonal antibodies also work in a second way. Interestingly, if the K-RAS gene is mutated, the tumor will not respond to cetuximab. Once they attach to a specific cancer cell, the body's immune system is activated to destroy that cell. Examples include rituximab, a

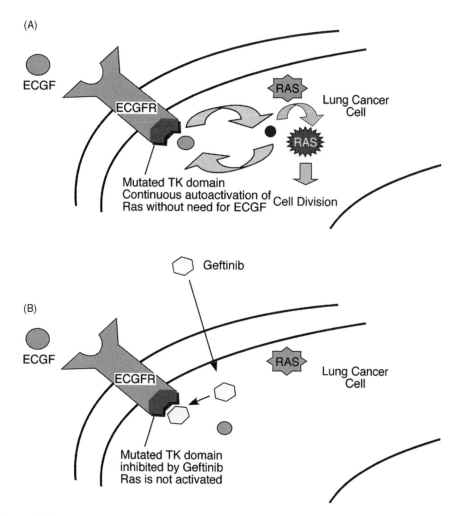

Figure 15. (A) Lung cancer cell: extracellular growth factor (ECGF) stimulates mutated receptor on cell. The tyrosine kinase enzyme (blue) located on the inner aspect of the receptor is mutated. It acts continuously to stimulate the RAS oncogene to be activated (red) and hence promotes continuous cell division (and tumor growth). (B) Geftinib inhibits the mutated form of the extracellular growth factor receptor (ECGFR), shutting off RAS activation and inhibiting cell growth. Gefnitinib is not effective on lung cancers that do not contain the mutation described above. (See insert for color representation.)

monoclonal antibody directed to attack the CD20 protein found on the surface of many B-cell non-Hodgkin's lymphoma patients. The front end of the antibody, called Fab, is engineered to attach to the CD20 protein and nothing else. The tail of the antibody (the Fc portion) activates the body's immune system against the tumor cell. An alternative approach has been developed to kill tumor cells more effectively. The Fc portion of the antibody or the tail can be fitted with a radioactive iodine molecule (^{131}I radioisotope) which emits high concentrations

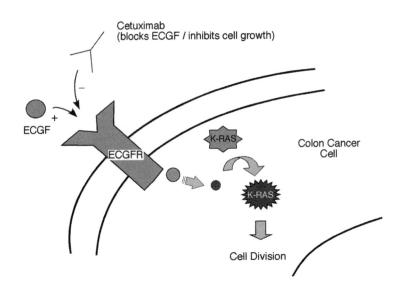

Figure 16. Colon cancer cell: ECGF is the normal growth factor stimulating normal cell growth. Colon cancer cells that express abnormal amounts of the ECGFR may be blocked by an antibody designed to attach specifically to the receptor. This antibody prevents stimulation by ECGF and reduces the ability of the cell to divide and grow. (See insert for color representation.)

of radiation in a crossfire pattern (Figure 17), affecting not only antibody-attached tumor cells but also other neighboring tumor cells. Bevacizumab is another monoclonal antibody that has been used to treat a variety of cancers based on its antiangiogenic properties.

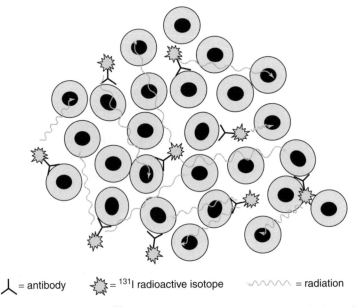

Figure 17. Radioimmunotherapy. ^{131}I-labeled antibodies (radioactive antibodies) attach to surface antigens on tumor cells. Radiation crossfires to other cells. (See insert for color representation.)

PALLIATIVE CARE AND INTEGRATIVE MEDICINE

Palliative care services help patients cope with the psychological and physical symptoms of cancer, usually at a point when the cancer is incurable. Pain and other symptom management, hospice care, and clarification of treatment goals with the patient and family are important contributions frequently made by the palliative care team. Palliative care teams should be used early in the management of patients and may even occasionally play a role assisting management of symptoms and expectations during complicated curative therapy.

Integrative medicine combines the benefits of medical science with other approaches that improve the physical, emotional, and spiritual aspects of patients' lives. *Complementary* and *alternative medicine* (CAM) describes a broad range of therapies, including naturopathy, traditional Chinese medicine (acupuncture), mind–body interventions (meditation, yoga), massage therapy, dietary and herbal treatments, and magnetic therapy. In treating cancer, CAM therapies are not substitutes for standard oncology care therapy. Integrative medicine combines standard medical therapies and some CAM therapies. Although CAM includes both proven and unproven therapies, the goal of integrative medicine is to incorporate complementary therapies that have a scientific basis for safety and effectiveness. In integrative medicine, evidence-based CAM approaches are used to help alleviate stress and anxiety, reduce pain, and promote a feeling of well-being. For instance, acupuncture helps relieve pain and nausea in some patients. Yoga, massage therapy, and meditation all have positive effects on attitude and mood. Some therapies may counteract conventional treatment, make side effects worse, or lead to infections. This is a concern mainly with specific herbal and nutritional supplements. Also, sometimes the use of CAM therapies can delay a patient from seeking effective cancer therapy. For example, garlic in large amounts together with antiplatelet agents can increase bleeding tendencies. Alternatively, St. John's wort, a common herbal treatment for depression, can decrease the potency of chemotherapy drugs such as cyclophosphamide. Patients who experience unusual side effects or experience no improvement with drugs known to be beneficial should raise a question to the physician about the possibility that a patient is taking herbal treatments.

Case 6

A 54-year-old female presents with a two-week history of pain on both sides of her abdomen and bloody bowel movements. She has had a 20-pound weight loss over the past six months. A colonoscopy reveals a large tumor in left bowel loop of her colon. A CT scan of her abdomen shows multiple spots in her liver (tumor nodules), consistent with spread of the tumor (Figure 18). The tumor appears to be blocking her bowel, and surgery is undertaken to remove the mass and relieve the obstruction. A biopsy of a tumor nodule is obtained at the time of her surgery.

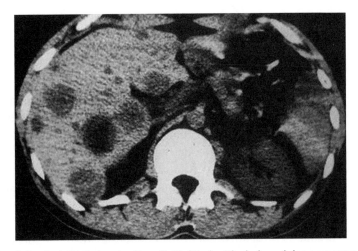

Figure 18. Abdominal CT shows the liver (left) filled with dark nodules or masses (metastatic colon cancer).

The pathology reports reveal an adenocarcinoma of the colon with spread to the liver. A palliative care consult is obtained. Following recovery from surgery, she is treated with chemotherapy, including bevacizumab, a monoclonal antibody to the pro-angiogenic protein, VEGF. Initially, her tumor responds and her symptoms of abdominal pain improve. Unfortunately, after eight months, the tumor progresses and fails to respond to therapy. Pain in the area of her liver becomes a significant problem and she is placed on long-acting narcotics, with some success. She has been followed by the hospital's palliative care service, which coordinates an approach to deal with her pain, depression, and the support she will need at home. An integrative medicine specialist is consulted and yoga and meditation are recommended for relaxation. Appropriate herbal supplements are prescribed in collaboration with her medical oncologist. The patient does not lose hope completely and is able to readjust her goals for spending quality time with her loved ones.

Discussion: This patient has metastatic colon cancer. The primary tumor in the colon caused intestinal obstruction. Although the cancer had spread to the liver, there was a role for surgery to relieve the immediate obstruction. Chemotherapy and radiation would be unlikely to do this as quickly and completely as surgery. Therefore, this example shows a palliative role for surgery in patients with metastatic disease. Occasionally, patients with slow-growing cancers that have spread to the liver or lung in the form of a single metastasis can be cured by removing the metastasis surgically. As this case shows, it is important to confirm by biopsy that the cancer had spread to the liver, since rarely, radiological abnormalities that appear to be cancer (e.g., a nodule that is presumed to be tumor but later found to be infection) are not cancer. Chemotherapy is the mainstay treatment for metastatic colon cancer. Many combinations are available but none will cure this disease. It is important to involve palliative care services early in the course of treatment to help clarify expectations and assist if needed in the treatment of symptoms. Once chemotherapy options have been exhausted, consultation with an integrative medicine specialist may be reasonable if desired by the patient. An integrative medicine specialist works closely with the oncologist to improve the patient's state of well-being using a variety of the methods discussed above.

CONCLUSIONS

Cancer therapy is complex, challenging, and continuously changing. Efforts to integrate multiple specialties in the treatment of these diseases is key to successful outcomes for both improved survival and quality of life. Clinical trials and continued pursuit of basic biological mechanisms of cancer development form the basis of future progress in these diseases.

RECOMMENDED READING

Imai K, Takaoka A. 2006. Comparing antibody and small molecule therapies for cancer. *Nat Rev Cancer* 6:714–727.

Weigner WA, Smith M, Boon H, Richardson MA, Kaptchuk TJ, Eisenberg DM. 2002. Advising patients who seek complementary and alternative medical therapies for cancer. *Ann Intern Med* 137:889–903.

Webb S. 2005. Intensity-modulated radiation therapy (IMRT): a clinical reality for cancer treatment *Br J Radiol* 78:S64–S72.

5

CLINICAL CHALLENGES FOR TREATMENT AND A CURE

Alan Rosmarin

Division of Hematology/Oncology and UMASS Memorial Cancer Center, University of Massachusetts Medical School, Worcester, Massachusetts

INTRODUCTION

The diagnosis of cancer can be among the most terrifying moments of your life. Every aspect of your physical, mental, spiritual, and family life may be affected. The diagnosis of cancer may provoke fears of death, disability, or pain, and it can challenge your notions about the meaning of life and your plans for the future. Naturally, when asked about their goals in cancer treatment, most people will respond that they hope to be cured. For many people, cure of their cancer is a reasonable goal.

More than one in three Americans is expected to develop cancer during his or her lifetime. Unfortunately, for most people with cancer, the goal of achieving a cure is not accomplished. Cancer kills more than half a million people in the United States annually, and it is second only to cardiovascular disease as the leading cause of death among Americans. In fact, cancer kills more Americans than strokes, emphysema, accidents, diabetes, and Alzheimer's disease combined. Sadly, for many patients afflicted with cancer, the goal of achieving a cure remains an elusive goal.

The Biology and Treatment of Cancer: Understanding Cancer
Edited by Arthur B. Pardee and Gary S. Stein   Copyright © 2009 John Wiley & Sons, Inc.

The term *cancer* represents many distinct diseases. In a sense, the word *cancer* is similar to a term such as *automobile*, which includes vehicles that range from VW Beetles to Formula 1 race cars. How can you describe the speed, mileage, performance, safety, and other features of an automobile without knowing what type of car is being discussed? Similarly, the term *cancer* refers to more than 100 distinct tumor types. Cancers differ based on the organ from which they arise, the microscopic appearance of the cancer cells, and the molecular defects that underlie the cancer. These characteristics also have important implications for the behavior of the cancer: to which organs it might spread, choices of effective therapy, and the probability that it will respond to treatment. Similarly, the likelihood that a cancer will be cured by treatment is strongly influenced by the specific type of cancer. For example, more than 90% of children with certain forms of pediatric leukemia can be cured, whereas fewer than one in ten patients with other types of cancer may be cured. Thus, inherent properties of the tumor have an important effect on treatment choice. In addition, characteristics of the affected person, including age and underlying medical ailments, may influence decisions regarding cancer treatment.

In this chapter we discuss what constitutes effective cancer therapy and the barriers to effective treatment and a cure. First, we define the terms that describe a response to treatment. We then examine barriers to effective treatment, including inherent properties of the tumor itself, patient characteristics that may influence treatment, limitations of current therapeutic approaches, and even societal and economic factors that lead to less that ideal outcomes.

ESSENTIAL DEFINITIONS: REMISSION, CURE, AND RELAPSE

In order to discuss what constitutes effective cancer treatment, we must first understand some of the terminology that is used to describe the response to therapy. The term *remission* is frequently used in cancer treatment, but what does this word mean? Remission signifies a shrinkage or reduction in the size or amount of tumor. However, the term *remission* alone is nonspecific. Defining a remission depends greatly on the approach and the methods that are used to document it. For it to be meaningful, it should be further defined as, for example, a clinical remission, a radiologic remission, a pathologic remission, or a molecular remission. This is not mere semantics. The ability to define a remission depends largely on the tools that are brought to bear on this question.

Let's examine more specifically how one might classify a remission. Consider the situation of a man with a lymphoma that is growing as a mass in the neck, in the spleen, and in the bone marrow. The same type of tumor cells are present at each of these sites, but different methods may be required to detect them. The neck mass may be visible to the naked eye and readily felt by an examining physician, the lymphoma in the spleen may only be apparent on a CT (computerized tomography) scan or a PET (positron emission tomography) scan, whereas involvement of the bone marrow may require specialized tests that are performed on a bone marrow biopsy.

For some patients of this types the large neck mass may shrink dramatically after even just one treatment cycle. Has this man achieved a remission? The disappearance of the neck mass by physical examination might, in fact, represent a clinical remission by physical examination, but has all tumor been eradicated by this single treatment cycle? Probably not, because the CT or PET scan is likely still to be positive in the spleen or other sites after only one treatment. Is this a pathological remission (disappearance of all detectable disease following a repeat biopsy) or a molecular remission (the absence of characteristic molecular abnormalities that are diagnostic of this type of tumor)? Again, the answer is probably "no," for it is likely that very sensitive molecular approaches such as PCR (polymerase chain reaction) or FISH (fluorescence in situ hybridization) may still detect traces of disease in the bone marrow after only one treatment. His tumor may not be detectable by physical examination, but he may still have disease that can be detected by radiological or molecular studies. Thus, the definition of remission is anything but semantics; a patient's future health may depend on the approaches that are used to define it.

This man would be described as having achieved a *complete clinical remission* if all sites of disease have disappeared completely by physical examination and radiological studies. What if the neck mass had shrunken but not disappeared entirely? Such a response of the tumor may suggest that it is responsive to treatment, but it may not have been fully eliminated. If all tumor masses have been reduced by 50% or more, it would be described as a *partial clinical remission*. If, instead, the tumor were unchanged by treatment, that might be described as *stable disease*. If the tumors actually grew during treatment, the situation would be described as *progressive disease*.

If CT scans, MRI (magnetic resonance imaging), PET scans, or other appropriate radiological imaging studies demonstrate a complete disappearance of tumor, the situation would be described as a *complete radiological remission*. Similarly, if a repeat biopsy demonstrated no evident tumor, this would be described as *complete pathological remission*. In certain diseases, molecular studies can detect exceedingly small quantities of tumor based on the presence of specific markers; if these abnormalities have normalized after treatment, the patient might be described as having achieved *complete molecular remission*. In summary, a remission is a description of the response of tumor to treatment. To be most meaningful, it should be defined by the approach (i.e., clinical, pathological, or molecular) and described further as partial or complete.

Many people assume that the terms *complete remission* and *cure* are one and the same. They are not! *Cure* represents a complete disappearance of tumor for the natural life of the patient. For example, chemotherapy treatment of an infant with leukemia may cure her if a complete pathological remission is sustained for the remaining decades of her life. Radiation treatment of prostate cancer may effectively cure a 90-year-old man of that disease if the remission is sustained for only a few years. Despite the different diseases, treatments, and durations of remission, both would be cured if the cancer never recurred during the natural lifespan of that person. Some oncologists are reluctant to describe a patient's response as a cure because this term can only be truly applied in retrospect. The patterns and most likely time for disease recurrence are well understood for most types of cancer. For example, nearly all testicular cancers that are destined to recur will happen within the first five years following treatment. Thus, if such a patient survives for five years without a recurrence of his testicular tumor, he is likely to be cured of that disease. Thus, many consider a sustained complete remission to be tantamount to a cure in many clinical situations. However, the duration of a sustained remission that would be considered to be equivalent to a cure depends importantly on the details of the tumor type.

Molecular and pathological approaches can detect microscopic or even lesser amounts of tumor. For example, certain molecular approaches, such as PCR, can detect individual cancer cells among millions of normal cells. In that sense, these molecular approaches are more sensitive than radiological or clinical approaches. For example, treatment might make a lymphoma mass disappear by physical exam and by even the most advanced radiological imaging techniques, but a biopsy might still demonstrate the presence of small amounts of residual malignant cells. Thus, molecular techniques are very powerful tools for documenting an effective complete remission in certain tumor types, such as leukemias and lymphomas. Because molecular techniques are generally more sensitive than clinical or radiological approaches, one might wonder why a molecular remission is not adopted as the standard for all tumor types. Unfortunately, diagnostic molecular tests are not yet available for many of the most common tumor types, such as breast cancer, lung cancer, and other solid tumors.

Unfortunately, some patients who achieve even a complete molecular remission may later have a regrowth of the cancer. Such regrowth is referred to as a *recurrence* or *relapse* of the tumor. Relapse of a tumor usually indicates that the cancer is unlikely to be cured by that treatment. However, there are some exceptions, most notably with certain leukemias, lymphomas, and testicular cancers. Even though most relapsed cancers are generally not curable after relapse, another treatment may still be effective against that cancer. For example, treatment may be very effective in relieving symptoms that are associated with the cancer. Nevertheless, it should be apparent that not every remission—even by the most sensitive techniques—will amount to a cure. However, without a complete remission, one cannot realistically hope to achieve a cure.

GOALS OF CANCER TREATMENT

Naturally, one hopes that every patient will benefit from his or her cancer treatment. However, in many cases it is not realistic to hope to cure a person's cancer. Thus, it is critically important for someone who has been diagnosed with cancer to discuss the goals of cancer treatment with his or her doctors. This is important whether the goal of treatment is to achieve a cure or to achieve something other than a cure.

Why would someone not seek to cure his tumor? Sometimes the nature of the cancer itself will make achieving a cure, or even a remission, an unrealistic goal. Some cancers are *metastatic* by the time they are diagnosed: that is, they have already spread beyond the organ from which they arose. In such situations, achieving a cure is unlikely or impossible. In other situations, the person is too frail or has other significant medical problems that will make potentially curative treatment unrealistic. In such a setting, the effects of treatment might risk the person's well-being and possibly even his or her life. For these reasons, or other reasons that are discussed below, the goal of treatment may be something other than a complete remission.

In some situations, the goal of cancer treatment is *palliation*, or relief from symptoms caused by the cancer. For example, a woman whose cancer has spread from a lung to her bones (i.e., a metastatic lung cancer) may be suffering from bone pain. Relief from the painful bone metastases may be the most important and realistic therapeutic goal. Treatment with radiation or chemotherapy may relieve symptoms even without achieving an objective improvement by radiological or other studies. Such treatment may be judged a success if it reduces her symptoms, even if it only achieves a state of stable disease. In this setting, the relief of symptoms may be the most important goal of all.

In other persons the goal of therapy is to delay the time when symptoms are likely to develop. For example, if a colon cancer has become metastatic before the time that it is detected, simply removing the tumor in the colon by surgery would not be expected to cure the disease. Even complete removal of the cancer in the colon would leave residual cancer in other organs. However, surgical removal of the tumor may still be recommended because it may prevent later complications, such as obstruction of the bowel or bleeding from the tumor. Even without prolonging that person's life, such treatment may be appropriate because it may improve the quality of his life.

Another goal of treatment may be to extend the person's life, that is, to delay the date when the cancer will take that person's life. Sometimes this goal can be achieved even without achieving a substantial remission of the tumor. The likelihood that a person's lifespan can be prolonged by treatment depends importantly on the type of cancer and the specific therapy that is planned. Generally, those types of cancers that respond well to therapy, often as measured by high rates of remissions, are more likely to be associated with a prolongation of survival.

There are some cancers for which treatment can induce a remission or relieve symptoms, without the expectation that therapy will cure the illness or even extend life. For example, chronic lymphocytic leukemia (CLL) is a slow-growing blood cancer that may be present in some people for many years without causing symptoms. Typically, CLL can respond effectively to many types of treatment. Chemotherapy, radiation therapy, biological therapies, and other approaches may reduce the elevated white blood cell counts, shrink swollen lymph nodes, or relieve symptoms of CLL, but it is likely that the disease will recur at a later date. Treatment in this setting may be warranted even without the expectation that it will extend the person's lifespan.

The effects of cancer treatment must be weighed carefully against the potential benefits, whether the goal of treatment is cure, remission, prolongation of life, delayed onset of symptoms, or palliation of symptoms. The perceived balance between the side effects of treatment—the costs—and the anticipated response— the benefits—are highly individual. A person may be willing to tolerate even severe side effects if it may result in a cancer cure. However, such side effects may not be acceptable if the goal is simply to delay the onset of symptoms. Decisions regarding cancer treatment deserve careful consideration and may involve discussion with family, trusted friends, physicians, and other caregivers. This may require balancing long-term goals against the possibility of short-term discomfort. Ultimately, these are highly individual decisions that benefit from honest and forthright discussion and self-reflection.

INTRINSIC PROPERTIES OF CANCERS THAT AFFECT TREATMENT

For more than 100 years, pathologists have examined cancers with microscopes in order to better understand them. The *morphology*, or microscopic appearance, of a tumor can be a powerful predictor of the growth properties of a cancer. Most cancer cells resemble—to a greater or lesser extent—the cells of the organ from which they arose. For example, breast cancer cells share many properties of normal tissues of the breast. The degree to which cancer cells resemble their normal cellular counterparts morphologically is referred to as the *grade* of a tumor. A *well-differentiated cancer* may look similar to its normal cellular counterpart, whereas a *poorly differentiated*, or *anaplastic* cancer bears little resemblance to normal tissues. This should not be surprising, because cancer cells arise from normal tissues through the sequential acquisition of mutations. All of the cells in a particular cancer arose from one original mutant cell, but as the cancer continues to grow, its cells may acquire additional mutations. Cancer cells that have acquired many mutations not only appear different from their normal counterparts, they also behave differently. For example, cancer cells may grow more rapidly or survive more effectively than corresponding normal tissues. The acquisition of additional mutations that alter the appearance or growth properties of cancer cells so that they increasingly lose their resemblance to normal cells is referred to as *clonal progression*.

A great deal is known about the growth properties and behaviors of cancer cells. Some of these findings have been translated into *prognostic tests* that can help to predict the response of certain tumors to treatments. For example, normal cells of the breast produce proteins that bind the female sex hormones, estrogen and progesterone. Expression of these estrogen and progesterone receptor proteins is an intrinsic property of breast tissue that permits normal breast tissue to respond to hormonal changes in the menstrual cycle and during pregnancy. Well-differentiated breast cancers not only resemble normal breast tissue morphologically but also share properties of their normal counterparts, such as expression of estrogen and progesterone receptors. Expression of these hormone receptors can offer prognostic information about the tumor. Importantly, it can also provide opportunities for effective and relatively well-tolerated treatment with drugs that can interfere with the functions of these hormones. Thus, understanding the patterns of gene and protein expression by a cancer can provide important prognostic information and may also provide opportunities for treatment.

In some types of cancer, the expression of *oncogenes* and other cancer-associated genes can yield important prognostic information about a cancer. For example, some breast cancer cells express high levels of a protein known as Her2/*neu*. This finding provides prognostic information regarding the cancer, but it also provides a therapeutic opportunity. Many women whose breast cancer exhibits amplification of Her2/*neu* are treated with trastuzumab, a therapeutic antibody that is directed against the protein that is encoded by Her2/*neu*. Because the Her2/*neu* protein can foster the growth of such cancer cells, interfering with its function by treatment with trastuzumab can block the growth of these cancers. The specific genes and proteins that provide prognostic information varies by the tumor type, and increasingly, this approach provides valuable information for decision making about cancer treatment.

In recent years, techniques have been developed that can analyze the expression of large numbers of genes and proteins by tumors. Microarray techniques can simultaneously examine the tumor's expression of many genes, including oncogenes. Similarly, proteomic approaches can analyze the production of proteins that may yield prognostic information. In certain tumors, these approaches can help to better define the nature of a cancer. Microarray and proteomic analysis have been applied to breast cancers and lymphomas, where they may be useful in classifying the tumor and providing prognostic information. These approaches may herald a new era in medicine in which treatment is more highly tailored to an individual cancer, based on its expression of critical target genes and proteins.

BARRIERS TO EFFECTIVE SURGICAL TREATMENT OF CANCER

Most human cancers are *solid tumors*, those they arise from organs such as the lungs, breast, colon, or prostate gland. A smaller number of cancers arise from blood and lymph tissues and give rise to leukemias, lymphomas, and related cancers. Cancer statistics usually exclude the common basal cell and squamous cancers of the skin, for only rarely do these cancers become metastatic or lethal.

Solid tumors are most effectively treated early in their development, especially when they are confined to the organ from which they arose. In such cases, the ability to remove the tumor surgically typically offers the greatest chance of cure. However, a cancer may already have spread from the *primary site* (the location from which it arose) to lymph nodes, the bloodstream, or other organs even before the time of diagnosis. Even if radiological studies and blood tests do not demonstrate spread of the tumor, microscopic quantities of cancer may already have lodged in other organs. They are likely to continue to grow if they remain untreated, and this would be described as a clinical relapse or recurrence of the cancer. If the recurrence occurs adjacent to the primary site from which it arose, it is described as a *local relapse*. If it occurs elsewhere, it is described as a *distant* or *metastatic relapse*.

Because solid tumors are most effectively treated before they have metastasized, determining if a solid tumor has spread beyond the primary site is a crucial part of the initial evaluation of a cancer. The extent of its spread is described as the tumor *stage*. Determining the stage of a cancer typically involves a physical examination, blood tests, and radiological studies (including x-rays, CT scans, and other evaluations). For example, staging studies for lung cancer may include physical examination, blood tests, a CT scan of the chest, and a PET scan. For prostate cancer, the staging may include a physical examination, special blood tests [such as the prostate-specific antigen (PSA)], a bone scan, and CT scans of the abdomen and pelvis. The particular studies that are used to stage a cancer clinically are determined by the specific type of tumor. Dramatic advances in radiological techniques have led to more accurate staging of tumors in recent years. This is particularly important because if staging demonstrates that a cancer has already spread, a person can be spared from undergoing surgery that would not cure the tumor.

Surgery may also play a role in the staging of some types of cancer. Unfortunately, clinical staging procedures are not always sufficiently sensitive to detect the microscopic spread of cancer cells. For example, if the clinical staging of a lung cancer indicates that it has not yet spread beyond the lung, additional studies may be warranted to determine if microscopic amounts of cancer cells are present in lymph nodes within the chest. Curative surgery to remove a primary lung cancer can carry substantial risks, and if the cancer is already present in those lymph nodes, surgery alone is unlikely to yield a cure. In such a setting, a smaller surgical procedure may be used to remove those lymph nodes and determine if cancer cells are present. The identification of cancer cells in the lymph nodes might alter the treatment recommendations. Sometimes, such *surgical staging* may be performed immediately prior to the planned surgical resection of the primary tumor. In other situations, the surgical staging may be performed as a separate surgical procedure. Surgical staging may be recommended if the findings would change the treatment plan, especially if it would avert a major operation that would expose the patient to the risks of surgery without providing the likelihood of curing the cancer.

Surgery is the primary means of curing most solid tumors, and we have discussed how surgery is most likely to be curative when the cancer is confined to the primary site. Thus, it stands to reason that the detection of cancers at an early stage leads to the highest rates of cure. The ability to detect cancers in asymptomatic persons is described as *cancer screening*. This approach has proven beneficial for several of the most common cancers. For example, mammography is recommended for most women over 40 or 45 years old, even in the absence of symptoms or a family history of breast cancer. Similarly, colonoscopy is recommended for all adults over 50 years of age. Certain blood tests can also be helpful for screening asymptomatic persons. For example, the PSA blood test is generally performed on men over 50, although this recommendation is somewhat controversial. For persons with a family history of certain cancers, screening studies may be performed at an earlier age or more frequently. Unfortunately, for the most common killer—lung cancer—the evidence that screening by chest x-ray or CT scan can save lives is not fully persuasive. Thus, one of the key barriers to effective treatment and cure of cancers is the failure to detect cancers at the earliest, and most curable, stages. More sensitive and accurate screening strategies for the most common forms of cancer could have an enormous impact on the number of people who die from cancer if they could detect more cancers at earlier stages.

Sometimes, a cancer may be confined to the organ from which it arose, but it is not surgically *resectable*; that is, it cannot be fully removed by surgery. For example, a lung cancer that is immediately adjacent to the aorta may not be resectable because of the risk that surgery might injure that critical blood vessel. In other cases, there may be concerns that a person may not tolerate the planned surgery. A patient with severe emphysema who has an early-stage lung cancer may not be considered *operable* if pulmonary function tests indicate that he would not have sufficient lung capacity after removal of the tumor and adjacent lung tissue. Similarly, severe heart disease or other medical problems may raise concerns that the patient would not tolerate the surgery. Thus, other medical conditions may restrict the possibility of achieving a surgical cure for some patients with apparent early-stage cancers.

Generally, when staging studies indicate that a cancer is metastatic, there are too many individual lesions to remove or destroy surgically. In addition to those metastases that are found by radiological studies, there are usually additional microscopic metastases that cannot be detected. Thus, cancers that are clinically metastatic are generally considered to be incurable by surgery alone. However, occasionally, a metastatic cancer generates only a few metastatic deposits. For example, a colon cancer that recurs with only a small number of metastatic lesions in the liver may occasionally be amenable to surgical removal or ablation (destruction) by techniques that use heating, freezing, or other approaches. However, this is a highly unusual situation and generally, solid tumors that have spread to sites beyond the organ from which they arose are not curable by surgery alone.

Surgery can have an important role even in situations where it is not expected to cure a cancer. For example, a colon cancer that has already spread to the liver before the time of diagnosis generally would not be considered curable by surgical removal of the primary tumor in the colon. However, even if that cancer has already metastasized, the colon tumor might still be removed surgically to prevent later bowel obstruction or bleeding. The prevention of such complications by appropriate surgical intervention can play an important role in improving the quality of life in patients who are battling cancer.

Surgery alone is generally not considered to be curative for most metastatic cancers, but it can play an important role in the management of certain cancers that have spread beyond the primary site. For example, ovarian cancers may spread within the abdominal cavity even early in the course of their development. Surgery is often used to "debulk" ovarian cancer, that is, to remove most of the larger tumor masses. However, surgery generally cannot remove all visible ovarian cancer, not to mention the additional microscopic deposits of tumor. Nevertheless, debulking surgery plays an important role in rendering ovarian cancer more curable by chemotherapy. There are other examples of tumors that can be cured when chemotherapy is used following surgery that is known to have left some detectable cancer behind. For example, testicular cancer can be cured even when it has spread to lymph nodes in the abdomen or chest.

There are some types of cancer for which surgery is not the primary treatment approach. Cancers that arise from blood- or lymph-forming organs generally are not treated with surgery. Such tumor cells may spread throughout the body even early in the course of their development because it is the nature of such cells to spread through the bloodstream or lymph vessels. For example, leukemias generally arise in the bone marrow. Because leukemia cells can spread throughout the body via the bloodstream even early in their course, surgical removal is not generally considered a means of curing such tumors. Surgery may still have a role in establishing the diagnosis of such blood-related cancers, in preventing certain complications, and even in the staging of certain lymphomas. However, other therapeutic modalities, including chemotherapy, radiation therapy, and biological approaches are more commonly used to treat these illnesses.

In summary, surgery is the primary therapeutic modality for most solid tumors. However, we have reviewed several factors that limit its effectiveness. Some patients cannot tolerate curative surgery because other medical illnesses, such as heart or lung disease, render them inoperable. Others have cancers that are unresectable, because the tumor lies too close to a critical organ, and it cannot be removed safely. Most important, the stage of a tumor can limit the curative potential of surgery. Except for cancers of the ovary, testis, and a few others, curative surgery is generally not undertaken if the cancer has already spread beyond the organ of origin. Even if clinical staging studies indicate that the tumor has not yet spread, a substantial number of patients will later relapse, either locally or distantly. This indicates that the cancer must have spread microscopically before the time of surgery. Thus, the understaging of tumors, the failure to detect the microscopic spread of tumor that occurred by the time of surgery, is an important barrier to surgical cure of cancer. Finally, more effective screening techniques that will accurately detect cancers in asymptomatic patients would have an enormous impact on cancer survival, because they can identify cancers at the earliest and most curable stages.

BARRIERS TO EFFECTIVE TREATMENT BY CHEMOTHERAPY

Chemotherapy refers to a large group of medicines that are used to treat cancer. There are dozens of types of chemotherapy. They differ based on the types of medicine, how they are administered, how they work, their likely side effects, and many other characteristics. Individual types of chemotherapy are discussed in greater detail in Chapter 4.

Judging the effectiveness of chemotherapy depends on the goals that have been set for treatment. Treatment with chemotherapy may be offered for a variety of reasons. Chemotherapy alone can cure some types of tumor, such as certain forms of lymphoma and leukemia. In other settings, chemotherapy may be used to relieve symptoms, to delay the onset of symptoms, or in an attempt to prolong a person's life. Chemotherapy may also be used as *adjuvant therapy* to prevent a later recurrence of tumor following surgery. For example, some people whose cancer has been surgically removed may have microscopic spread of the tumor that was not detected by clinical staging studies. Left untreated, it may cause a clinical relapse at a later date. However, in some situations this recurrence can be prevented by the administration of adjuvant chemotherapy. This strategy is often applied to the treatment of breast cancer, colon cancer, and others following surgical removal of the tumor.

From decades of experience, we know that specific tumor types are killed by particular chemotherapeutic compounds, but not by others. In general, chemotherapy acts by interfering with basic properties of a cancer cell, such as growth and proliferation, deoxyribonucleic acid (DNA) synthesis, metabolism, and other essential cellular functions. Regardless of the specific mechanism by which chemotherapy acts, it generally kills a cancer cell by activating the process known as programmed cell death, or *apoptosis*. This process can be envisioned as a form of cell suicide that is stimulated by chemotherapy.

In some situations it is easy to understand why a particular chemotherapeutic agent kills a specific tumor type. For example, compounds that block the effects of estrogen may effectively kill breast cancer cells, because these cells are dependent on this hormone for their growth. Rapidly growing lymphomas are often sensitive to agents that block the synthesis of DNA, which must be duplicated every time that these fast-growing cells divide. However, in most circumstances it is not clear why a specific cancer is especially sensitive to a particular chemotherapeutic compound. For example, it is not clear why ovarian cancer cells are especially sensitive to chemotherapeutic agents such as paclitaxel. In most situations, chemotherapy recommendations are based on clinical trials and other studies that have shown that a certain cancer type is sensitive to particular therapeutic agents.

Treatment choices are strongly influenced by the likely sensitivity of that tumor to a particular type of chemotherapy. These decisions must also consider the likely side effects of the treatment. Many forms of chemotherapy will damage any rapidly dividing tissues in the body and render them susceptible to the effects of chemotherapy. The impact of chemotherapy on rapidly dividing tissues of the skin, mouth, and gastrointestinal tract accounts for some of the hair loss, mouth ulcers, and gastrointestinal effects that occur with many forms of chemotherapy. Increasing knowledge of how these normal body tissues are affected by chemotherapy has led to improved efforts to minimize the side effects of treatment.

Choices of chemotherapy must also consider the patient's other illnesses. Particularly for elderly patients, heart disease, lung problems, or kidney disease may limit the amount and the type of treatment that is available. For instance, some drugs can have serious effects on the heart, and a patient with heart failure might not be able to tolerate such agents. Other drugs may not be well tolerated by people who have significant lung, liver, or kidney problems. Thus, the choice of chemotherapeutic agents must consider not only the likelihood of success against a particular tumor type, it must also consider probable side effects and the patient's other medical ailments.

For many types of cancer, several types of chemotherapeutic agents are administered at the same time. This approach is known as *combination chemotherapy*. Often, these combinations of drugs will utilize medications that kill cancer cells by different mechanisms of action and which have different profiles of side effects. The simultaneous administration of a combination of drugs that have similar toxicities might cause intolerable side effects. For example, if several drugs that tend to suppress the bone marrow, are administered simultaneously, severe anemia or severe infections due to low white blood cell counts might result. In contrast, if one agent affects predominantly the bone marrow while another affects primarily the kidneys, it may be possible to administer both agents safely without causing intolerable effects on either organ.

The severity of side effects may influence whether treatment with that agent is tolerable. For example, certain platinum-related chemotherapy compounds affect the function of nerves. This may be acceptable if, for example, it causes only mild numbness and tingling in the hands and feet. However, if more severe nerve problems interfere with activities of daily living, such as the ability to open buttons or handle small objects, it may not be acceptable and treatment may have to be altered. The willingness to tolerate side effects may be influenced by the goals of treatment. For example, side effects that may be acceptable if the ultimate goal is to cure a cancer may not be appropriate when the goal is simply to palliate symptoms.

There are many strategies that can be applied to lessen the side effects of chemotherapy. In some situations, side effects may be alleviated simply by reducing the dose of chemotherapy. Sometimes, symptoms can be relieved by increasing the interval between treatments to allow more time for recovery from the side effects. Medications can relieve the symptoms of certain side effects. For example, many forms of chemotherapy cause anemia, low white blood cell counts, or low platelet counts. Administration of certain medications can lessen the effects of chemotherapy on blood cells and prevent or relieve related symptoms. Similarly, there are numerous drugs that can effectively relieve chemotherapy-associated nausea. However, sometimes side effects are so severe that they require the discontinuation of a particular form of chemotherapy. In such a situation, an agent that does not cause similar side effects may be recommended as an alternative. Just because one type of chemotherapy causes severe side effects does not mean that other agents will not be tolerable. Thus, treatment decisions should include the sensitivity of the tumor to a particular type of chemotherapy, but should also consider the probable side effects and the patient's other medical conditions.

Thus, chemotherapy may be administered to cure a cancer, palliate symptoms, or shrink a tumor. What determines if chemotherapy will be ineffective in any of these roles? The ability of a cancer to survive or grow in the face of chemotherapy treatment is referred to as chemotherapy *resistance*. Drug resistance is a complex and dynamic process that is related to cell cycle and apoptotic pathways, the cancer's microenvironment, metabolism of the drug, and other factors. To some extent, you can envision a cancer cell as being in a Darwinian struggle to survive. It will use any possible trick or tool that it has to avoid being killed by the chemotherapy.

Perhaps the most important reasons why chemotherapy does not achieve its intended goal relate to intrinsic properties of the cancer. For example, some types of lymphomas seem to respond to many different agents. In contrast, certain forms of solid tumors seemingly will not respond to any type of treatment. Certain characteristics can be useful in predicting a response to treatment. For example, as described earlier, breast cancers that express the estrogen receptor are likely to respond to treatment with hormonal agents. Unfortunately, there is no surefire way of predicting whether a given person's tumor will respond to a specific agent.

Some cancers grow in the face of treatment with various chemotherapeutic agents and combinations. When this occurs, it may still be possible to control symptoms with other approaches, such as radiation therapy. In some situations, a cancer may initially respond to treatment, but later relapse despite continued use of the agents that were effective previously. For example, a lymphoma may respond initially to a single medication or to a combination of drugs, but the tumor masses may later grow again despite continued treatment. In such a situation, the tumor may respond to other agents or other approaches.

What accounts for chemotherapy resistance? Some cancers develop the ability to remove the chemotherapeutic agents from their cells. The ability of cancer cells to pump out the chemotherapy agent can reduce drug levels to a point where they are no longer lethal to the cells. Prolonged exposure to chemotherapy may induce a cancer cell to increase its production of such molecular pumps and survive in the face of previously effective treatment. Sometimes, increasing the chemotherapy dose can overcome this form of resistance. In other situations, the use of different agents that are not affected by this mechanism may overcome this form of drug resistance.

There are many other specific types of chemotherapy resistance that relate to the mechanism by which a particular type of chemotherapy kills cancer cells. Regardless of the particular mechanism of resistance, the physician may recommend treatment with another drug or another approach. Sometimes drugs that work by a different mechanism of action can overcome such resistance. At other times, a cancer may be resistant to all available forms of chemotherapy, but another therapeutic modality, such as radiation treatment, can be effective. However, there are situations in which cancers do not respond to any treatment. In such situations, the most appropriate treatment may be to focus on the relief of symptoms with medications or other approaches that relieve pain, nausea, fatigue, or other cancer-associated symptoms.

Increased knowledge of the molecular defects that cause particular cancers is leading to wholly new approaches to cancer treatment. Treatments that target the specific molecular defects that cause certain cancers are transforming the way that cancer is treated. Such approaches differ from conventional chemotherapy because they can often exploit cellular targets that are present in cancer cells but not in normal cells. We have discussed the fact that conventional chemotherapy can affect both cancer cells and normal cells, and may cause side effects as a result of the effects on normal tissues. *Targeted therapies* are aimed at specific molecular defects that contribute to the growth of cancer cells, and in some situations, these targets are not present in any normal tissues.

Perhaps the best known example of molecularly targeted therapy is the use of imatinib in chronic myelogenous leukemia (CML). In this disorder, a rearrangement of chromosomes 9 and 22 in certain blood cells generates an abnormal protein, called Bcr-Abl, that is unique to the malignant cells. Imatinib is specifically targeted against Bcr-Abl, and because this abnormal protein is not found in any normal tissues in the body, it has only limited effects on other tissues. As a result, it causes very limited side effects compared with conventional chemotherapy. Imatinib can normalize the blood counts in the vast majority of people with CML and even induce molecular remissions. As remarkably effective as this drug is, some patients with CML ultimately develop resistance to its effects and their leukemia will recur. In most of these patients, new mutations develop in the Bcr-Abl oncogene that alter its binding by imatinib. As a result, the drug loses its effectiveness and the leukemia can regrow. Newer generations of agents are being developed that can overcome this resistance and again induce remissions in many of these patients. Nevertheless, this illustrates that even molecularly targeted medicines are vulnerable to the ability of tumors to evade the effects of chemotherapy.

In recent years, it has been recognized that the growth of tumors can be altered by targeting the milieu in which cancer cells grow rather than only by attacking the cancer cells themselves. For a tumor to grow, it must continue to obtain adequate nutrients and oxygen. In a sense, the cancer is acting as a parasite that places nutritional demands on the host. These increased needs require the development of an ever-enlarging blood supply that is provided by adjacent normal tissues. A strategy to use antiangiogenic agents that block the formation of new blood vessels has proven to be effective in certain clinical settings. This approach is distinct from the conventional strategy of attacking cancer cells directly.

In summary, chemotherapy is used in a variety of settings to achieve cure of some cancers, as adjuvant treatment to prevent the recurrence following surgical treatment of some cancers, and to relieve or prevent symptoms. The specific choices, schedules, and combinations of medications vary depending on the nature of the cancer and the goals of therapy. These choices are also influenced by the patient's other medical conditions and his or her ability to tolerate the side effects of the medications. In any of these settings, a tumor may develop resistance to the treatment by a variety of mechanisms. Nevertheless, changes in the dose, schedule, or choice of medications can sometimes overcome this resistance.

BARRIERS TO EFFECTIVE TREATMENT BY RADIATION THERAPY

Radiation is another treatment modality that can be used to treat cancer. Like surgery and chemotherapy, radiation may be used to cure cancers in certain clinical settings. In contrast to chemotherapy, which is a systemic therapy, radiation is a local therapy that affects tumors in the region of the body that is radiated. It may also be used as adjuvant therapy following surgery, either alone or in combination with chemotherapy. Finally, it may be utilized to palliate symptoms associated with cancer or to prevent complications. The choice of when and how to utilize radiation treatment depends on the type and stage of the cancer, among other factors.

Radiation treatment is administered in a variety of ways, including by various energetic subatomic particles and gamma waves. Radiation may be generated by radioactive compounds or by linear accelerators, and it may be delivered by external beams, by placement of radioactive sources within the body, or attached to compounds that selectively target tumor cells. These issues are discussed in more detail in Chapter 4.

Regardless of the source and type of radiation, these treatments generally kill cells by damaging DNA, which ultimately leads to apoptosis. Just as conventional chemotherapy kills both cancer cells and normal tissues, radiation will damage normal cells of the body. The tolerance of various tissues to radiation plays an important role in the choices of dose, source, treatment field size, and other factors. Recent advances in the administration of radiation include the ability to conform or shape a beam of radiation so that it matches the tumor precisely. The use of multiple beams that converge on the tumor can reduce the toxicity to surrounding tissues while delivering lethal radiation doses to the tumor itself.

Different tumors have specific sensitivities to radiation. For example, lymphomas are generally sensitive to even modest doses of radiation, whereas many types of solid tumor require high radiation doses to kill the tumor. There are important limits to the amount of radiation that can be delivered to a tumor, because radiation can have harmful effects on surrounding tissues. For example, radiation of the pelvis for a prostate cancer may include significant amounts of pelvic bones in the radiation field. Because of the effects of radiation on the blood-forming bone marrow that lies within these bones, a patient may develop anemia, or other low blood counts following treatment. Thus, an important barrier to effective treatment by radiation is the amount that is tolerated by surrounding tissues. Knowledge of the doses that are required to kill a specific type of tumor can reduce treatment to the smallest effective dose while sparing adjacent normal tissues. Refinements in shaping the radiation field can also reduce such side effects.

Radiation damages tumors and other tissues by causing DNA damage. The interaction of radiation with oxygen products can create reactive oxygen species. Thus, for radiation to kill cancer cells, a tumor should receive adequate amounts of blood flow. In some large tumors, there is insufficient delivery of oxygen because of limited blood supply. Such hypoxic tumors may not be killed effectively by radiation. However, there are some ways to make radiation more effective, such as concurrent use of low doses of chemotherapy along with radiation.

The decision to use radiation therapy is influenced by the type of cancer and its stage. For some cancers, radiation alone, or radiation combined with chemotherapy, is as effective as surgery for management of a cancer. For example, certain forms of cancer of the head and neck are managed very effectively with radiation and chemotherapy. This approach may prevent the disfigurement or disability that might result from such surgery. Radiation therapy plays an important role in the management of many forms of cancer, but the specific choices of approach must take into account the goals of treatment, the possible side effects, and other medical conditions.

SOCIAL BARRIERS TO EFFECTIVE CANCER TREATMENT

The barriers to effective cancer treatment that have been discussed up to this point reflect aspects of the individual and his or her specific type of tumor. We have discussed how intrinsic properties of a tumor can be an important determinant of the effectiveness of a treatment. For example, lymphomas may be considerably more sensitive to chemotherapy than are certain forms of solid tumors, such as kidney cancers or melanomas. The extent of the spread, or stage, of a tumor can also figure importantly in its response to treatment. A metastatic lung cancer may be considerably more challenging to treat than a small surgically resectable lung cancer. Regardless of the tumor type and planned treatment, a person's general health may also affect the effectiveness of treatment. Someone with severe congestive heart failure may not be able to tolerate certain medications that would otherwise have the potential to cure his cancer.

In addition to these characteristics of a patient and his or her cancer, there are social aspects to medicine that may have an important impact on the ability to treat the illness effectively. In many ways, American medicine is the most advanced in the world. However, there are significant inequities in American health care that prevent some patients from receiving optimal care. A shocking number of uninsured Americans have only limited access to optimal medical care. The rapidly escalating costs of medical care make it unaffordable to many who lack insurance. Even the remarkable safety nets of Medicare and Medicaid do not cover many diagnostic tests and treatments. We discussed how earlier detection of cancers by effective screening strategies has the potential to greatly improve cancer outcomes if cancers can be identified early in their course. Despite the proven benefit of some such screening approaches, many Americans lack the insurance coverage to make them affordable. Such social barriers are further magnified in other countries with more limited medical, financial, and social resources. In much of the developing world, even the basics of medical care are lacking. The realities of contemporary medical care are but a dream in such settings.

SUMMARY

Advances in our understanding of cancer biology and improvements in medical technology have led to remarkable progress in the fight against many forms of cancer. For many of the cancers of children and for certain adult tumors, most of the persons affected can expect to be cured. However, for many of the most common cancers, the goal of a cure remains elusive. More precise understanding of cancer biology allows more accurate prognostication that can focus treatment on those who will benefit the most. Greater understanding of the molecular processes that initiate cancers and support their growth has begun to provide more precise and effective treatments. Further progress should yield treatments that are targeted to the cancer while sparing normal tissues, and provide more effective and safer approaches to the eradication of cancer.

III

CANCER BIOLOGY

6

UNDERSTANDING THE BIOLOGY OF CANCER

Laura A. Lambert

Department of Surgical Oncology, M.D. Anderson Cancer Center, University of Texas, Houston, Texas

Donald H. Lambert

Department of Anesthesia, Boston University Medical School, Boston Medical Center, Boston, Massachusetts

Khandan Keyomarsi

Department of Experimental Radiation Oncology, M.D. Anderson Cancer Center, University of Texas, Houston, Texas

NORMAL CELL BIOLOGY

Cells are the building blocks of all living things, whether a unicellular bacterium or a multicellular human being. Cells were first described in 1665 by the English scientist Robert Hooke, who saw tiny boxlike structures in a piece of cork through the microscope. It took nearly two centuries following this remarkable discovery to recognize that all living things consist of cells. This formed the basis of the *cell theory*. The theory was expanded when the cell was determined to be the smallest

The Biology and Treatment of Cancer: Understanding Cancer
Edited by Arthur B. Pardee and Gary S. Stein   Copyright © 2009 John Wiley & Sons, Inc.

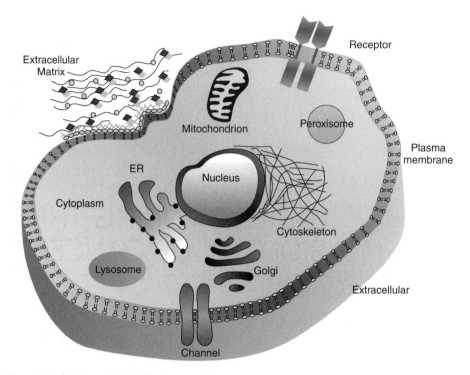

Figure 1. Overview of a cell. The most common structures of a cell, including a variety of organelles (i.e., mitochodria, peroxisome, Golgi apparatus). The most prominent organelle is the nucleus. Most of the cell's metabolic activity occurs in the cytoplasm. ER, endoplasmic reticulum. (See insert for color representation.)

structure capable of all the activities that define life. Paramount among such cellular activities is the transfer of an exact copy of genetic material to the next generation in a cell line. For these reasons, the cell theory now states that all living things are cellular and that all cells come from cells. In other words, all living things are generated through the replication and division of a single progenitor cell.

All cells share a member of basic features (Figure 1):

1. Cells are surrounded by a *plasma membrane* that functions as a selective barrier allowing passage of essentials such as oxygen, nutrients, and wastes needed to maintain the life of the cell.

2. Within the plasma membrane is a semifluid known as *cytosol*.

3. The cytosol contains a variety of subcellular *organelles* such as energy-producing *mitochondria* and other structures responsible for cellular functions.

4. Most cells, except bacteria and some other single-celled organisms, possess a membrane-bound organelle known as a *nucleus*.

5. All cells carry a full complement of genetic information known as *deoxyribonucleic acid* DNA.

6. DNA is stored in the nucleus. (In cells lacking a nucleus, the DNA is stored in the cytoplasm.)

7. The entire region between the nucleus and the plasma membrane is known as the *cytoplasm*.

Cell replication of a unicellular bacterium generates an entirely new organism. However, the creation of a multicellular organism is significantly more complicated. In addition to replicating and dividing, cells of a multicellular organism must also mature into particular types of cells, which then form organs that perform specialized functions such as conducting nervous impulses. Cells must communicate with, and respond to, neighboring cells and their environment. Sometimes they must sacrifice their own existence for the preservation of the organism. Finally, and perhaps most important, cells must regulate and coordinate precisely all of these processes. Loss of control of these processes can have severe consequences: the development of cancer.

The Cell Cycle

The purpose of cellular reproduction is the passing on of genetic information to the next generation. To produce two genetically identical *daughter cells*, a cell must first create a perfect copy of its entire genetic (DNA) content. The DNA of a typical human cell placed end to end is roughly 3 meters long. For the nucleus to accommodate all this material, the deoxyribonucleic acid (DNA) is folded precisely and packaged with special proteins which when combined in this compact manner form a substance known as *chromatin*. In addition, during cellular replication, the amount of DNA must double temporarily. To accommodate this increased volume, the chromatin becomes even more efficiently packaged by forming structures known as *chromosomes*. During replication, every cell packages its chromatin into a specific number of chromosomes. Human cells package their DNA into 46 chromosomes (23 pairs). Replication of the chromosome DNA molecules produces two sister *chromatids*. Each chromatid is an identical copy of the chromosome DNA molecule. By faithfully distributing one complete chromatid to each daughter, cells are able to maintain the entire DNA content, without dilution, between generations of cells. This entire process is referred to as *cell proliferation* (Figure 2).

In embryos, cell division is the means by which the cell mass of the organism increases. However, as development proceeds, additional regulation of cell division becomes crucial for normal growth and development. Left unregulated, the organism will grow out of proportion and forever! Fortunately, regulatory mechanisms ensure the accuracy of genetic transfer and restrict cell division appropriately. The major regulatory mechanism of cell proliferation is the *cell cycle*.

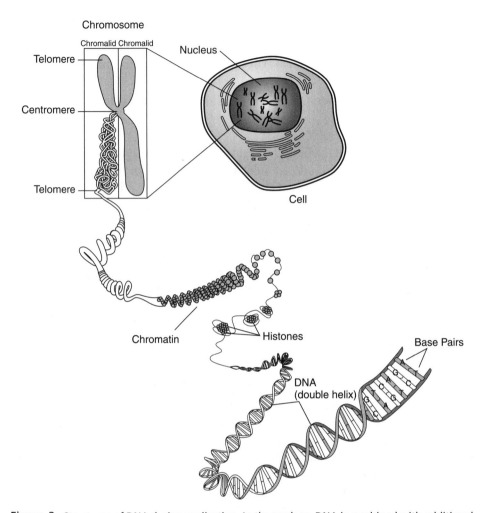

Figure 2. Structures of DNA during replication. In the nucleus, DNA is combined with additional proteins to form *chromatin*. To accommodate the increased volume of DNA during cell replication, chromatin packages itself into *chromosomes*. Replication of the chromosome DNA molecules produces two sister *chromatids*. (Courtesy of the National Human Genome Research Institute.)

The cell cycle is the orderly sequence of events by which cell replication and division are accomplished precisely (Figure 3). The two major divisions of the cell cycle are interphase and mitosis. The cell spends most of its time in *interphase*, during which it grows, doubles its contents, and copies its DNA chromosomes in preparation for dividing. Interphase is divided into subphases: the G1 phase (first gap), the S phase, and the G2 phase (second gap).

- The *G1 phase* precedes the S phase. G1's length depends on the type of cell and the growing conditions.

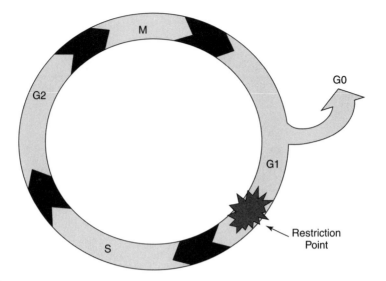

Figure 3. The cell cycle. The cell cycle is divided into four major phases. Cells in G1 can either progress through the cell cycle or exit to G0 (quiescence). Passage of the cell from the G1 phase to the S phase is controlled by an important biochemical switch known as the restriction point. Once through the restriction point, the cell is committed to DNA replication, which occurs in the S phase. The G2 phase ensures that the newly replicated DNA is ready for segregation into daughter cells. In the M phase, the nucleus and then the cytoplasm divide.

- The G1/S transition is controlled by a biochemical checkpoint known as the *restriction point*. This checkpoint prevents cell cycle progression until all the conditions are appropriate for cell replication.
- When conditions are inappropriate for cell replication, cells are delayed in G1. Depending on the reason for the delay, cells can either enter another phase known as *G0* or *quiescence*, or they can self-destruct (*apoptose*). Once in G0, cells can either reenter the cell cycle at an appropriate time or remain in G0 indefinitely.
- The *S phase* is the time when DNA replication (synthesis) occurs. In a human cell the S phase requires approximately 8 hours. Unlike G1, the S phase is relatively constant in length.
- The second gap phase, the *G2* phase, follows the S phase. The time a cell spends in G2 is also relatively constant (approximately 2 hours). G2 ensures that the cellular components needed to complete the following phase (*mitosis*) are available and that the newly synthesized DNA is undamaged and appropriate for segregation into the daughter cells.

Mitosis is the second major division of the cell cycle (M phase). Here the cell's nucleus is physically divided and its DNA segregated. Mitosis is normally

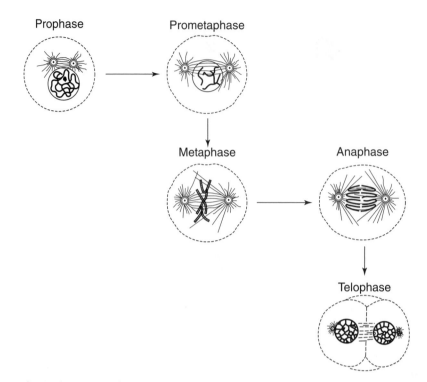

Figure 4. The five stages of mitotic division. During *prophase*, nuclear chromatin condenses into chromosomes and the mitotic spindle begins to form. In *prometaphase*, the nuclear envelope dissolves and the chromosomes interact with the mitotic spindle. During *metaphase*, the chromosomes convene at the metaphase plate. *Anaphase* involves the separation and migration of the sister chromatids toward the spindle poles. In *telophase*, the daughter nuclei form at the two poles of the cell and the chromosomes uncoil to re-form chromatin. Mitosis is complete and cytokinesis is under way. (Images from online version of lithograph plate from *Gray's Anatomy of the Human Body*, 20th U.S. edition, 1918.)

completed in about 1 hour. Mitosis is divided into five subphases: prophase, prometaphase, metaphase, anaphase, and telophase (Figure 4):

- In *prophase*, an organelle in the cytoplasm known as the *centrosome* organizes the cell for division of the nucleus. After duplicating itself in interphase, the "sister" centrosomes, initially located near the nucleus, move away from each other. During the move, the centrosomes create a new structure known as the *mitotic spindle*, which is made up of thin filaments known as *microtubules*. Eventually, the centrosomes reach opposite poles of the cell and are now referred to as *spindle poles*.

- In *prometaphase*, the membrane around the nucleus dissolves and the mitotic spindle microtubules interact with the DNA chromatids.

- *Metaphase* is the alignment of the duplicated chromosomes at the *metaphase plate* (an imaginary plane equidistant between the spindle poles).

- *Anaphase* begins with the migration of one chromatid of each of the duplicated chromosomes along the mitotic spindle toward their spindle pole. At the end of anaphase, the two spindle poles have equal and complete collections of chromosomes.
- During *telophase*, daughter nuclei re-form at each spindle pole by recycling fragments of the parent cell's nuclear membranes. At that point, mitosis is complete. *Cytokinesis*, the division of the cytoplasm, occurs through the formation of a cleavage furrow, which divides the original cell into two daughter cells.

Because of the high degree of precision required for faithful DNA replication and cell division, the events of the cell cycle are regulated by an independent biochemical control system that possesses a number of important features. These control features are termed *checkpoints*. The checkpoint system acts as a clock or timer turning on each event at a specific time and providing adequate time for their completion.

1. It initiates events in the correct order so that later events (mitosis) do not occur before earlier events (DNA synthesis)
2. It triggers each event only once per cycle.
3. The control system contains a series of internal checks and balances that respond to a variety of signals, so that cell cycle progression can be arrested when the cell either fails to complete an essential process or encounters an unfavorable environment.

The journey through the cell cycle checkpoints requires the activation and coordinated function of a family of important proteins known as *cyclin-dependent kinases* (Cdks). At least 11 different Cdks have been identified (Cdk1 through 11). *Kinases* are proteins that attach phosphate groups to other proteins. This process, known as *phosphorylation*, causes either activation or inactivation of the *phosporylated* protein. Like falling dominos, phosphorylation of one protein leads to the activation or inactivation of another protein, and so on. Ultimately, this causes either transition to the next phase of the cell cycle or cell cycle arrest. This type of protein–protein interaction, referred to as *signal transduction*, is a common theme for many types of cell regulation.

Because the control of cell cycle events is so important, Cdk activity is tightly regulated. Hence, the activity of individual Cdk types is restricted to specific phases of the cell cycle. In addition, the activity of these phase-specific Cdks is controlled by other cell cycle regulatory proteins, both positive and negative. Negative regulation is controlled by proteins known as *Cdk inhibitors* (CKIs). For positive regulation, Cdk activity is mostly dependent on its association with a regulatory subunit protein called a *cyclin* (Figure 5). Cyclins, as the name suggests, are proteins that undergo a cycle of synthesis and degradation in each cell cycle. Unlike

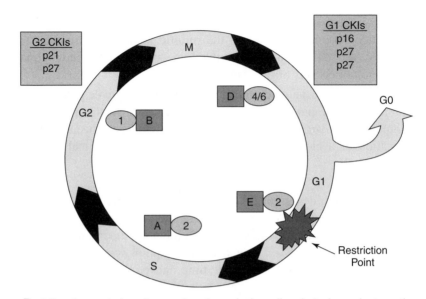

Figure 5. Cell cycle regulation. Progression through the cell cycle is dependent on the cyclin-dependent kinase (Cdk) proteins (ovals). Cdk function is both negatively and positively regulated. Cyclin-dependent kinase inhibitors (CKIs), block the function of the Cdks. Cdks are active only when bound to a phase-specific cyclin protein (squares).

the Cdks, which are present throughout the entire cell cycle, cyclins are synthesized in each cell cycle phase. Once synthesized, a phase-specific cyclin then assembles with the phase-specific Cdks, creating a *cyclin–Cdk complex*. This complex is then phosphorylated by yet another kinase, the *Cdk-activating kinase* (CAK). This phosphorylation activates the cyclin–Cdk complex. The "cycling" of cyclin levels and the assembly and activation of cyclin–Cdk complexes directs the cell cycle events. This system controls two of the most important points in the cell cycle, the G0/G1 transition and the restriction point.

In normal cells, the cell cycle events are very tightly regulated (Figure 6). As discussed above, cells in G0 can be induced to reenter the cell cycle and proliferate. This reentry into the cell cycle is a transition that requires activation of specific cyclins and specific Cdks. A *mitogen* is a protein signal that causes cells to divide. When a cell in G0 receives a signal from a mitogen, a cyclin protein of the D-type (cyclin D) is created and assembled with two Cdks that are specific to both cyclin D and the G1 phase. These cyclin D-specific Cdks are Cdk4 and Cdk6. These cyclinD–Cdk complexes then phosphorylate and *deactivate* an important cell cycle regulatory protein known as the *retinoblastoma tumor suppressor protein* (pRb). In normal cells, pRb is a continuously expressed protein whose function is to prevent the cell from progressing through the G1 phase. pRb deactivation by the cyclinD–Cdk complexes allows the synthesis of other proteins involved in cell cycle progression, including the next cyclin, *cyclin E*. Once synthesized, cyclin E complexes with its late G1 phase-specific

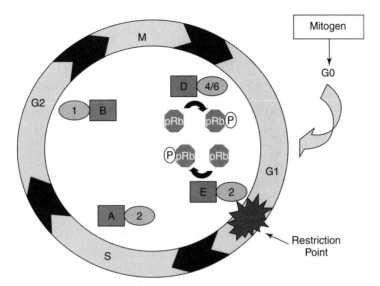

Figure 6. Cell cycle and the restriction point. After mitogen stimulation of a G0 cell, cyclin D assembles with the G1-specific Cdks: Cdk4 and Cdk6. The cyclin D–Cdk complexes phosphorylate and deactivate the retinoblastoma tumor suppressor protein (pRb). pRb deactivation allows the synthesis of cyclin E. Cyclin E complexes with Cdk2, and the cell progresses through G1 into the S phase. These events form the basis of the restriction point.

Cdk, Cdk2, and the cell progresses from G1 into S phase. These events form the basis of the most important checkpoints of the cell cycle, known as the *restriction point*. The restriction point is considered to be one of the most important checkpoints because after passing through it, the cell is committed to DNA replication, even if the signals that stimulated cell division are removed. Other major cyclin–Cdk checkpoints, such as the *G2-phase DNA damage checkpoint* and the *M-phase spindle checkpoint*, ensure the precise replication and segregation of the cell's DNA. Cancers can occur with loss of control of the regulation of any part of the cell cycle.

Programmed Cell Death (Apoptosis)

Although the rate of cell division and proliferation contributes to the growth and development of an organism, the rate of cell death is equally important. In one day, the adult human produces 50 to 70 billion cells. To maintain a status quo, an equal number of cells must be destroyed. Fortunately, multicellular organisms have a mechanism of *programmed cell death*, known as *apoptosis*, to accomplish this.

Cell death can occur in one of two ways. First, it can die as a consequence of a lethal injury such as exposure to excessive heat, a sustained lack of oxygen or essential nutrients, or a traumatic injury. Under these circumstances, the lethally injured cell dies by swelling and bursting, a process known as *necrosis*. The second method of cell death is programmed cell death (apoptosis). Unlike necrosis, apoptosis is a much cleaner process by which a cell shrinks and condenses rather than exploding and damaging its neighbors by discharging its toxic contents.

In addition to maintaining the appropriate cell number, the ability of every cell to undergo apoptosis protects the organism from cell division that would be detrimental. For example, if a cell suffers irreparable DNA damage prior to the restriction point, or DNA replication is not perfect at the G2/M checkpoint, it would be better if the cell underwent apoptosis than proceed through the cell cycle. Thus, apoptosis and cell proliferation are closely linked.

The signal for apoptosis can be initiated externally or internally. External signals are transmitted to the cell through activation of *death receptors* on the cell membrane. Under conditions of damage or stress, internal mechanisms of apoptosis can be triggered by the release of the protein *cytochrome c* from an organelle known as the *mitochondrion*. Once triggered, either externally or internally, the intracellular chemicals responsible for apoptosis, known as *caspases*, cleave target proteins. Caspases are synthesized in the cell as inactive precursors or *procaspases*. Activation of procaspases is triggered by *adapter proteins* that bring together specific procaspases, known as *initiator procaspases*. Once in close proximity, the procaspases activate one another either through structural changes or by cleavage of other procaspases. These actions result in the cleavage and activation of more caspases and procaspases. This amplification or cascading of activated caspases causes the cleavage of other key proteins in the cell. Eventually, the cell is dismantled. Activation of apoptosis is an all-or-none phenomenon that is amplifying, self-destructive, and irreversible. As it is with the cell cycle, the cell's capacity for programmed death is highly regulated to ensure that it occurs when needed but only when needed. Not surprisingly, abnormal resistance to apoptosis is another characteristic of most cancers.

Cell Differentiation

The large variety of cell types required by a complex organism demands cells of special form and function. These specialized cells obviously differ from the original cell that arose from the union of sperm and egg. The DNA sequence of every cell contains genes, which are in essence a blueprint for how the cell will specialize (i.e., nerve, heart muscle, etc.) or *differentiate*. The activation of a particular set of instructions or genes is known as *gene expression*. Each gene contains the DNA code for a specific protein. When a gene is "expressed," the protein encoded by that particular gene is produced. The exact pattern of gene expression depends simultaneously on the cell's embryonic lineage, the developmental stage, the tissue and cellular environment, and the functions that the particular cell is destined to perform. Maturation of a cell toward its ultimate form and function, known as *cell differentiation*, is the result of the comprehensive interaction of the cell's expressed genes.

Like apoptosis, cell differentiation is intimately linked to the cell cycle. After reaching complete or *terminal differentiation*, most cells enter G0. While in G0, terminally differentiated cells can actively perform their function (i.e., making mucus, secreting hormones, absorbing nutrients, etc.). As with cell proliferation and apoptosis, elaborate mechanisms regulate precise patterns of gene expression and maintain the cell's differentiated status. Loss of cell differentiation, whether due to a genetic mutation or an alteration in gene expression, can alter a cell's specialization, its metabolism, and ultimately the cell's function. Loss of cell differentiation can also result in abnormal cellular functions, including functions that help the cell become less dependent on its environment and more resistant to other regulatory mechanisms, including apoptosis. All cancer cells exhibit some loss of differentiation. Thus, loss of differentiation is considered a hallmark of cancer.

CANCER CELL BIOLOGY

As described above, precise functioning of the cell's regulatory systems is essential to maintain the delicate balance of cell division, cell differentiation, and cell death. Unfortunately, many factors can cause any of these regulatory mechanisms to malfunction or prevent a cell from responding appropriately to internal and/or external regulatory signals. The most devastating consequence of upsetting this delicate balance is the development of cancer.

Altered regulation of the cell cycle can result in faster cell division, excessive cell division, or both. With uncontrolled cell division, the result is a *neoplasm*, which is a relentlessly growing mass (tumor) of identically abnormal cells. When these abnormal cells remain clustered together in a single mass, the neoplasm is considered *benign* or noncancerous. Depending on where it is located, a benign neoplasm is often completely treatable by surgical removal alone.

An important concept to understand is that all cancers are neoplasms, but not all neoplasms (or tumors) are cancers. Cancers are neoplasms, because like benign tumors, they all have some loss of cell cycle regulation. However, benign neoplasms are not cancers because they are incapable of *invading* the tissue in which they reside. Cancers are defined as *malignant* because of the ability of individual cells to escape from the tumor mass and invade the surrounding tissue. Once the cancer cells have invaded, they can then spread to distant sites by invading other body cavities, the bloodstream, or the lymphatics. New tumors arising in other parts of the body as a result of invasion are known as *metastases*. Metastases are the main reason that malignancies are harder to treat than benign neoplasms and why removing the main tumor surgically is not enough to effect a cure. Tumors that have metastasized usually require *chemotherapy* to treat them. More often than not, it is the metastatic cancer cells that are lethal, not the original or *primary tumor.*

Benign neoplasms and cancers are classified according to the tissue and cell type from which they originate. Most complex organisms are composed of three different tissue types: epithelial (tissues that form the outer surface of the body, line the body cavities, and form the secreting portions of glands and their ducts), mesenchymal (connective tissues, such as muscles, nerves, and bones), and endothelial (tissues that line vascular structures, such as blood vessels and the heart). The names of benign neoplasms often reflect the tissue type of origin and end in the suffix: *oma* (e.g., lipoma for a benign fatty tumor, leiomyoma for a benign uterine fibroid tumor). Benign neoplasms originating from *epithelial* gland-forming tissues are called *adenomas.* Malignant neoplasms are referred to as *carcinomas,* and those originating from gland-forming epithelial tissues (such as breast or colon) are referred to as *adenocarcinomas.* Cancers that originate from *mesenchymal* tissues are known as *sarcomas.* Most cancers are derived from epithelial tissues, which is probably related to the fact that mesenchymal tissues are much less proliferative than epithelial tissues. Consequently, sarcomas are much less common than adenocarcinomas.

Regardless of the tissue type, however, it is now understood that most cancer cells are derived from a single abnormal cell. Ultimately, it is an alteration or *mutation* in the cell's DNA that transforms a normal cell to a cancerous cell. Mutations can result in an increase or decrease in the mutated gene's activity or a change in its function. Genes in which a mutation results in a gain of function that pushes the cell toward cancer are called *proto-oncogenes,* while the mutant, overactive forms of the gene are known as *oncogenes.* Conversely, genes in which a mutation results in a loss of function that pushes the cell toward cancer are known as *tumor suppressor genes.*

Cell Cycle Deregulation

Restriction Point

Because all cancers have some form of cell cycle deregulation, gene mutations that affect the cell cycle play an important role in cancer development. One place where loss of cell cycle control frequently occurs is at the *restriction point.* The restriction point is the key checkpoint in the late G1 phase where the cell commits to replicating its DNA before dividing. Errors at this checkpoint have important consequences. First, loss of control of this checkpoint commits cells to abnormal replication. Second, this checkpoint also is the nexus of two pathways that are important in cancer formation. The *pRb pathway* is named for the pRb *tumor suppressor protein.* The *c-Myc pathway* is named for the *c-Myc proto-oncogene* (Figure 7).

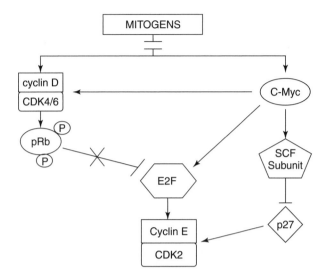

Figure 7. Cyclin E and the restriction point. The restriction point is the key checkpoint in the late G1 phase where the cell commits to replicating its DNA. This molecular switch revolves around the activity of Cdk2 and its G1-associated cyclin, cyclin E, and the point of convergence of the pRB (p16-Cdk4/6-cyclin D-pRb) tumor suppressor pathway and c-Myc proto-oncogene pathway.

pRb Pathway

pRb (p for *protein*) is considered a *tumor suppressor protein* because mutations resulting in the loss of its function can cause cancer. In fact, mutations found in the pRb pathway are the most common in all human cancers. Loss of pRb function can result in the development of cancer because pRb's primary function is to *prevent* inappropriate cell division while *allowing* normal cell division. Under normal circumstances pRb accomplishes this through its ability to exist in either an *active* or an *inactive* state. The active or inactive status of the pRb protein is determined by whether or not it has been phosphorylated. Normally, pRb exists in an unphosphorylated and active state (unphosphorylated active Rb protein is designated pRb). In its active state, pRb prevents cell division. When pRb protein is phosphorylated (ppRb), it becomes inactive and it allows cell division. In the G1 phase, active pRb is *inactivated* when the cyclin D/Cdk4/Cdk6 complex phosphorylates it (adds a phosphate ion to it). This typically occurs late in the G1 phase and results in the up-regulation of the next cell cycle cyclin, cyclin E.

pRb regulation of cyclin E is an important part of the G1/S transition. Active pRb prevents the transition from G1 to S by repressing cyclin E production. Once pRb is phosphorylated to ppRb, it no longer inhibits cyclin E production. The cyclin E then complexes with its specific Cdk (Cdk2) and the cyclin E/Cdk2 complex further phosphorylates pRb. This additional production of ppRb then causes up-regulation of the next cell cycle cyclin, cyclin A. Thus, ppRb accumulation allows the cell cycle to progress to mitosis. Mutations that generate ppRb are equivalent to a persistent pRb inactivation. Cells with this mutation have no functional G1 restriction point. They are incapable of remaining in G1 or of entering G0, and they undergo continual and inappropriate replication (Figure 8).

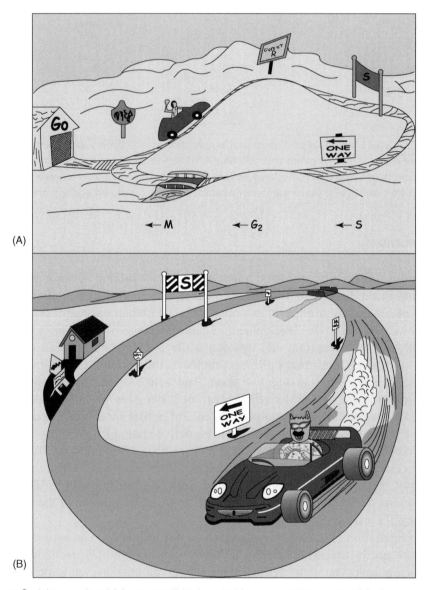

Figure 8. (A) Normal and (B) cancer cell biology. Without a restriction point (B), the cancer cell (as depicted by the car) progresses through the cell cycle in a completely uncontrolled manner and is no longer able to exit to G0.

In addition to pRb inactivation, other cell cycle control system changes related to the pRb pathway can increase cell proliferation. For example, mutations can cause increased production or function of cyclin D or its Cdks, which inappropriately promote ppRb accumulation and thereby, cell division. Also, errors that occur during cyclin E production can result in a hyperactive form of cyclin E. The increased activity of this type of cyclin E (known as the low-molecular-weight (LMW) form of cyclin E) results in faster cell division, decreased cell size, and loss of growth factors required for proliferation—all are signs of cancer.

c-Myc Proto-oncogene Pathway

Cell cycle deregulation also occurs through mutation in the c-Myc proto-oncogene pathway. The c-Myc pathway is activated when the cell is stimulated by a mitogen (something that causes mitosis, i.e., cell division). The product of the c-Myc gene is a transcription factor, which is a protein that functions as a signal for other genes to be expressed (start functioning). One of those is the cyclin E gene. Production of cyclin E by the c-Myc signal can then result in the phosphorylation and inactivation of pRb and inappropriate cell cycle division. c-Myc is called a proto-oncogene because mutations that increase c-Myc activity can lead to increased cell division and cancer (*proto-* meaning before, *onco-* meaning cancer).

Although these are just a few examples, functional alterations at almost every step in the pRb and c-Myc pathways can contribute to cancerous transformations. Thus, the pRb and c-Myc pathways illustrate a salient point in our understanding of cancer. *It is possible to alter the cell cycle control system in more than one way and at the same time produce the same effect (or defect).* It demonstrates that the same cancer can be caused by oncogenes, which become *activated* by mutation (i.e., c-Myc), or by tumor suppressor genes, which become *inactivated* by mutation (i.e., ppRb). This is possible because both types of mutations increase cell division. This also illustrates that individual cancers can have similar characteristics even when they arise from different mutations. Finally, because different mutations can produce the same types of cancers but by dissimilar mechanism, this may explain why the same types of cancers often respond so differently to the same anticancer therapy.

Resistance to Apoptosis

It takes more than just abnormal cell division for a cell to undergo a complete malignant transformation. In fact, a malignant transformation requires multiple gene mutations, which affect not only the cell cycle, but also cell differentiation and apoptosis. These mutations usually accumulate over time. During this interval, the mutant clone generation with the greatest growth advantages (i.e., fastest division, least apoptosis, least dependence on environment) takes over.

Resistance to apoptosis is an extremely important characteristic of cancer cells. The lack of programmed cell death contributes to the development of cancer by more than merely tipping the balance in favor of cell accumulation. Defective apoptosis allows cells to survive beyond their normal lifespan, lowers their dependence on external factors, and protects against some stresses associated with tumor expansion, such as decreased nutrients and oxygen. Resistance to apoptosis also abets genetic changes that promote cell proliferation, differentiation, and cell invasiveness during tumor progression. It also allows cells to continue replicating their DNA despite DNA damage that would otherwise cause them to die rather than divide. Furthermore, it has been shown to enhance the cell's ability to metastasize, avoid destruction by the immune system, and resist chemotherapy and radiation treatment.

Loss of Differentiation

Compared with a normal cell of the same origin, all cancer cells show changes in their differentiation. As with the loss of regulation of the cell cycle and the increased resistance to apoptosis, altered differentiation is usually due to abnormal gene expression or to mutations. Cancer cells tend to be less differentiated than their normal counterparts. Technically, the degree of differentiation is determined by how much the cancer cells resemble their normal counterparts *morphologically* (i.e., how they look under the microscope) and functionally. *Well-differentiated cancers* closely resemble the mature normal cells of the tissue from which they are derived. *Poorly differentiated* or *undifferentiated cancers* have a less organized appearance and lack specialization or functionality. Generally, benign neoplasms are well differentiated. Malignant neoplasms, however, can range from well to undifferentiated. Cancers composed of undifferentiated cells are said to be *anaplastic*.

Anaplasia is characterized by great variations in the size and shape of cells and nuclei. The nuclei become disproportionately large in relation to the rest of the cell. This variation, referred to as *polymorphism*, is an easily visualized (under the microscope) departure from normal cells, which maintain a relatively consistent size and shape with each new generation. In addition, poorly differentiated cancers contain large numbers of cells that are undergoing mitosis, a sign of the heightened proliferative activity of the cancer cells. There are other problems with poorly differentiated cells. They lose their ability to progress normally through mitosis, resulting in erroneous DNA segregation and transfer during cell division. In addition, loss of differentiation affects cell–cell interactions. Most normal cells, and even benign neoplastic cells, depend on physical contact with surrounding cells to initiate and progress through cell division. This is known as *anchorage dependence*. As cells become less differentiated, they become *anchorage independent*, a characteristic that gives these cells the ability to proliferate in the absence of physical contact with other cells and the potential to metastasize to other parts of body.

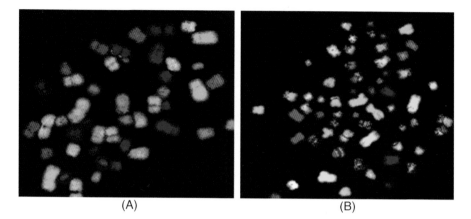

(A)   (B)

Figure 1.1 Cancer-related chromosomal aberrations. In early stages of cancer, chromosomes break and join with segments of other chromosomes that are not adjacent in normal cells (chromosomal translocations). As a consequence, genes that control cell growth and specialized properties of cells are frequently rearranged. Other cancer-related alterations that result from reorganization are in cell adhesion and motility as well as in capacity to invade and grow in tissues at distant sites from the initial tumor (metastasis). (A) normal chromosomes (note that each chromosome is a single color); (B) chromosomes in cancer cells that contain fused segments of multiple chromosomes (note multicolored chromosomes).

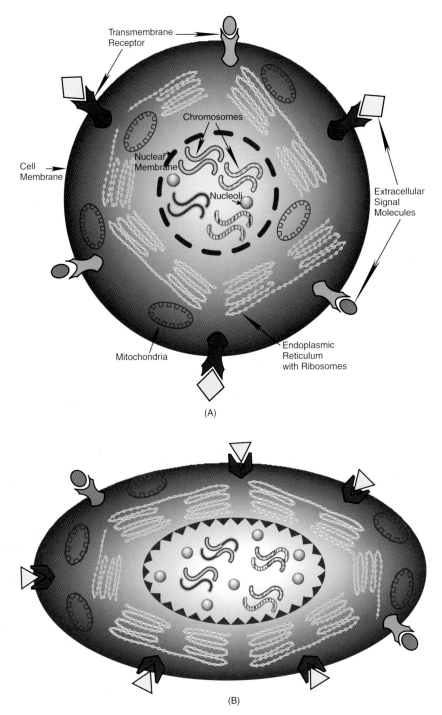

Figure 1.2a,b Structure and organization of regulatory machinery in (A) normal and (B) cancer cells. The organization and location of machinery that controls genes is modified during the onset and progression of cancer. (*See text for full description*).

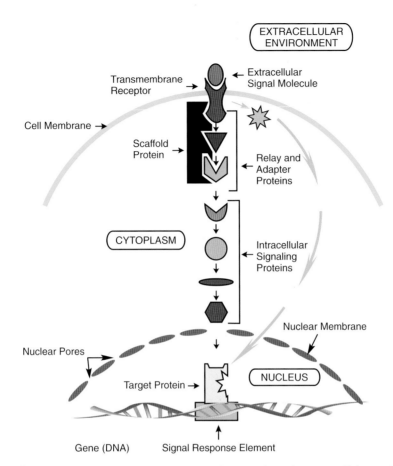

Figure 1.3 Cell signaling. Cells communicate and respond to the extracellular environment through a process designated *signal transduction*. Signal molecules bind to transmembrane receptors that span the cell membrane. The interaction of signal molecules with components of receptors located outside the cell modifies the intracellular components of the receptors. An environmental signal is thereby transduced into a cascade of regulatory steps that control genes which control cell proliferation and specialized properties of cells.

In some signaling pathways, scaffold proteins assemble signaling molecules into complexes for the initial passage of information from the transmembrane receptor to relay and adaptor proteins. Subsequent steps in the signaling process amplify and integrate signals. A chain of intracellular signaling proteins processes regulatory information through the cytoplasm and into the cell nucleus to activate or suppress genes. In other signaling pathways the regulatory cascades are abbreviated. The transduction of regulatory information from the intracellular component of the transmembrane receptor is more direct, circumventing intermediary steps in information transfer. At an early stage in the signaling process a signaling protein enters the nucleus and interacts directly with genes to modify expression.

Many cancer cells exhibit defects in one or more steps of signaling cascades that alter control of cell growth, specialized cell properties, cell–cell communication, cell motility, and cell adhesion. The components of signaling pathways that are modified in tumor cells are targets for treatments that are effective and specific.

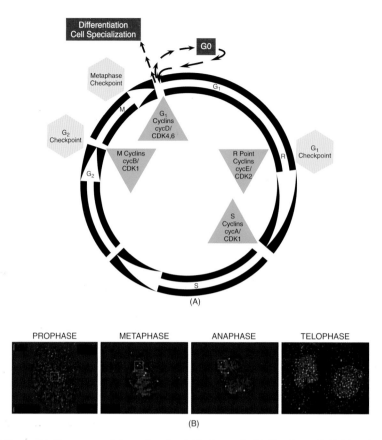

Figure 1.4a,b (A) The stages of the cell cycle. G1 is the period following cell division (M; mitosis) and precedes the S phase, the period when genes (DNA) are duplicated to provide an identical set of genes for progeny cells. (*See text for full description*).

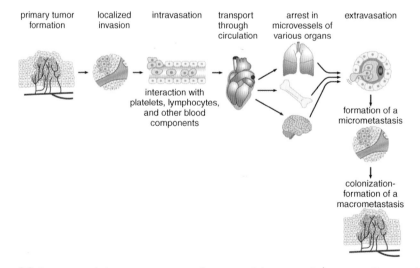

Figure 2.3 Summary of the steps necessary for successful metastasis. Cancer cells must break down the tissue surrounding them, invade their environment, and attract a blood supply. (*See text for full description*).

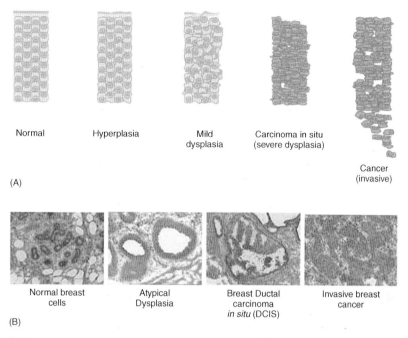

(A)

(B)

Figure 2.4 Formation of tumor. As the normal cells mutate and divide, they start to pile up (hyperplasia): (A) artists drawing; (B) actual pictures of this occurring in the breast. Over time, these cells develop added mutations and begin to look abnormal (atypical dysplasia). If this process occurs in an organ with ducts, such as the breast, they fill in the normal breast ducts before they come invasive (ductal carcinoma in situ). Overall, this process is thought to take years to occur. [(A) From ref. 40.]

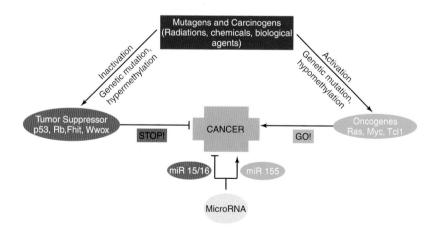

Figure 3.1 Schematic representation showing the complex relationships among genetics, epigenetics, and environmental factors (radiations, chemicals, and microorganisms) in causing cancer. Oncogenes and tumor suppressors are protein-coding genes, whereas microRNA genes are noncoding genes (see the text).

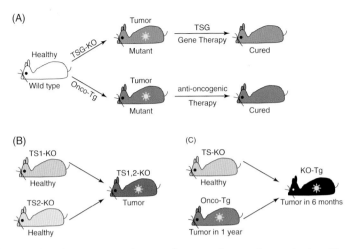

(A)

Healthy
Wild type

TSG-KO

Tumor
Mutant

TSG
Gene Therapy

Cured

Onco-Tg

Tumor
Mutant

anti-oncogenic
Therapy

Cured

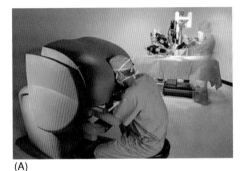

(B)
TS1-KO
Healthy

TS2-KO
Healthy

TS1,2-KO
Tumor

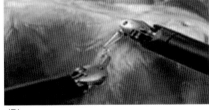

(C)
TS-KO
Healthy

Onco-Tg
Tumor in 1 year

KO-Tg
Tumor in 6 months

Figure 3.3 Examples of cancer genetics experiments using engineered mice. (*See text for full description*).

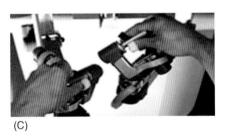

(A)

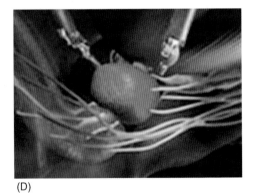

(B)

(C)

(D)

Figure 4.2a–d (A) Surgeon operates from a console located adjacent to the patient and the operative field. (B,C) Robotic arms are used to transect the tumor. Hand controls offer stability and precision in movement. (D) Simulated surgical approach to prostate cancer: robotic arms allow careful separation of nerves away from site of tumor/prostate resection, preserving urinary and sexual function. (Images © 2008 Intuitive Surgical, Inc.)

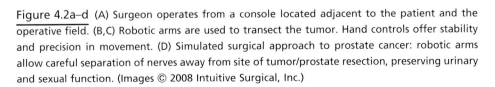

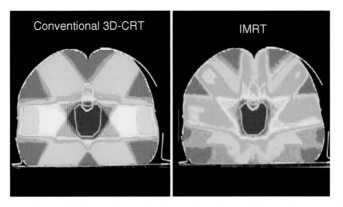

Figure 4.5 Comparison of three-dimensional conformal radiation therapy with intensity-modulated radiation therapy for prostate cancer (red). IMRT utilizes greater number of beams (yellow) tailored with various shapes and intensities to deliver more radiation to the tumor and less to the normal tissues.

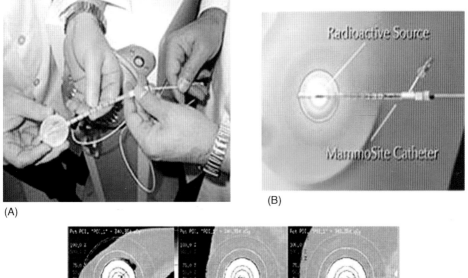

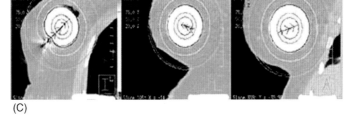

Figure 4.7a–c Brachytherapy for breast cancer. (A) Special balloon and catheter prior to insertion into tumor site following lumpectomy. (B,C) Radioactive seeds introduced into balloon through the catheter and removed after various time intervals. Extent of radiation effects show by concentric circles. (Image 7A used with permission of The University of Toledo Medical Center. Images 7B and 7C courtesy of Hologic.)

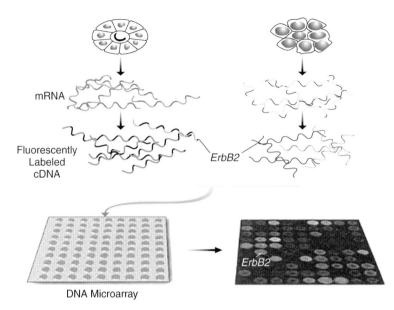

Figure 4.8 Microarray analysis used to detect abnormal expression of *ErbB2*. Flurorescent-labeled cDNA for the *ErbB2* gene combines specifically with a patient's mRNA containing *ErbB2*. If a patient with breast cancer (right) has a large amount of *ErbB2* in her cells, it will appear as a bright fluorescent spot on the array plate.

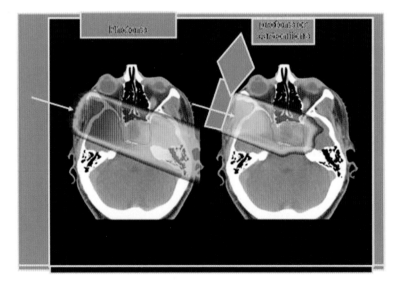

Figure 4.9 Comparison of photon delivery by linear accelerator and proton therapy by cyclotron to a brain tumor. (A) Photon radiation passes through normal tissue, tumor (center, circular structure), and more normal tissue. (B) Proton beam released in the tumor stops at the far edge if the tumor, sparing normal tissue.

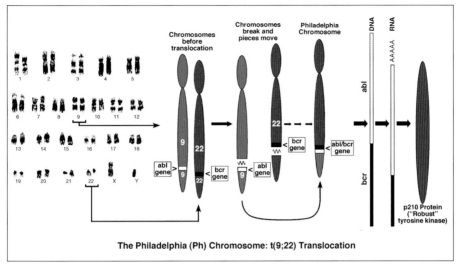

Chromosomes before translocation

Chromosomes break and pieces move

Philadelphia Chromosome

DNA

RNA

abl

bcr

9

22

22

abl gene

bcr gene

bcr gene

abl gene

abl/bcr gene

p210 Protein ("Robust" tyrosine kinase)

The Philadelphia (Ph) Chromosome: t(9;22) Translocation

Figure 4.12 Philadelphia chromosome translocation. (*See text for full description*).

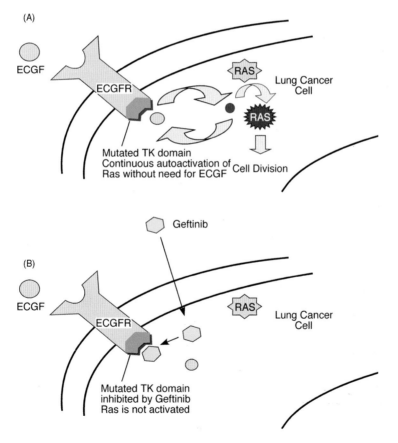

(A)

ECGF

ECGFR

RAS

RAS

Lung Cancer Cell

Mutated TK domain
Continuous autoactivation of Ras without need for ECGF

Cell Division

Geftinib

(B)

ECGF

ECGFR

RAS

Lung Cancer Cell

Mutated TK domain
inhibited by Geftinib
Ras is not activated

Figure 4.15a,b (A) Colon cancer cell: extracellular growth factor (ECGF) stimulates mutated receptor on cell. The tyrosine kinase enzyme (blue) located on the inner aspect of the receptor is mutated. (*See text for full description*).

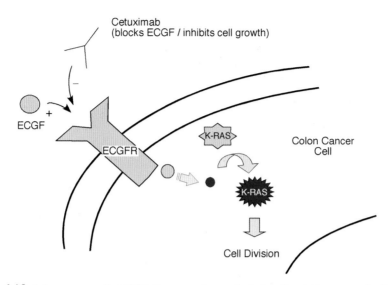

Figure 4.16 Colon cancer cell: ECGF is the normal growth factor stimulating normal cell growth. Colon cancer cells that express abnormal amounts of the ECGFR may be blocked by an antibody designed to attach specifically to the receptor. This antibody prevents stimulation by ECGF and reduces the ability of the cell to divide and grow.

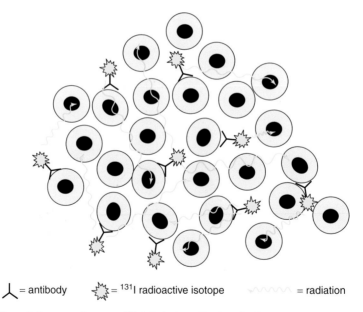

Figure 4.17 Radioimmunotherapy. ^{131}I-labeled antibodies (radioactive antibodies) attach to surface antigens on tumor cells. Radiation crossfires to other cells.

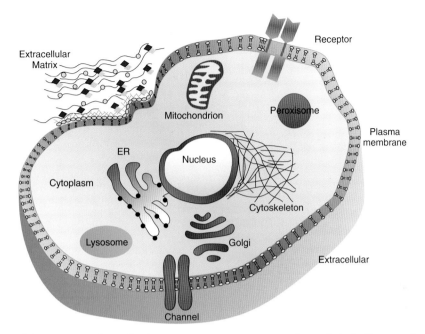

Figure 6.1 Overview of a cell. The most common structures of a cell, including a variety of organelles (i.e., mitochodria, peroxisome, Golgi apparatus). (*See text for full description*).

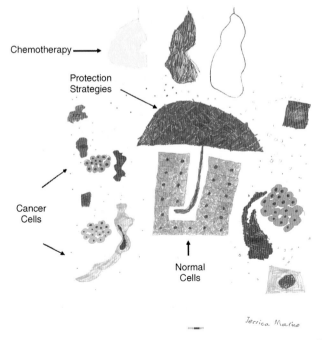

Figure 6.9 Protection of normal cells against the toxic affect of chemotherapy. (*See text for full description*).

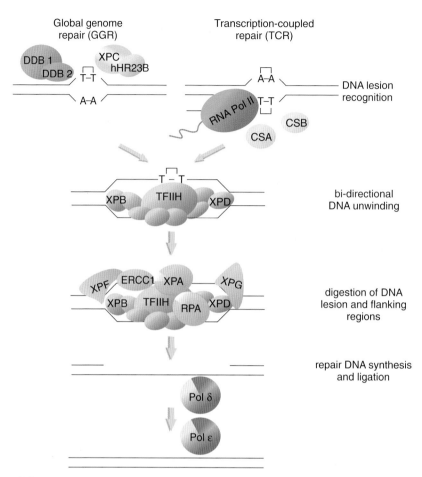

Figure 7.6 Nucleotide excision repair pathway (NER). NER recognizes and repairs DNA lesions that distort the overall structure of double-helical DNA. Two subpathways have been identified: global genome repair (GGR), which surveys the entire genome for such lesions, and transcription-coupled repair (TCR), which acts on DNA that is actively being decoded into RNA.

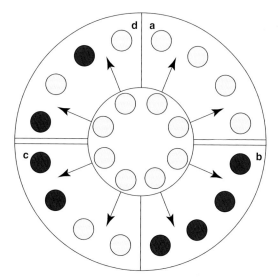

Figure 7.10 Outcomes of stem cell division. (*See text for full description*).

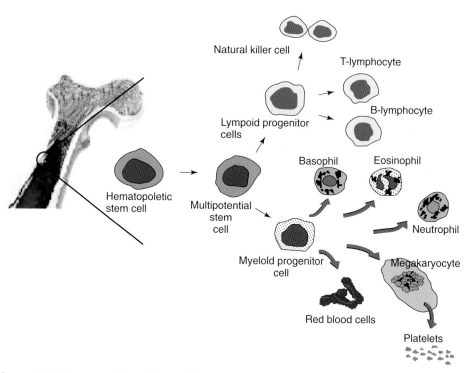

Figure 7.11 Hematopoietic and stromal stem cell differentiation. (*See text for full description*).

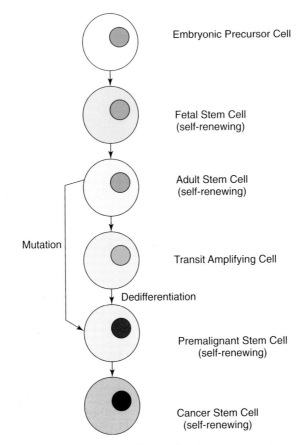

Figure 7.12 Mutations in normal stems cells can give rise to cancer stem cells. Fetal stem cells and normal adult stem cells derive from embryonic precursor stem cells. Further division of adult stem cells will result in self-renewal (more copies of the stem cells themselves) or will proceed down a pathway of differentiation, creating cells termed *transit amplifying cells* that will go on to maintain adult tissues. A premalignant stem cell can arise by mutation of an adult stem cell, or a change in a transit amplifying cell that leads to dedifferentiation and the acquisition of self-renewal properties. These can give rise to aggressively proliferating cancer stem cells that self-renew unabated by normal control signals.

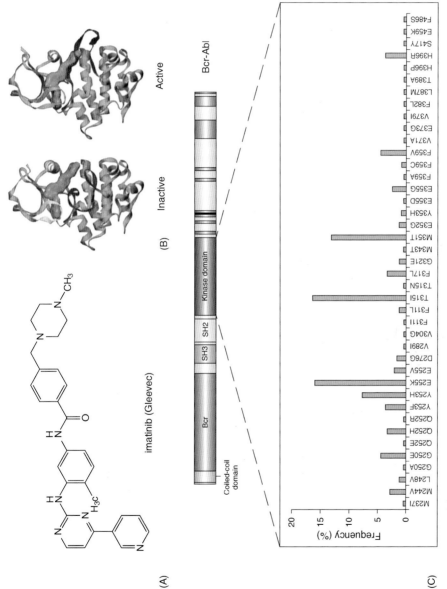

Figure 12.2 Imatinib binding and clinical resistance profile. (A) Chemical structure of imatinib. (B) Imatinib (blue) binds the inactive conformation of the Abl kinase domain. The p-loop (represented in yellow and orange) and the activation loop (magenta and red) are shown in the context of each conformation. (C) Organization of select domains of Bcr-Abl. The spectrum and clinical frequency of kinase domain point mutations reported in imatinib-resistant patients are shown expanded below.

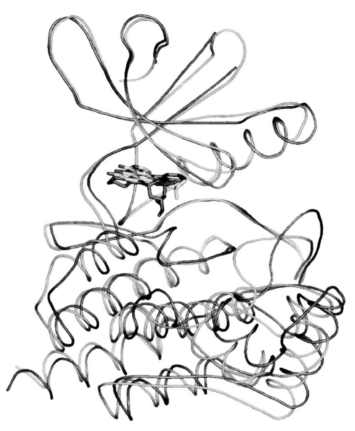

Figure 12.6 Crystallographic comparison of JAK2 and JAK3. The tyrosine kinase domains of JAK2 (blue) and JAK3 (green) bound to the specific small-molecule pan-JAK inhibitor CMP6 (yellow) and staurosporine analog AFN941 (magenta), respectively, feature a high degree of homology and are shown superimposed above. (Image graciously provided with permission from J. Rossjohn [46].)

Cancer Cell Biology and Novel Treatment Strategies

Tumor resistance to anticancer therapy is the main cause of failure of cancer treatment. The cancer-killing mechanisms of most conventional chemotherapeutic agents used today are attributable to their effects on DNA. However, as illustrated by the high rate of resistance, this approach is limited in a number of ways. First it is highly nonspecific, damaging normal as well as tumor cells. Second, it is only the very imprecise, higher rate of cell division in cancer cells that makes them relatively more susceptible than normal cells to these agents. Another limitation is the partial lethality of the drug, with the ultimate outcome (susceptibility versus resistance) dependent on the the cell's mechanisms of cell cycle arrest, DNA repair and apoptosis. Discovering ways of overcoming tumor cell resistance to chemotherapy is an important area of active investigation. Potential targets for new types of therapy include the mechanisms of deregulation of the processes of the cell cycle, apoptosis and differentiation.

One target of particular interest for this approach is the cyclin E–Cdk2 complex, and the restriction point of the cell cycle is an exceptionally attractive target for novel cancer therapy. In particular, the tumor-specific LMW forms of cyclin E provide both a unique means of determining differential expression of the potential chemotherapy target in tumor versus normal cells and a way of increasing the selective lethality to cancer cells. In addition, because these LMW forms of cyclin E occur only in tumors, assays of their levels may provide a more objective measure of both tumor aggressiveness and therapeutic response.

To target these cancer-specific forms of cyclin E, the reasons for their differential expression need to be understood. These include either increased levels of the enzyme that alters the cyclin E (*elastase*), increased *elastase-like* activity in tumor cells, *decreased elastase inhibitor* levels in *tumor* cells or *increased elastase inhibitor* levels in *normal* cells. One therapeutic option currently under investigation includes the development of elastase inhibitors that could prevent the formation of the altered forms of cyclin E in tumor cells.

Another potential target at this nodal point in the cell cycle is Cdk2. Because of their central role in cell cycle regulation, Cdks are attracting significant interest as targets for anticancer therapy. Over 50 chemical Cdk inhibitors with various degrees of Cdk specificity have been described. Most of these compounds work by interfering with the kinase activity of the Cdk. Both in the laboratory and in patients, Cdk-specific cell cycle and antitumoral effects have been described for three Cdk inhibitors: flavopiridol, R-roscovitine, and BMS 387032. One major limitation of these agents, though, is their inability to actually damage the cell instead of just inducing cell cycle arrest. Preclinical evidence that these agents induce tumor cell apoptosis has not held up in clinical trials. However, it is possible that combining these agents with more conventional chemotherapeutics would overcome some forms of chemoresistance. For this reason, results of ongoing combination chemotherapy trials are eagerly awaited.

Other potential indirect inhibitors of Cdk2 activity worth considering include the naturally occurring *cyclin-dependent kinase inhibitors* (CKIs) known as p27 and p21. As mentioned above, a relative loss of function of any cell cycle regulators, including negative regulators such as p27 and p21, can result in loss of cell cycle control and increased cell proliferation. Possible strategies for targeting these types of CKIs include increasing their expression through gene therapy or increasing their amount through administration of a tumor-targeted synthetic version of the CKIs or similar peptides that inhibit Cdk activity. Another strategy includes decreasing the degradation of these CKIs by inhibiting their breakdown by a cell organelle known as the *proteosome*. Although these examples are related to cell cycle deregulation, alterations in the regulation of apoptosis and cell differentiation provide equally exciting targets for novel anticancer treatment strategies.

We can also use our knowledge of the ways in which normal and tumor cells differ in cell cycle regulation to design strategies and identify novel targets to increase the therapeutic index and to protect normal cells from the toxic effects of chemotherapeutic agents, and by doing so, minimize the dose-limiting toxicity.

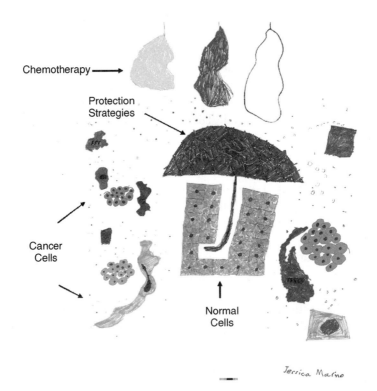

Figure 9. Protection of normal cells against the toxic affect of chemotherapy. A schematic drawing of how normal cells (under the umbrella) can be protected (umbrella) against the toxic affects of chemotherapy (different-colored bags and the "raindrops"). Notice that normal cells are all uniform in shape and size, whereas tumor cells are all different. (See insert for color representation.)

Modification by a drug of an effect specific to a normal cell can raise the therapeutic index, thereby permitting administration of a higher dosage of a drug that is lethal to the cancer cells. If the normal cells in the body are reversibly stopped from cycling, the toxic effects of cycle-dependent chemotherapy should be diminished (Figure 9).

SUMMARY

Cells are the building blocks of all living creatures. Creation and maintenance of any multicellular organism requires a delicate balance between cell proliferation, cell differentiation, and cell death. Elaborate control systems exist to regulate and coordinate these essential processes. Cancer is the most devastating consequence of loss of control of these processes.

Most cancers arise from a single cell that has undergone a growth-promoting mutation. Over time, the progeny of this original cell acquire additional mutations and the tumor becomes malignant through a natural selection process that favors the most rapidly dividing and aggressive cells. Eventually, the cancer cells undergo deregulation of the normal processes of cell proliferation, cell death, and cell differentiation. Identification of the exact changes that result in the cancer cell's ability to defy normal proliferation controls, resist apoptosis, or differentiate are providing new targets for cancer therapy. In theory, these targets are cancer cell–specific, thus sparing normal cells from negative anticancer therapy effects. Only through continued study and increased understanding of the abnormal properties that distinguish cancer cells from normal cells can we hope to develop truly effective cancer treatments.

Acknowledgments

The authors would like to thank Jessica Marino for the generous donation of her artwork illustrating the concept of protecting normal cells from the toxic effects of chemotherapy (Figure 9).

RECOMMENDED READING

Akli S, Keyomarsi K. 2003. Cyclin E and its low molecular weight forms in human cancer and as targets for cancer therapy. *Cancer Biol Ther* 2(4 Suppl 1):S38–47.

Blagosklonny MV, Pardee AB. 2002. The restriction point of the cell cycle. *Cell Cycle* 1(2):103–110.

Druker BJ, Mamon HJ, Roberts TM. 1989. Oncogenes, growth factors, and signal transduction. *N Engl J Med* 321(20):1383–1391.

Evan GI, Vousden KH. 2001. Proliferation, cell cycle and apoptosis in cancer. *Nature* 411(6835): 342–348.

Hanahan D, Weinberg RA. 2000. The hallmarks of cancer. *Cell* 100(1):57–70.

Hartwell LH, Weinert TA. 1989. Checkpoints: controls that ensure the order of cell cycle events. *Science* 246(4930):629–634.

Reed JC. 1999. Dysregulation of apoptosis in cancer. *J Clin Oncol* 17(9):2941–2953.

Shapiro GI. 2006. Cyclin-dependent kinase pathways as targets for cancer treatment. *J Clin Oncol* 24(11):1770–1783.

Thornberry NA, Lazebnik Y. 1998. Caspases: enemies within. *Science* 281(5381):1312–1316.

Weinberg RA. 1995. The retinoblastoma protein and cell cycle control. *Cell* 81(3):323–330.

7

MUTATIONS AND CELL DEFENSES

Otto S. Gildemeister, Jay M. Sage, and Kendall L. Knight

Department of Biochemistry and Molecular Pharmacology,
University of Massachusetts Medical School, Worcester, Massachusetts

INTRODUCTION

The information required for the development and growth of an organism is encoded in its deoxyribonucleic acid (DNA), the genetic material. In human cells, the entire DNA content, or *genome*, is packaged in 46 chromosomes that reside in the cell's nucleus. Because this information is critically important for all biological processes occurring during the lifetime of an organism, evolution has resulted in many and various means by which a cell can either avoid damage to this information, or repair damage once it has occurred. DNA is a double-stranded helical ribbon, with each strand consisting of a continuous sequence of bases. Bases can be considered as the letters of words that are strung together to make up the information code (Figure 1). Remarkably, only four bases—adenine, guanine, cytosine, and thymine (A, G, C, and T)—are required to generate the amazingly diverse information encoded in the human genome, and it is the varying, ordered sequence of these bases that creates all the different bits of information along the DNA strand. For the purposes of our discussion in this chapter, remember that genetic information is decoded by the following general path: DNA codes for

The Biology and Treatment of Cancer: Understanding Cancer
Edited by Arthur B. Pardee and Gary S. Stein   Copyright © 2009 John Wiley & Sons, Inc.

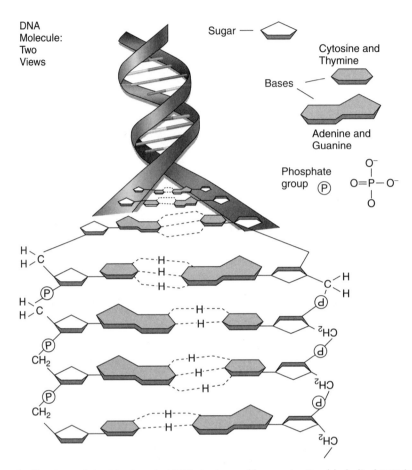

Figure 1. Structure of double-stranded DNA duplex and base pairs. Double-helical DNA is made up of two antiparallel strands of polymerized bases. The fundamental repeating unit of DNA, a deoxyribonucleoside monophosphate, consists of a sugar moiety (ribose), a base (either A, G, C, or T), and a phosphate group (see also http://en.wikipedia.org/wiki/DNA). (From http://www.accessexcellence.org/RC/VL/GG/images/dna_molecule.gif.)

ribonucleic (RNA), acid which in turn codes for protein molecules, whose amino acid sequence derives from the DNA sequence. Although this is an oversimplification of the complex information contained within DNA, it suffices for our appreciation of how changes in the DNA sequence (*mutations*) may adversely effect cellular function. The bases in each of the two DNA strands form what are referred to as *base pairs*, and each strand is polymerized in an orientation opposite relative to its partner (Figure 1). The chemical composition of the bases dictates that A always pairs with T on the opposite strand, and G with C. Hence, normal DNA contains only A : T and G : C base pairs. Mutations defined as changes in the sequence of the bases, can occur by a number of means: for example, single base substitutions that might result from errors during DNA replication (copying of the DNA prior to cell division; see below), or deletion of larger pieces of a chromosome or translocation events (swapping pieces from one chromosome to another).

It is also important to note that mutations can be grouped into two general categories, germline and somatic. *Germline mutations* are those that we inherit from our parents and will pass on to our children, while *somatic mutations* are those that occur during our lifetime and are not passed on to our descendants. Most mutations have no effect on our health and lifespan because they result in changes to DNA base sequences that do not alter the coded genetic information. However, those mutations that make changes to the genetic information such that cells no longer can control their growth are the hallmark of cancer. The discovery of the structure of DNA in 1953 by James Watson and Francis Crick initiated a rapid increase in the study of how the information encoded in the double-helical fibers of DNA was copied and passed from generation to generation. It has been estimated that the human genome carries approximately 35,000 sequences whose codes are read to produce protein molecules with specific metabolic functions. In cells that are growing and dividing, and even in those cells in a resting phase, mutations occur at an alarmingly high rate, both from normal cellular processes (e.g., copying of the DNA strands prior to cell division) and from exposure to environmental or chemical carcinogens [e.g., the ultraviolet rays in sunlight or especially cigarette smoke (at least 40 different carcinogens are found in a typical cigarette)]. However, all cells use remarkably effective strategies to either avoid mutations or to repair them when they occur.

MUTATIONS THAT RESULT FROM NORMAL METABOLIC PROCESSES

Cells grow and eventually divide, and must therefore create an exact copy of their DNA so that both daughter cells contain exactly the same genetic information. The process of copying the DNA strands (DNA replication) prior to cell division can be considered as a molecular assembly line, and the most important machines in this process are the replicative DNA polymerases. Of course, as with all assembly lines, occasional errors do occur. However, DNA polymerase and its associated proteins do a remarkably good job of minimizing the damage. One of the most studied DNA polymerases is the bacterial DNA Pol III, whose catalytic functions are very similar to those of human DNA polymerases. DNA replication requires that the two DNA strands be separated, permitting the polymerase to read the base sequence of each strand (the template strand) and produce a complementary copy (the daughter strand), thereby creating a new double-stranded DNA. As the polymerase reads the template and incorporates complementary bases into the daughter strand, on average it will incorporate the wrong base every 1 in 10,000 times ("misincorporation" in step 1, Figure 2). However, the polymerase has an editing function that allows it

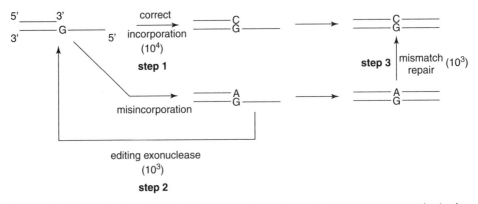

Figure 2. DNA replication fidelity. Three important steps occur during DNA synthesis that minimize the errors made by polymerases as they create duplicate copies of the DNA: (1) correct incorporation of a new base, (2) backward editing of occasional errors, and (3) correction of errors by the mismatch repair system. In this figure the bottom strand is shown as a template and the polymerase inserts the corresponding complementary base into the growing daughter strand (top strand); in this case, C should be inserted opposite G (step 1). In those instances where the wrong base is mistakenly inserted, the polymerase can detect the mistake, back up, and remove the incorrect base and move forward again to insert the correct base (step 2). For those errors that escape this process, another detection and correction system, mismatch repair, will act to make the correction.

to recognize mistakes, back up, and remove the misincorporated base. This editing exonuclease function (step 2, Figure 2) will let mistakes go through only once in 1000 times. Mistakes that slip through this step will be recognized by the DNA mismatch repair system (discussed below in more detail), which misses errors only once in 1000 times (step 3, Figure 2). Taking these steps into account, on average only one mistake occurs for every 10 billion bases copied. The human genome consists of approximately 6 billion bases, and using a loose estimate that growing cells on average will divide 100 times per year (there are large variations in rates of division for cells from different tissues), we approximate that 60 base changes (mutations) will escape detection per year per starting cell. This is an extremely low mutation rate and underscores the incredible precision and fidelity with which DNA polymerases operate. An additional remarkable feature of DNA replication is that this low error rate occurs while the polymerase is zipping along at an incredible speed, approximately 500 to 1000 new bases are added per second. In a 1998 review article, Stephen Bell and Tania Baker provide a striking analogy (Baker and Bell, 1998). With the DNA polymerase incorporating 1000 new bases per second into the growing daughter strand, if we imagine the double-stranded DNA to be 1 meter wide, the polymerase moves at 375 mph, and the protein complex that includes the polymerase and its associated proteins would be the size of a FedEx truck. This machinery will make only one mistake every 106 miles!

In addition to the DNA polymerases that make duplicate copies of the entire genome, cells can invoke the use of a family of DNA polymerases referred to as *error-prone polymerases*. In contrast to the extremely high fidelity with which replicative DNA polymerases operate, error-prone polymerases are inherently sloppy and misincorporate bases into a newly synthesized DNA strand at frequencies ranging from 1 in every 1000 bases to an incredibly high rate of 1 in every 10 bases (Goodman, 2002). Error-prone DNA polymerases are most often used in situations requiring the synthesis of only very short stretches of DNA (e.g., in some DNA repair pathways; see below).

Base mispairs that may lead to mutations can also arise if DNA bases become chemically altered. How might this occur in a normally growing cell? Actually, there are a number of normal cellular metabolic processes that give rise to side products that can damage DNA. For example, the oxidative metabolic processes carried out by mitochondria (the cellular compartment responsible for generating energy) give rise to reactive forms of oxygen known as *reactive oxygen species* (ROS), which can move through the cell and chemically modify any number of biomolecules, including DNA. A first line of defense available to the cell are enzymes that can detoxify ROS: for example, catalase, superoxide dismutase, and glutathione-S-transferases (GSTs). In fact, the increased risks of cancer resulting from defects in GSTs derive from the weakening of this defense mechanism such that a higher percentage of naturally occurring ROS escapes detoxification, thereby resulting in higher levels of DNA damage.

DNA REPAIR MECHANISMS

Many types of DNA damage escape the avoidance mechanisms described above, and the cell must then call upon various DNA repair pathways to fix the mutated genetic material. As we begin our discussion of the cellular mechanisms that repair DNA damage, it is important to note that different types of damage are recognized specifically and repaired by different repair pathways. We will also make specific note of defects in the function of certain DNA repair proteins (resulting from mutations in the genes encoding these proteins) that have been linked to increased risks in developing cancers. It is proposed that human cells have five distinct DNA repair pathways: (1) base excision repair (BER), (2) nucleotide excision repair (NER), (3) mismatch repair (MMR), (4) nonhomologous end joining (NHEJ), and (5) homologous recombinational repair (HRR). Examples of specific types of DNA damage, or lesions, that are recognized and repaired by each of these pathways is shown in Figure 3. Each of the pathways described next (BER, NER and MMR) operates using a series of ordered and regulated steps by first recognizing the specific type of DNA damage, then removing the damaged base and sometimes several flanking bases, followed by resynthesis of the missing DNA by specialized DNA polymerases. Defects in any

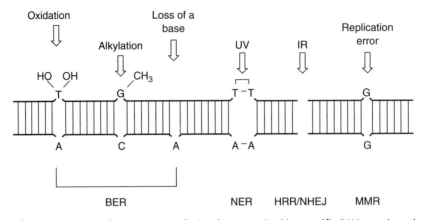

Figure 3. Specific types of DNA damage (lesions) are repaired by specific DNA repair pathways. Base excision repair (BER) acts on lesions that do not disrupt the overall double helical structure of DNA (e.g., small chemical modifications such as oxidation or methylation, and missing bases). Nucleotide excision repair (NER) acts on lesions that disrupt the structure of DNA (e.g., cross-linked bases). The nonhomologous end joining (NHEJ) and homologous recombinational DNA repair (HRR) pathways fix double-strand breaks: in the case shown, those resulting from exposure of cells to ionizing radiation. Mismatch repair (MMR) acts on base pair mismatches and small insertions that may occur on one of the strands.

of these steps can lead to a decreased efficiency of DNA repair that will inevitably result in higher frequencies of persistent mutations, thereby increasing the risk of cancer development.

The *BER pathway* recognizes DNA bases that have been chemically altered but that do not distort the overall structure of the DNA double helix. The example in Figure 4 shows a U base paired with a G on the opposite strand. Although U is commonly found in RNA, it does not normally exist in DNA, but can result when C base-paired with G undergoes a chemical reaction referred to as *deamination*. This changes the normal C : G base pair to a U : G pair. Because U pairs most frequently with A, an unrepaired U : G base pair results in a C : G-to-T : A mutation during the next round of DNA replication, and this mutation will be carried forward in all subsequent DNA copies. Therefore, to avoid creating this mutation, it is critically important to return the U back to the original C. BER accomplishes this by using specialized enzymes referred to as DNA glycosylases that recognize specific base pairs containing chemically modified bases and cutting the bond that holds the modified base to the DNA backbone [in this case, uracil DNA glycosylase (UDG)]. Remarkably, there are at least four different uracil DNA glycosylases in human cells, each of which removes U from mispairs in different DNA sequence contexts (Krokan et al., 2002), and recent evidence suggests that defects in some if not all of these enzymes results in an increased risk of cancer. Next come specialized enzymes that recognize the DNA structure left behind and cleave the DNA backbone at precisely the spot where the base has been

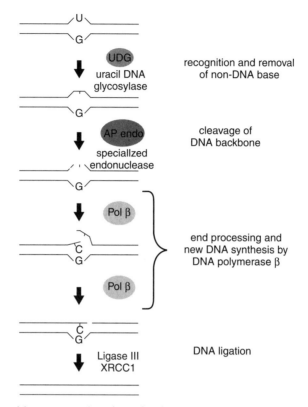

Figure 4. Base excision DNA repair pathway (BER). BER recognizes base pairs in DNA in which one of the bases has suffered some form of chemical modification that will lead to mutations in the subsequent round of DNA replication if not repaired.

removed. Then a special DNA repair polymerase, here DNA polymerase β, uses the undamaged base as a template to put the normal C back in. The last step involves resealing, or ligating, the DNA backbone using a DNA ligase. Figure 4 also shows a protein called Xrcc1, which serves as a scaffold of sorts by interacting with polymerase β and DNA ligase. Xrcc1 functions to coordinate the action of these other enzymes, and defects in Xrcc1 activity have been associated with increased risk of various cancers (Divine et al., 2001). The BER pathway is the main defender against DNA damage resulting from normal by-products of cellular metabolism, very frequently ROS (Mol et al., 1999; Hoeijmakers, 2001). A common example of this type of oxidative damage is 8-oxo-G, which can occur when reactive oxygen reacts with G bases in DNA. Unlike a normal G base, which will pair only with C during the next round of DNA replication, 8-oxo-G frequently pairs with A, thus generating a G : C-to-T : A mutation in the newly replicated DNA. Therefore, as for the U:G mispairs described above, it is critical that the BER pathway remove 8-oxo-G before the next round of DNA replication occurs. There are also several DNA glycosylase enzymes that recognize 8-oxo-G,

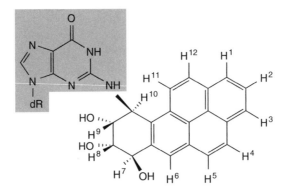

Figure 5. Benzo[a]pyrene dG structure. Benzo[a]pyrene is a potent environmental carcinogen commonly found in cigarettes and car exhaust. It will react with a G base in DNA to create a large, bulky chemical modification that disrupts the double-helical DNA structure. Left uncorrected, this lesion leads to mispairs in subsequent rounds of DNA replication. (From http://www.nyu.edu/its/pubs/connect/archives/98spring/broydedna.html.)

and defects in some, for example, the MutY homolog protein, correlate with an increased risk of colorectal cancer (Sampson et al., 2005).

The *NER pathway* serves to repair damaged DNA that has been chemically modified to the point where it is distorting the normal helical structure of the DNA duplex, and this structural distortion is key to the initial step in the pathway, recognition of DNA damage (De Silva et al., 2000; Hoeijmakers, 2001; Fuss and Cooper, 2006). Benzo[a]pyrene is a potent carcinogenic chemical found in cigarettes and car exhaust, and its chemical reaction with G bases in DNA creates a large, bulky modification (Figure 5) that is recognized by proteins in the NER pathway. Another commonly occurring mutation repaired by NER results from chemical cross-linking of neighboring T bases, which also distorts the local DNA structure. This is one of the most frequent chemical changes in DNA caused by exposure to sunlight (we will see below that defects in NER can give rise to conditions in which victims show an extreme sensitivity to sunlight). The overall process of NER can be divided into two distinct subpathways (Figure 6), global genome repair (GGR), which surveys all chromosomes for structurally distorting damage, and transcription-coupled repair (TCR), which is activated specifically in regions of DNA that are in the process of being decoded by RNA polymerase (remember that DNA codes for RNA, which in turn codes for a protein whose amino acid sequence derives from the DNA sequence). In the TCR pathway the stalled RNA polymerase is displaced from the DNA by the CSB and CSA proteins, whereas in the GGR pathway distorting damage is recognized by the XPC/hHR23B protein pair and/or the DDB1/DDB2 protein pair. From this initial recognition step, the pathways converge and there is a sequential recruitment of proteins to the site of damage, with each protein performing a specific function. TFIIH is a multiprotein complex containing XPB and XPD, each of which serves

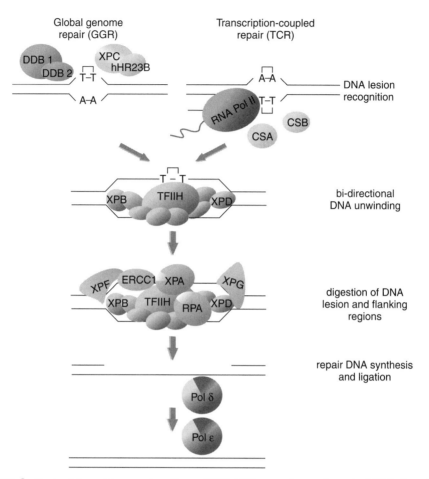

Figure 6. Nucleotide excision repair pathway (NER). NER recognizes and repairs DNA lesions that distort the overall structure of double-helical DNA. Two subpathways have been identified: global genome repair (GGR), which surveys the entire genome for such lesions, and transcription-coupled repair (TCR), which acts on DNA that is actively being decoded into RNA. (See insert for color representation.)

to unwind the DNA duplex in opposite directions, creating a bubble of about 25 to 30 base pairs. The XPG protein and XPF/ERCC1 protein pair are endonuclease enzymes that position themselves at opposite ends of the bubble and cut the DNA backbone. XPA and RPA serve to stabilize the bubble structure by binding to DNA and also help to position the endonucleases. Once the DNA strand containing the damage has been cut, this protein–DNA complex is released and the gap is filled in by DNA polymerases (e.g., Pol δ, Pol ε), thus restoring the original DNA sequence to the damaged area.

Many of the initials used to define specific proteins in these subpathways come from the names of diseases that result if that protein is defective. For example, defects in the function of various XP proteins result in the condition xeroderma pigmentosum (XP), a rare disease (1 in 250,000 in the United States) in which victims suffer an extreme sensitivity to sunlight and a very high incidence of skin cancer (xeroderma = mild, abnormal dryness and roughness of skin; pigmentosum pigmented areas of the skin). Defects in either CSA or CSB result in Cockayne syndrome (CS), which also causes sensitivity to sunlight but does not increase the risk of cancer. CS, however, unlike XP, results in severe mental retardation and premature aging (Hoeijmakers, 2001; Fuss and Cooper, 2006).

As noted above, the *MMR pathway* performs in conjunction with DNA polymerases as they work to make a complete duplicate of the DNA prior to cell division. Here we provide a brief description of some of the proteins involved in MMR and note that identification of mutations in MMR genes from colon cancer tumors was the first time that cancer had been linked to defects in any DNA repair pathway (Fishel et al., 1993; Fishel and Kolodner, 1995). As for BER and NER, the first step in the MMR pathway is specific recognition of the damage (Hoeijmakers, 2001; Jascur and Boland, 2006). The example in Figure 7 shows that the MSH2/MSH6 protein pair recognizes a mismatched G:T base pair. Different protein pairs in the MMR pathway can recognize DNA damage resulting from insertion or deletion of several bases on one strand, but for the sake of brevity

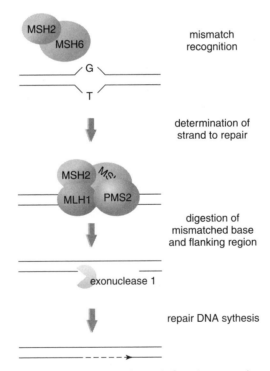

Figure 7. Mismatch repair pathway. Mismatch repair functions together with DNA polymerase to ensure high-fidelity copying of the genetic material, and can recognize mismatched base pairs in the genome independent of DNA polymerase.

we consider simple mismatches that occur when DNA polymerase makes one of its rare errors. Interestingly, once bound to DNA at the site of the mismatch, the structure of the MSH2/MSH6 pair changes to form a closed ring that can then slide along the DNA. It is likely that multiple MSH2/MSH6 pairs recognize the mismatch and undergo this structural change. The MSH2/MSH6 complexes recruit yet another protein pair, MLH1/PMS2, which assists in displacing the stalled DNA polymerase from the growing daughter strand as well as in recruiting an exonuclease that will remove all the DNA in that strand from the point where the mismatch proteins encounter the DNA polymerase back to the DNA mismatch itself, a distance that could be as much as 1000 bases. The final step is resynthesis of the missing stretch of DNA, which again restores the original DNA sequence.

In the early 1990s researchers followed genetic clues suggesting that defects in the MMR pathway may be linked to a specific cancer called *hereditary non-polyposis colorectal cancer* (HNPCC). Indeed, they discovered a clear association between mutations in the MSH2 gene that rendered its protein nonfunctional and the occurrence of HNPCC (Fishel et al., 1993). This was a dramatic verification of an idea that had been percolating for some time: that defects in a cell's ability to deal with commonly occurring mistakes made by DNA polymerases increased the overall mutation frequency to the point where critical regulatory genes controlling cell proliferation themselves suffered mutations, thereby significantly increasing the risk of getting cancer. At the present time, defects have been identified in each of these three DNA repair pathways (BER, NER, MMR) that correlate with increased risks in the occurrence of specific cancers (Table 1).

TABLE 1. Cancers Resulting from Defects in Repair Pathways

Repair Pathway	Gene(s)	Cancer Type	Disease
Base excision repair	MUTYH	Colorectal	
	XRCC1	Lung	
Nucleotide excision repair	XPC, XPE, XPF, XPV, XPA, XPG, XPD, XPB	Skin	Xeroderma pigmentosum
	CSA, CSB	None	Cockayne syndrome
Mismatch repair	MLH1, MSH2, 3, 6, PMS2, MSH6	Colorectal and others	Hereditary nonpolyposis colon cancer
	XRCC4	Breast	
Nonhomologous end joining	NBS1	B-cell non-Hodgkin's lymphoma	Nijmegen breakage syndrome
	LIG4	Breast	Lig 4 syndrome
Homologous recombination	BRCA1, BRCA2, CHEK2	Breast and ovarian	Familial breast cancer
	WRN	Multiple	Werner syndrome
DNA damage signaling	ATM	Multiple	Ataxia telangiectasia
	ATR	Breast, ovarian, and lung	Seckel syndrome

The final two DNA repair pathways, *NHEJ* and *HRR*, specialize in repairing a particularly devastating form of DNA damage, a *double-strand break* (DSB). DNA DSBs arise from a number of different insults that cells must contend with: for example, exposure to ionizing radiation, x-rays, free radicals resulting from certain chemical reactions (remember ROS, mentioned earlier), as well as during normal DNA replication across a single-stranded DNA break. In fact, the intentional creation of DNA DSBs is an important aspect of two critical events that take place in specific cell types: (1) the generation of antibodies by immune cells in response to invasion by a foreign substance, and (2) the segregation of chromosomes during meiotic division to produce gametes (i.e., sperm and egg cells). However, our focus here will be on the repair of unwanted DSBs, and how defects in specific components of these two pathways increase the risk of developing certain cancers.

The choice of whether to use the NHEJ or HRR pathway to repair a double-strand break depends largely on at what stage in its life cycle a cell finds itself in. During and immediately after the cell has copied its complete DNA content in preparation for the next division, it will typically use the HRR pathway. This is because duplicate copies of each chromosome lie immediately next to each other, and if one has suffered a double-strand break, the information in the undamaged partner (typically referred to as its *sister chromatid*, or more simply, *sister*) can be used to replace the missing information in the damaged chromosome (for this short period of time the cell actually carries four copies of all chromosomes). However, for most of a cell's life the chromosome pairs are not in close proximity, and the cell typically uses the NHEJ pathway under these circumstances.

Because double-strand breaks are such a severe form of DNA damage, cells have evolved sophisticated DNA damage-signaling systems that slow or stop the progression of cell growth in order that enough time is available for DSB repair to finish. Two important signaling molecules that work in the very early stages of the cell's recognizing the occurrence of DSBs are the ATM and ATR proteins. Defects in the ATM protein that inhibit its function cause the radiation-sensitive, cancer-prone disorder ataxia telangiectasia (AT), hence the derivation of the name ataxia telangiectasia mutated (ataxia = loss of coordination; telangiectasia enlargement of blood vessels, causing redness of the skin). Defects in the ATR protein (ataxia telangiectasia related) also result in a disorder that is prone to increased genome instability, referred to as Seckel syndrome. Both ATM and ATR belong to a family of enzymes referred to as protein kinases. Kinases are enzymes that chemically modify other proteins by attaching a phosphate group to specific amino acids, thus altering their activity in a manner that promotes the overall function required. Once ATM and ATR sense the presence of DNA breaks, their kinase function is activated, resulting in their phosphorylating numerous other proteins that serve to slow cell growth and activate the NHEJ and HRR pathways.

The NHEJ pathway gets its name *nonhomologous end joining* because it simply involves pasting the broken ends of DNA back together and does not require that the two chromosomes share any homology. However, because the broken ends always suffer some processing (e.g., deletion or addition of one or several bases), the sequence of the repaired DNA will not be the same as the original. Hence, NHEJ is referred to as an error-prone pathway. The Ku70/Ku80 protein pair has a very high affinity for binding to the ends of the DNA break, and this binding is the first step in NHEJ. Once on board, this complex assists in recruiting the DNA-PKcs protein. DNA-PKcs is the catalytic subunit of a DNA-dependent protein kinase. Although we do not currently know all the details of how the kinase activity of DNA-PKcs is used to promote NHEJ, it is clear that DNA-PKcs phosphorylates itself after the repair process is finished and this leads to disassembly of the Ku70/Ku80/DNA-PKcs complex. Prior to recruitment of the Xrcc4/ligaseIV protein pair that seals the break (designated X4 and IV in Figure 8), the DNA ends can be processed by a number of enzymes, which result in unwinding of the DNA duplex (Werner helicase) and either the removal of a number of bases (via the activity of the Werner and/or MRN complex endonuclease) or possible addition of bases by certain DNA polymerases (e.g., Pol μ). The MRN complex noted in Figure 8 consists of the Mre11, Rad50, and Nbs1 proteins, and this complex has many diverse roles in both the signaling events following detection of DNA damage as well as direct involvement in DNA repair. The Nbs1 protein (or nibrin) is named for the Nijmegen breakage syndrome, in which defective Nbs1 causes an AT-like disorder characterized by increased

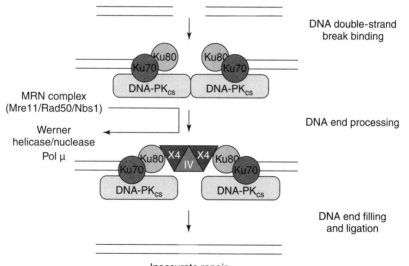

Figure 8. Nonhomologous end-joining pathway (NHEJ). NHEJ is one of two major pathways that specifically repair DNA molecules that have suffered a double-strand break. NHEJ is considered an error-prone pathway because the fragmented DNA ends are processed (bases are added or deleted) prior to re-sealing the ends. Therefore, the DNA sequence following repair is not the same as the original undamaged DNA (center piece in final product).

radiation sensitivity and an increased risk of cancer. Similar diseases result from defects in either the Xrcc4 or ligaseIV protein (Table 1).

As noted at the beginning of this chapter, human cells contain 46 chromosomes, and these reside in the cell's nucleus as 23 pairs. The two chromosomes in each pair carry essentially identical sets of information and thus are referred to as *homologs*. Repair of DNA damage by the HRR pathway involves the physical exchange (or recombination) of DNA sequences from an undamaged chromosome to replace the DNA sequences that have been removed from the damaged homolog: hence, the term *homologous recombinational repair*. Therefore, unlike NHEJ, which is an error-prone mechanism, HRR is considered to be an error-free mechanism. The first step in HRR involves removal of several hundred to thousands of bases from only one strand of the DNA at the site of the break (Figure 9), and currently it is thought that the MRN protein complex carries this out. Although there are many proteins involved in binding to this stretch of newly exposed single-stranded DNA, which play roles in either DNA damage signaling or repair of the break, we focus here on the BRCA2 and Rad51 proteins. Rad51 binds to the single-stranded DNA at the site of the break and uses this DNA sequence to find the complementary sequence in the undamaged homolog (Figure 9, catalysis of DNA crossover). This results in the formation of crossover structures that allow DNA polymerase to synthesize new DNA using the undamaged DNA as the template (as described in Figure 2). Hence, the missing information removed from the damaged chromosome is restored. In 1994, a defective form of the *BRCA2* gene was identified in a number of cases of early-onset breast cancer (Wooster et al., 1994, 1995), and later studies showed that a specific function of the Brca2 protein involved loading the Rad51 protein onto the single-stranded DNA at the site of a double-strand break. As a note, defects in a related gene, *BRCA1*, were identified around this same time in a number of cases of breast and ovarian cancers (Castilla et al., 1994). At the present time it is not known whether the Brca1 protein plays a specific role in the HRR pathway, but it clearly has complex roles in both DNA damage signaling and repair. Although the majority of breast cancers result from sporadic mutations occurring during the course of one's life, of the 200,000 new cases diagnosed in women in the United States each year, anywhere from a 5 to a 27% result from inherited mutations, the majority of which occur in either *BRCA1* or *BRCA2*. In fact, inheriting mutations in these genes results in a 40 to 85% lifetime risk of developing breast cancer. Thus, additional genetic defects relating to DNA repair have been shown to predispose individuals to higher incidences of cancer.

In summary, defects in all DNA repair pathways have been shown to contribute to various types of cancers (Table 1). While specific defects in the repair proteins themselves do not necessarily cause cancer, the fact that DNA damage will accumulate and persist as a result of these repair defects greatly increases the risk that mutations will occur in genes and their encoded proteins that are critical controls of cell proliferation. As an example, the retinoblastoma protein (Rb), discussed further in Chapter 3, is one such important component of cell growth

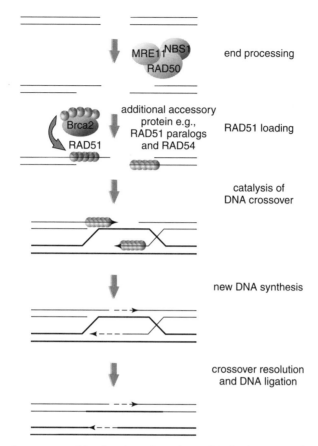

end processing

additional accessory
protein e.g.,
RAD51 paralogs
and RAD54

RAD51 loading

catalysis of
DNA crossover

new DNA synthesis

crossover resolution
and DNA ligation

Figure 9. Homologous recombinational repair pathway (HRR). The HRR pathway involves physical exchange of DNA between homologous chromosomes. If a double-strand break occurs in one
homolog or sister chromatid immediately following DNA replication, the HRR machinery will find
the equivalent sequence of DNA in the undamaged homolog and use it to restore the missing
information in the damaged chromosome.

control. Survival of an organism relies heavily on precise regulation of cell
division and proliferation. As a cell grows it proceeds through several defined
stages, and specific molecular events must occur and reach completion during
each stage before the next can begin. Together these growth stages are referred as
the cell cycle. Progression of the cell cycle depends on timely activation and
inhibition of Rb (first identified in a retinal tumor), which normally prevents a cell
from dividing (Giacinti and Giordano, 2006). If defects in DNA repair systems
result in Rb mutations that would otherwise be repaired successfully but now give
rise to a nonfunctional Rb protein, the cell cycle progresses in an unregulated
manner, resulting in uncontrolled cell growth with the concomitant appearance of
a tumor. This is one of many examples of the catastrophic consequences that can
result when the cellular DNA repair machinery is compromised.

CELL DEATH AND STEM CELL RENEWAL AS A
CANCER DEFENSE MECHANISM

In addition to the mechanisms of mutation avoidance and DNA repair described above, there are other specific strategies used by multicellular organisms that contribute to the defense against the development of cancer and protection of the genetic material. Although stem cell biology and the process of programmed cell death (apoptosis) are described in more detail in Chapter 6, we introduce both of these ideas here only to emphasize their roles in limiting the cancer potential of tissues and organs that suffer accumulated DNA damage through normal metabolic processes or exposure to external carcinogens.

From the moment that a new organism starts developing, there are systems in place to protect the integrity of the dividing cells and the genetic information they contain. During the earliest stages of development, the embryo contains an inner cell mass that includes *embryonic stem cells*, unspecialized cells that have the power of self-renewal without differentiating and also have the potential to proliferate and differentiate into any kind of tissue (Molofsky et al., 2004). As the development of the organism proceeds, a subset of stem cells that begin specific differentiation patterns on the way to forming distinct tissue types will remain in a tissue-committed but undifferentiated state. Termed *adult stem cells*, these can proliferate to replenish cells lost due to tissue-specific cell death. Upon division, these adult stem cells can generate two stem cells, two differentiating daughter cells, or one of each. The outcome will depend on the existing needs of the particular tissue or organ: that is, balance between maintenance of the tissue-specific stem cell population versus the need for tissue replenishment via terminal differentiation (Figure 10). Daughter cells, which upon further divisions produce different cell lineages, are called *progenitor cells*. They have some ability to renew themselves during proliferation, but their cell division potential is limited. This hierarchy is exemplified by the hematopoietic system, which generates all blood and lymph cell lines (Figure 11). All cells in this system arise from *hematopoietic stem cells* (HSCs), a small pool of adult stem cells that reside in the bone marrow (Reya et al., 2001). Upon cell division, each HSC will generate larger populations of additionally differentiated progenitor cells. These divide and differentiate further into mature cell lines that perform specific tasks (immune response, carrying oxygen to tissues, aid in blood clotting) but have no ability to divide further. A practical consequence of these different cell populations is observed when HSC or their descendants are transplanted into mice whose bone marrow has been destroyed by radiation: If the transplant consists of progenitor cells, hematopoiesis is restored for a few weeks before the transplanted cells die out; when hematopoietic stem cells are transplanted, the hematopoietic system is restored for the remaining lifetime of the animal.

In a grown living organism, most cells that make up tissues and organs are highly differentiated and have normally defined functions and short life spans. Mutations in their DNA will accumulate as a result of continued exposure to toxic

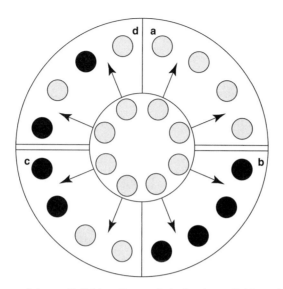

Figure 10. Outcomes of stem cell division. Stem cells (yellow) can divide and result exclusively in copies of themselves, thereby maintaining their original stem cell properties (sector a), a process referred to as self-renewal. Alternatively, their division can initiate a differentiation pathway that results in the formation of adult stem cells, progenitor cells, and/or terminally differentiated tissue-specific cells (blue; sector b). Because each stem cell division gives rise to two daughter cells, the division can proceed through the self-renewal and differentiation pathways, resulting in mixes of stem cells and differentiated cells (sectors c and d). (See insert for color representation.)

agents and physical insults, as well as multiple rounds of DNA replication and cell division. For example, epithelial cells in the colon live on average for 7 days before they undergo apoptosis, with the dead cells being sloughed off and removed from the body. Certain skin cells, having suffered exposure to environmental carcinogens, whether chemicals or sunlight, live for approximately 30 days before undergoing cell death and shedding. These cells are replaced using the tissue-specific adult stem cells described above. Thus, the body uses this system to replenish cells that have suffered DNA damage to the point where they could become cancerous (remember that XP victims exposed to sunlight will suffer from accumulated DNA damage, leading to skin cancer that would occur well before this 30-day time frame).

Two additional considerations are important to note regarding how stem cells avoid the accumulation of mutations. First, stem cells divide only occasionally, thereby avoiding the inevitable mutations resulting from errors made by DNA polymerase. Second, adult stem cell populations frequently reside in discrete, well-protected tissue compartments that are shielded from toxic agents (stem cell niches). However, the unique metabolic properties of stem cells create an intriguing dilemma regarding their relationship to the development of cancer. On the one hand, their features, described above, show how they contribute to cancer prevention. In contrast, it has become apparent in recent years that some types of cancer probably derive from stem cells. In these cases the cancerous cells

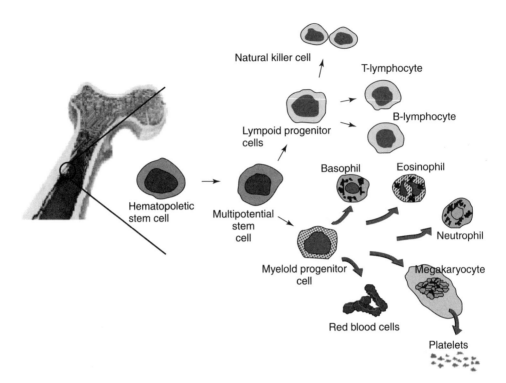

Figure 11. Hematopoietic and stromal stem cell differentiation. Differentiation of hematopoietic stem cells in the bone marrow gives rise to all forms of cells found in the blood. These include cells functioning in the immune response (natural killer cells, T-and B-lymphocytes, basophils, eosinophils, neutrophils), cells that carry oxygen from the lungs to all peripheral tissues (red bloods cells), and cells involved in clotting following tissue injury (platelets). (From http://stemcells.nih.gov/info/basics/basics4.asp.) (See insert for color representation.)

share many of the attributes of stem cells. Small populations of tumor-originating cells have been identified in cancers of the hematopoietic system [chronic myelogenous leukemia (CML); acute myelogenous leukemia (AML); acute lymphoblastic leukemia (ALL)], as well as in some breast and brain cancers. Because of their stem   cell–like properties, these cells have been named cancer stem cells (Reya et al., 2001; Pardal et al., 2003; Jordan et al., 2006). They may originate through mutations of normal stem cells or by transformation of progenitor or differentiated cells, which have acquired the potential for self-renewal and subsequent uncontrolled proliferation that is characteristic of tumor cells (Figure 12). Similar to normal stem cells that express higher drug resistance and greater antiapoptotic characteristics relative to differentiated cells, cancer stem cells are typically resistant to chemotherapy to an extent greater than are more differentiated cancer cells. This would explain the observation that treatments resulting in complete remission of some primary tumors rarely prevent metastasis (i.e., cancer stem cells avoid destruction by initial chemotherapy regimens only to proliferate and metastasize when treatment is stopped). Because

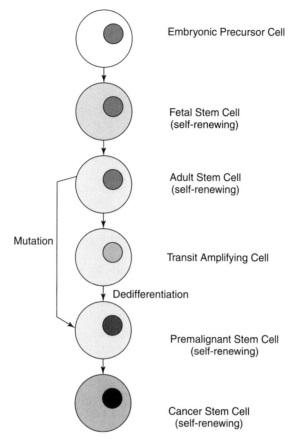

Figure 12. Mutations in normal stems cells can give rise to cancer stem cells. Fetal stem cells and normal adult stem cells derive from embryonic precursor stem cells. Further division of adult stem cells will result in self-renewal (more copies of the stem cells themselves) or will proceed down a pathway of differentiation, creating cells termed *transit amplifying cells* that will go on to maintain adult tissues. A premalignant stem cell can arise by mutation of an adult stem cell, or a change in a transit amplifying cell that leads to dedifferentiation and the acquisition of self-renewal properties. These can give rise to aggressively proliferating cancer stem cells that self-renew unabated by normal control signals. (See insert for color representation.)

the signaling pathways associated with malignancy also appear to regulate stem cell self-renewal, research on therapeutic strategies targeting cancer stem cells exclusively have become a matter of utmost importance.

REFERENCES

Baker TA, Bell SP. 1998. Polymerases and the replisome: machines within machines. *Cell* 92:295–305.

Castilla LH, Couch FJ, Erdos MR, Hoskins KF, Calzone K, Garber JE, Boyd J, Lubin MB, Deshano ML, Brody LC, et al. 1994. Mutations in the *BRCA1* gene in families with early-onset breast and ovarian cancer. *Nat Genet* 8:387–391.

De Silva IU, McHugh PJ, Clingen PH, Hartley JA. 2000. Defining the roles of nucleotide excision repair and recombination in the repair of DNA interstrand cross-links in mammalian cells. *Mol Cell Biol* 20:7980–7990.

Divine KK, Gilliland FD, Crowell RE, Stidley CA, Bocklage TJ, Cook DL, Belinsky SA. 2001. The *XRCC1 399* glutamine allele is a risk factor for adenocarcinoma of the lung. *Mutat Res* 461:273–278.

Fishel R, Kolodner RD. 1995. Identification of mismatch repair genes and their role in the development of cancer. *Curr Opin Genet Dev* 5:382–395.

Fishel R, Lescoe MK, Rao MR, Copeland NG, Jenkins NA, Garber J, Kane M, Kolodner R. 1993. The human mutator gene homolog *MSH2* and its association with hereditary nonpolyposis colon cancer. *Cell* 75:1027–1038.

Fuss JO, Cooper PK. 2006. DNA repair: dynamic defenders against cancer and aging. *PLoS Biol* 4: e203.

Giacinti C, Giordano A. 2006. RB and cell cycle progression. *Oncogene* 25:5220–5227.

Goodman MF. 2002. Error-prone repair DNA polymerases in prokaryotes and eukaryotes. *Annu Rev Biochem* 71:17–50.

Hoeijmakers JH. 2001. Genome maintenance mechanisms for preventing cancer. *Nature* 411:366–374.

Jascur T, Boland CR. 2006. Structure and function of the components of the human DNA mismatch repair system. *Int J Cancer* 119:2030–2035.

Jordan CT, Guzman ML, Noble M. 2006. Cancer stem cells. *N Engl J Med* 355:1253–1261.

Krokan HE, Drablos F, Slupphaug G. 2002. Uracil in DNA: occurrence, consequences and repair. *Oncogene* 21:8935–8948.

Mol CD, Parikh SS, Putnam CD, Lo TP, Tainer JA. 1999. DNA repair mechanisms for the recognition and removal of damaged DNA bases. *Annu Rev Biophys Biomol Struct* 28:101–128.

Molofsky AV, Pardal R, Morrison SJ. 2004. Diverse mechanisms regulate stem cell self-renewal. *Curr Opin Cell Biol* 16:700–707.

Pardal R, Clarke MF, Morrison SJ. 2003. Applying the principles of stem-cell biology to cancer. *Nat Rev Cancer* 3:895–902.

Reya T, Morrison SJ, Clarke MF, Weissman IL. 2001. Stem cells, cancer, and cancer stem cells. *Nature* 414:105–111.

Sampson JR, Jones S, Dolwani S, Cheadle JP. 2005. *MutYH* (MYH) and colorectal cancer. *Biochem Soc Trans* 33:679–683.

Wooster R, Neuhausen SL, Mangion J, Quirk Y, Ford D, Collins N, Nguyen K, Seal S, Tran T, Averill D, et al., 1994. Localization of a breast cancer susceptibility gene, *BRCA2*, to chromosome 13q12–13. *Science* 265:2088–2090.

Wooster R, Bignell G, Lancaster J, Swift S, Seal S, Mangion J, Collins N, Gregory S, Gumbs C, Micklem G. 1995. Identification of the breast cancer susceptibility gene *BRCA2*. *Nature*, 378:789–792.

IV

CANCER DIAGNOSIS AND TREATMENT

8

CANCER DETECTION AND BIOMARKERS

Arthur B. Pardee

*Harvard Medical School, Dana-Farber Cancer Institute,
Boston, Massachusetts*

Peng Liang

*Vanderbilt-Ingram Cancer Center, Vanderbilt University,
Nashville, Tennessee*

EARLY DETECTION

Cancer treatment can become ineffective as the disease progresses and it has a greater chance of success if applied early (Suzuki et al., 2006). Cancers progress, going from bad to worse. Mutations increase repeatedly, produced from errors that are made during duplication of the genetic material [deoxyribonucleic acid (DNA)] and from damage caused by chemicals or radiation. As a result, the many cells in a tumor develop very different properties. Their multiplication and ability to spread through the patient's body (metastasize) become increasingly uncontrolled. Metastasis is the major cause of cancer death. It makes surgery ineffective. Other mutations change the targets of therapeutic drugs, and resistance appears to drugs that initially were effective (Sorlie et al., 2003). These changes make killing all the cancer's cells very difficult.

The Biology and Treatment of Cancer: Understanding Cancer
Edited by Arthur B. Pardee and Gary S. Stein   Copyright © 2009 John Wiley & Sons, Inc.

Most cancers are diagnosed when they have advanced. A symptom or change is noticed, such as pain, an unusual lump, bleeding (such as blood in the feces), or changes in bowel behavior that raise the suspicion of colon cancer. A skin mole that grows or changes color may signal melanoma. But even if one reports these warning signs to a physician immediately, the tumor may already be a clump of 100 million cells or more and too advanced to be treated successfully.

Earliest possible detection of the disease should improve the chance of successful therapy. Early detection has saved many people's lives. The Papanicolaou (Pap) smear test identifies early cervical cancer by distinguishing differently stained cancerous cells that form abnormal tissue architecture. Unfortunately, this test often gives incorrectly positive results. Novel inexpensive techniques that are equivalent to the Pap smear have been developed.

Breast cancer is tested by frequent physical mammary examinations. Mammography for premenopausal women and ultrasound examinations for postmenopausal women are the most effective methods for breast cancer detection, and indeed mammography is the only screening test shown by clinical trials to reduce death by 30% (Houssami et al., 2006). Mammograms, colonoscopies, and so on, can be of high value in practice. But a more reliable screening method is needed because mammography produces false positive results. Newer techniques include examination of fluid collected from the several independent ducts of the breast, where cancers can begin. Ultrasound imaging or biopsy sampling with a needle can help make a more informed decision about whether to have surgery.

Prostate cancer is tested for by determining prostate-specific antigen (PSA) in the blood (Constantinou and Feneley, 2006). This protein can increase 5 to 10 years before clinical symptoms appear, and an average of 17 years before death. But this test is not an accurate indicator that cancer is present because PSA is also elevated by an enlarged noncancerous prostate, and so can give a false positive result. Increases in PSA during a period of "watchful waiting" may indicate that treatment is advisable, because it indicates tumor progression. Elevated PSA can be followed by biopsy sampling of the prostate.

Other cancers are found less effectively. Colon cancers may be seen by colonoscopic examination and by looking for blood in fecal samples. Neither test is very sensitive, and only three-fourths of advanced colon cancer patients were positive for both of them. Lung, colon, ovarian, and pancreatic cancers do not show early symptoms and so are often discovered at an advanced stage, when they are very difficult to treat successfully.

X-ray photography shows advanced tumors, but it is not sensitive enough to reveal early cancers. Imaging methods with x-rays are being developed to allow tumor localization and identification of enzymes that influence their properties (Weissleder, 2006). Spiral computerized tomographic (CT) screening is a more sensitive method, and another is positron emission tomography (PET). New computerized systems are used to examine results of mammography, but it is not yet clear that they improve detection, and false alarms and biopsies are increased. Ovarian cancer may be treated effectively only in stage I, but very unfortunately is usually found at an advanced stage. Its screening with high sensitivity by mass spectroscopy reveals patterns from proteins or of protein fragments. The methods are being improved to decrease their error rates and to simplify their application. Currently recommended guidelines for cancer surveillance techniques are available at websites such as the American Cancer Society or NCCN.

DETECTION WITH BIOMARKERS

For the reasons just discussed, we are actively searching for much earlier abnormalities, such as biomarker molecules that are released from tumor cells into the blood, where they can be identified. Molecules that differ between cancer and normal tissues are being discovered by several techniques (Chanin, 2004; Dalton and Friend, 2006). There are three main classes of biomarker molecules: the modified DNA sequences, proteins for which they code, and messenger ribonucleic acids (mRNAs) which are the intermediates between DNA and protein (Chatterjee and Zetter, 2005).

DNA

Markers can be revealed by determining changed sequences of DNA bases in cancer cells (Sjoblom et al., 2006). Mutated DNAs are found in genes that cause hereditary cancers, and these are valuable for early detection in persons with a family history of frequent cancer. Examples are the mutated p53 gene responsible for the Li–Fraumeni cancer syndrome, and the *BRCA1* and *BRCA2* genes, which are mutated in 15% of breast cancers. Another is hereditary retinoblastoma, caused by a mutated gene in one of the two chromosomes. Its nonhereditary mutation in the second gene of a cell produces cancer. Appearance in the patient's blood of cells with retinoblastoma mutations show the disease's appearance. Some African-Americans have inherited a DNA sequence that makes them likely to have prostate cancer.

Attachment of methyl groups to DNA changes gene expressions and can lead to cancer. These were found to provide biomarkers in lung cancer patients' sputum up to three years before clinical diagnosis of high-risk individuals who are smokers and/or had been exposed to radon, and also in prostate cancer patients. Methylation is in addition to DNA base changes.

Messenger RNA

mRNA molecules are copied from DNA into the closely related ribonucleic acid. They are working blueprints of the 15% or so of the cell's genes that are being used. They provide excellent molecular markers because many of them differ between normal tissue and cancers. And they can be measured very sensitively because their amounts can be increased greatly by a repetitive reaction named *reverse transcriptase–polymerase chain reaction* (RT-PCR). A technique for their specific recognition is named *microarrays*. Tens of thousands of short known base sequences are attached at specific locations on a solid surface. mRNAs isolated from cells are revealed by their binding at these locations. The patterns produced from normal tissues differs from those from major cancers, including leukemia, lymphoma, and adenocarcinoma of lung, breast, and prostate. This technique might change the way in which cancer is diagnosed, classified, and treated in the clinic, although it requires refinements in reliability.

Differential display (DD) is an alternative method to identify differentially expressed mRNAs. It is used widely to study differential gene expression between normal and cancerous cells, and many changes have been identified with it (Liang et al., 2007). One that is produced from the *ras* oncogene was shown to encode secreted protein IL-24, which is being investigated as a potential cancer diagnostic marker in blood. A systematic search revealed 13 candidate mRNA markers in blood samples from the vast majority of breast cancer patients (Martin et al., 2001). DD integrates two of the most powerful and commonly used molecular biological methods to amplify random sets of mRNAs and then separate the products. The high sensitivity of DD is valuable because little cancer material may be available, sometimes only a few cells.

Proteins

Protein biomarkers can be discovered by a variety of sensitive methods. One is binding of specific antibodies to them, which can be shown with color or radioactive labeling or a size change. These immunological tests give somewhat variable results that depend in part on the concentration of antibody used. Protein biomarkers can be discovered by combining immunology with mass spectrometry. *Proteomics*, a microarray technology, is another method for determining the multiple proteins in a biological specimen (Posadas et al., 2005). Proteomic signatures of numerous differences of sets of markers are seen, and these can distinguish early- versus late-stage disease. Proteins that are involved in cell proliferation indicate metastases of prostate cancers. New studies that propose detection of cancer by applying proteomics to serum specimens are promising but need confirmation.

SAMPLING

A small surgically removed sample of a cancer, a *biopsy*, can be used to detect molecular abnormalities. Lymph nodes can be biopsied for biomarkers of metastases. A problem arises as to the choice of locations for biopsy sampling in a nonuniform cancer. As examples, disseminated tumor cells were frequently identified by the presence of mRNA for the structural protein cytokeratin 20 in lymph nodes and less often in bone marrow, but not by conventional pathology after surgery for early colorectal cancer. A signature composed of multiple selected mRNAs from the bone marrow of untreated breast cancer patients indicated a 3.5-fold greater risk of death. The risk was 2.9-fold greater as estimated immunochemically by specific binding of an antibody to the target protein.

Microarrays from uterine tissue predict metastasis to lymph nodes. As several examples, markers that include collagen XXIII and thymosine b15 proteins are being developed clinically. Several markers detected by immunological protein microarrays predict distant spreading of early-stage breast cancer in young women. CA125 is an early ovarian cancer marker. Early cervical cancer has been detected immunologically from overexpression of the negative regulatory p16^{INK4A} protein. α-Fetoprotein is used widely in the detection of liver (hepatocellular) carcinoma caused by hepatitis virus, the second most common cause of death in Southeast Asia.

Bodily fluids, especially blood and urine, can contain biomarkers for cancer. Some are located in escaped tumor cells. Others, such as PSA, are soluble molecules. Biomarkers for early detection of lung cancer are being sought in serum, sputum, and exhaled breath. Peripheral blood of colon cancer patients contains tumor-related mRNAs, which might provide an analysis to replace colonoscopy. Proteins unique to bladder cancer patients are found in blood or urine samples (van Gils et al., 2005). Mutated mRNA of PSA has been found in prostate cancer cells from the blood of prostate patients, as well as PSA protein. The *PTEN* and *BRCA1* genes and chromosome region 7q22–23 are commonly altered in higher-grade prostate cancer patients' blood, and correlated with early death. The cells usually come from only one of the many tumors that have developed, and these can be small (0.2 cm^3), indicating that primary tumor cells frequently escape into blood after they have lost *PTEN*.

Many tumor-related proteins have been identified in serum from patients with a variety of cancers. As examples, antigens are found in the blood of breast cancer patients, of which the most common are protein CA 15-3 and carcinoembryonic antigen (CEA), used to monitor therapy of patients with advanced breast cancer. Numerous other markers, including oncofetal antigens, glycoprotein antigens, enzymes and isozymes, genes, and cytokines, are also promising. The fecal blood test for detection of colon cancer has limited sensitivity, and DNA markers were identified in feces and blood samples from patients. Genomic approaches are being taken to cancers of blood cells. Advantages of noninvasive sampling include safety, convenience, low bias of sampling, and lower cost.

PROBLEMS OF EARLY DETECTION

Although biomarkers could permit early detection of cancers, they would not necessarily show that there is immediate danger. Pancreatic cancer remains a very lethal disease because current screening methods are unable to detect it while still localized and treatable by surgery. Many small cancers remain microscopic and do not progress. This is because they do not produce the new blood vessels (angiogenesis) required for their growth. Special biomarkers for these micro-metastases have been identified in tissues, blood, and urine (Naumov et al., 2006). They do not pose a threat to life, so their treatment is questioned.

Lung cancer is usually metastatic before it is found and only a few percent of patients survive for a few years; and the surgery can be lethal. The value of early detection is questionable. In one trial, CT scans showed it in 1 of 60 randomly selected individuals, 80% of whom survived for 10 years after immediate treatment. But another recent study reported that lives were not saved by detecting lung cancers with CT scans; the same fraction of people died in a control group as in the group who had CT scans (Bach et al., 2007). An explanation for these different conclusions is that CT scans reveal many early cancers that are not lethal. Many lives could be saved with more powerful techniques that focus on early abnormal events in lung cells that, for example, have been shown to precede cancer—amplified or missing genes. Designer drugs could potentially target these abnormalities.

So the decision as to whether or not to use therapy is important because risk from surgery or chemotherapy might outweigh possible benefits. Techniques that have the sensitivity to reveal early cancer must also be capable of identifying whether or not they will progress to malignancy. We need biomarkers that distinguish lethal from less dangerous early cancer. These could include mutations of the *p53* gene that is central to killing cancer cells, indicators of shorter survival, and indicators of resistance to chemotherapy. Prognostic factors for failure in early-stage breast cancer in young women included the progesterone receptor and protein Ki- 67, as well as tumor stage and lymph node status. Patients whose cyclin E protein in advanced breast cancers has changed were no longer responsive to any chemotherapy. Proteins such as phosphorylated Akt kinase and CXCR4 appeared in metastatic cancers and could indicate that the cancer probably has spread and therefore that surgery is less likely to be curative.

TECHNICAL PROBLEMS

Biomarkers could be applied today (Bild et al., 2006). Routine cancer detection tests should be possible during periodic checkups if they are noninvasive and use sets of established biomarkers. Perhaps 1000 commercial genetic tests are being developed for medical problems, including cancer. Although some of these are promising, their reliability has not been determined, nor are they yet closely legally regulated (Ransohoff, 2005). Furthermore, effective treatment methods are necessary if early detection can improve survival.

But realizing the potential of biomarkers is a challenge. Several problems need to be overcome. Research is necessary to determine whether cancer can be found sufficiently early to improve treatment. An earlier detection method's usefulness will depend on whether subsequent treatments are effective. The decision as to whether to proceed with therapy is a question of benefit versus risk. As discussed above, a tumor that is detected might not be lethal, so additional biomarkers would be valuable that identify cancers with higher risk of further growth and metastasis. Techniques must be standardized and optimized. Sensitivity should be improved. Although noninvasive tests recently showed the K-*ras* oncogene DNA to be present in eight of nine cases of both benign and malignant colon cancer patients, the majority of cancers found by colonoscopy were not revealed.

A difficulty is that a multitude of random changes are present in advanced cancers. There are far more mutations of random genes than of the genes that contribute to cancer (Sjoblom et al., 2006). These conceal the few biomarkers that frequently distinguish cancer from normal cells. A single marker is therefore not often applied clinically. Sets of the markers that are usually altered are needed. Cancer signatures have been identified as sets of mRNAs selected from small blood samples taken from breast or colon cancer patients. Such an entire group of markers can be examined by an array technique (Martin et al., 2001). Signatures have been found composed of 76 mRNAs from stored frozen specimens of early lymph node negative cancers (Foekens et al., 2006). A problem is to find these rare common biomarkers. Pooling multiple tumor samples dilutes infrequent markers, whereas it can retain strong signals for markers that are present in most of the samples. A rapid high-throughput screening method has been developed for finding mutations in the oncogenes of many cancers.

FURTHER APPLICATIONS OF BIOMARKERS

Prevention Trials

Cancer prevention trials can reach a clinical endpoint only after a very long time, and their results can then be inconclusive. Five different trials of breast cancer prevention with raloxifene or tamoxifen versus placebo produced mixed clinical results, probably because of heterogeneity of the patients' tumors. The biomarkers designed for earlier detection should permit results to be seen earlier.

Therapy Decisions

Cancers are not produced by changes of the same genes, and their responses to therapies are different. Breast cancers have different clinical properties. The receptor protein for estrogen stimulates excessively the growth of 70% of breast cancers whose estrogen receptor is elevated (ER+). Tamoxifen is an antagonist of estrogen that specifically acts against these cancers. Most other breast cancers have many copies of HER2, receptor for a human epidermal growth factor protein present in blood, and these express a different set of markers. These patients may benefit from a different treatment, with an antibody named herceptin. The choices of therapy can be more complex, for invasive breast cancers can have different clinical properties and show five different main patterns of proteins, as identified by immunochemistry. Selected markers that show the presence or absence of response could predict an individual cancer patient's response to treatments. For example, prostate cancer might respond initially to an antiandrogen therapy to which a more advanced cancer would fail to respond. Many prostate cancers require androgen for growth and can be treated with drugs that decrease or inhibit androgen, but others are hormone independent and therefore require chemotherapies.

Individualizing Therapy

The goal is to provide each patient with a specific most effective treatment rather than applying a one-fits-all general therapy. A personalized therapy could be guided by determining selected biomarker expressions in that patient. Prediction of what drugs could be effective against an individual patient's cancer are being developed from biomarkers that identify oncogenic pathways in subtypes of responding tumors (Bild et al., 2006). A set of biomarkers may be helpful in addition to the criteria of cancer stage and grade now used, especially for intermediate-grade (stage II) cancers. An initial aim could be to predict whether or not to apply chemotherapy following surgery. In one study, patients who did not have metastasis to lymph nodes were divided into positive versus negative groups as determined by expression of 70 genes in the tumors that had been removed. Twenty-three percent of those with a positive pattern had recurrence within five years versus only 5% of the negatives.

Surveillance of Patients

Other uses could come from following changes in biomarkers after treatment. The results could be estimated before the clinical reappearance of cancer by measuring biomarker patterns, which should change back toward normal if a treatment was effective. The protein fibrinogen reverted to normal after surgery; mRNA for the protease inhibitor maspin reappeared in the blood after chemotherapy.

Conversely, detection of any cancer-related gene or gene product, such as an mRNA or protein in the patient's blood, would indicate progression of disease and recurrence (Baker, 2004). Proteins CA 15-3 and carcinoembryonic antigen are used to monitor the therapy of patients with advanced breast cancer. The time before clinical recurrence is detected can vary from two to nine months, and breast cancer recurrence has been found by looking in bone marrow and lymph nodes for an antibody specific to cytokeratin. Reappearance of biomarkers could give an earlier indication of recurrence. Patients with long versus short times to recurrence and survival have been identified with microarrays of sets of mRNAs from the original breast tumors. Many practical problems will have to be addressed, however, before selective and sensitive genomic tests can be applied clinically. Use of such markers will require a database connecting profiles with the results of clinical treatment. A first genetic test to predict risk of relapse of breast cancer (MammaPrint) has been approved by the U.S. Food and Drug Administration. Ideas similar to those presented here have recently been published (Mol et al., 2007).

REFERENCES

Bach PB, Jett JR, Pastorino U, et al. 2007. Computed tomography screening and lung cancer outcomes. JAMA 297:953–961.

Baker SG, Kramer BS, Prorok PC. 2004. Development tracks for cancer prevention markers. *Dis Markers*. 20:97–102.

Bild AH, Yao G, Chang JT, et al. 2006. Oncogenic pathway signatures in human cancers as a guide to targeted therapies. *Nature* 439:353–357.

Chanin TD, Merrick DT, Franklin WA, et al. 2004. Recent developments in biomarkers for the early detection of lung cancer: perspectives based on publications 2003 to present. *Curr Opin Pulm Med* 10:242–247.

Chatterjee SK, Zetter BR. 2005. Cancer biomarkers: knowing the present and predicting the future. *Future Oncol* 1:37–50.

Constantinou J, Feneley MR. 2006. PSA testing: an evolving relationship with prostate cancer. *Prostate Cancer Prostatic Dis* 9:6–13.

Dalton WS, Friend SH. 2006. Cancer biomarkers: an invitation to the table. *Science* 312:1165–1168.

Foekens JA, Atkins D, Zhang Y, et al. 2006. Multicenter validation of a gene expression–based prognostic signature in lymph node–negative primary breast cancer. *J Clin Oncol* 24:1665–1671.

Houssami N, Cuzick J, Dixon JM. 2006. The prevention, detection, and management of breast cancer. *Med J Aust* 184:230–234.

Liang P, Meade JD, Pardee AB. 2007. A protocol for differential display of mRNA expression using either fluorescent or radioactive labeling. *Nat Protocols* 2:457–470.

Martin KJ, Graner E, Li Y, et al. 2001. High-sensitivity array analysis of gene expression for the early detection of disseminated breast tumor cells in peripheral blood. *Proc Natl Acad Sci USA* 98:2646–2651.

Mol AJ, Geldorf AA, Meijer GA, Van der Poel HG, van Moorselaar RJ. 2007. New experimental markers for early detection of high-risk prostate cancer: role of cell–cell adhesion and cell migration. *J Cancer Res Clin Oncol.* Epub.

Naumov GN, Akselen LA, Folkman J. 2006. Role of angiogenesis in human tumor dormancy: animal models for the angiogenic switch. *Cell Cycle* 5:1779–1787.

Posadas EM, Simpkins F, Liotta LA, et al. 2005. Proteomic analysis for the early detection and rational treatment of cancer—realistic hope? *Ann Oncol* 16:16–22.

Ransohoff DF. 2005. Bias as a threat to the validity of cancer molecular-marker research. *Nat Rev Cancer* 5:142–149.

Sjoblom T, Jones S, Wood LD, et al. 2006. The consensus coding sequences of human breast and colorectal cancers. *Science* 314:268–274.

Sorlie T, Tibshirani R, Parker J, et al. 2003. Repeated observation of breast tumor subtypes in independent gene expression data sets. *Proc Natl Acad Sci USA* 100:8418–8423.

Suzuki T, Toi M, Saji S, et al. 2006. Early breast cancer. *Int J Clin Oncol* 11:108–119.

van Gils MP, Stenman UH, Schalken JA, et al. 2005. Innovations in serum and urine markers in prostate cancer current European research in the P-Mark project. *Eur Urol* 48:1031–1041.

Weissleder R. 2006. Molecular imaging in cancer. *Science* 312:1168–1171.

9

CLINICAL CHALLENGES FOR TREATMENT AND A CURE

Eleni Efstathiou and Christopher J. Logothetis

*Department of Genitourinary Medical Oncology,
M.D. Anderson Cancer Center, University of Texas, Houston, Texas*

INTRODUCTION

Cancer replaced cardiovascular disease as the leading cause of deaths in the United States in 2005, a shift that had been forecast in the past few years by the National Cancer Institute (NCI) and the Centers for Disease Control and Prevention. While age-adjusted death rates for cardiovascular disease have been slashed by an extraordinary 60% during the last half-century, the war on cancer declared 35 years ago with the signing of the National Cancer Act in 1971 is definitely not won. Admittedly, testicular cancer, Hodgkin's disease, some leukemias, carcinomas of the thyroid, and most childhood cancers currently have impressive cure rates, these account for only a small fraction of malignancies. These success stories, together with the introduction of revolutionary targeted therapeutics such as Gleevec, Herceptin, Iressa, Erbitux, Avastin, and others, have ignited much needed enthusiasm, yet these cannot account fully for the impressive financial and scientific resources recruited over the years. More important, we have no therapy other than palliation to offer those diagnosed with metastatic disease, and even in

The Biology and Treatment of Cancer: Understanding Cancer
Edited by Arthur B. Pardee and Gary S. Stein   Copyright © 2009 John Wiley & Sons, Inc.

locally advanced disease we are still striving for some degree of certainty. And all this is still offered at the cost of considerable toxicity.

In this chapter we review the various therapeutic modalities used currently and strategies applied to improve efficacy, some of the challenges met in the process of testing a new drug in the clinic, and the pharmacogenomic approach and particular difficulties in the treatment of metastatic disease.

THERAPEUTIC MODALITIES

The standard treatment modalities for patients with cancer include surgery, radiotherapy, and chemotherapy. Radiotherapy and chemotherapy are cytotoxic therapies; they kill tumor cells by affecting deoxyribonucleic acid (DNA) synthesis directly or by damaging microtubules. Their mechanism of action implies that they do not have any selective destructive effect against cancer cells. They destroy all rapidly dividing cells, including normally dividing cells in vital tissues such as hematologic precursors, gonads, hair follicles, and the lining epithelium of the gastrointestinal tract and mouth. Other toxicities may also be a result of organ-specific toxicity (e.g., the cardiotoxicity of anthracyclines or mediastinal radiotherapy). With regard to clinical efficacy, there are at least two other limitations of cytotoxic therapies besides those related to dosing. First, many tumors have moderate or little chemo- or radiosensitivity. This may be inherent or acquired (e.g., as a result of the hypoxia that is common in larger tumors, especially in their center). Second, cancer cells tend to develop drug resistance rapidly during treatment. Cytotoxic agents have been supplemented by hormonal agents, while in recent years the focus of anticancer drug development has shifted dramatically to targeted agents that modulate proteins such as kinases, whose activities are more specifically associated with cancerous cells. However, conventional cytotoxic agents remain the mainstay of medical treatment. The challenge still faced with this cytotoxic approach is how to minimize toxicity and maximize anticancer activity. Improvement in clinical efficacy includes overcoming therapy resistance and inhibiting regrowth of cancer as a result of the limitations incurred to treatment duration in order to avoid lethal toxicity.

Strategies to overcome drug resistance and inhibit tumor repopulation must be relatively specific for tumor cells, compared with their effects on normal tissues, to improve therapeutic outcome without increasing toxicity. Monoclonal antibodies and small-molecule compounds currently introduced in the clinic are promising tools for target cancer therapy. Promising strategies also include those that modify the dose schedule of treatment (e.g., accelerated radiotherapy and dose-dense chemotherapy) and introduction of therapeutic combinations based on a biologically relevant rationale.

CHEMOTHERAPY

The use of drugs to cure or control cancer is relatively new compared to the use of surgery and radiation. During studies performed for the possible military use of nitrogen mustard gas in 1942, people exposed to the agent were found to have low white cell counts. This finding was associated with a potential for lowering high white blood cell counts in patients with leukemia. The first patient to receive it had a response, even though brief. This experiment initiated the era of cancer treatment with chemotherapeutic agents.

While single-agent chemotherapy is sometimes employed, the combination of two or more agents has clearly achieved a therapeutic advantage and expanded the use of chemotherapy. The use of drug combinations to circumvent tumor resistance is a well-established principle of therapy. Malignant cells are not of uniform composition within a given tumor. Since different classes of chemotherapy affect the cells differently, combination chemotherapy has a greater chance of destroying a larger number of cancer cells. With few exceptions, effective drug treatments for cancer are due to combining agents of known activity, with different mechanisms of resistance and minimally overlapping spectra of toxicity, at their optimal doses and according to schedules that are compatible with normal cell recovery.

As already mentioned, chemotherapy comes at a toxicity cost that may range from mild to lethal. Conventional cytotoxic therapy chiefly affects proliferating cells such as those in the bone marrow, gastrointestinal tract, gonads, and hair follicles. Therefore, the prevalent side effects of chemotherapy include myelosuppression, nausea, vomiting, mucositis, infertility, and alopecia. The introduction of growth factors that accelerate the regeneration of blood cells and antiemetics has allowed the use of higher and more frequent than initially sustained doses of chemotherapy and has partially helped relieve some side effects, thus improving quality of life.

The effectiveness of chemotherapy is limited by primary and acquired resistance to the drug administered, and possibly by tumor cell repopulation during therapy intervals mandated to avert lethal toxicity. Cancer cells acquire resistance to chemotherapy by a range of mechanisms, including the mutation or overexpression of the drug target, inactivation of the drug, or elimination of the drug from the cell.

Intervals between courses of chemotherapy are required for the repopulation of blood by white cells and platelets produced in the bone marrow before the next treatment cycle. This is necessary to minimize the chance of infection or bleeding. Adequate repopulation proliferating of hematological precursor cells in the bone marrow takes about 3 weeks. As mentioned, the introduction in the clinic of growth factors that accelerate this process, such as granulocyte-colony stimulating factor (G-CSF, also known as filgrastrim), has enabled faster repopulation of the bone marrow. Thus, courses of chemotherapy can be given safely at 2-week instead of 3-week intervals. Randomized clinical trials for which 2-week schedules with growth factors were compared with standard 3- or 4-week schedules have shown improved survival when used as adjuvant treatment for breast cancer and for treatment of non-Hodgkin's lymphoma, as well as possibly advanced bladder cancer, without an increase in normal tissue toxicity compared with conventional schedules.

High-dose chemotherapy with autologous stem cell support has been another attempt to circumvent bone marrow toxicity and thus deliver higher doses of chemotherapy. In this case, patient's stem cells are removed and stored prior to chemotherapy and reintroduced after it. Thus, they are not exposed to the toxic effects of chemotherapy and they soon reestablish themselves in the blood marrow and restore the body's ability to produce blood cells. The benefits of this highly toxic approach across the spectrum of malignancies are still debatable, even though it has become important for the consolidation of treatment in some advanced disease states, such as multiple myeloma or high-risk advanced testicular cancer, after successful initial treatment. Successful use of available drugs depends on the ability to design clinical trials to assess optimally the activity of the combination in the most appropriate patient population.

RADIOTHERAPY

Radiotherapy originates from two nineteenth-century scientific discoveries: the discovery of x-rays by Röentgen in 1895 and then of radioactivity by Becquerel in 1896. Over the years, treatment and treatment units have evolved to allow for efficient delivery of radiation. Radiotherapy offers a realistic possibility of improving local control of disease, although it is ineffective in controlling metastatic disease.

Traditionally, radiotherapy used to treat cancer is administered in small doses [1.8 to 2.0 gray (Gy)], which are given, often daily on weekdays, for 5 to 7 weeks. This standard of care was established to allow for the recovery of normal tissues from sublethal radiation damage between treatments and the repopulation of surviving cells in normal tissues during the prolonged overall treatment time. Severe toxic reactions might thereby be avoided. This approach, while mandated to prevent lethal toxicity, also allows the surviving and possibly more resistant tumor cells to repopulate, thereby increasing the number of tumor cells that must be eradicated. There is evidence that these surviving cells may actually proliferate more rapidly in this state. The detrimental effects of extending overall treatment time for tumor control is established for many malignancies, including squamous cell carcinomas of the larynx and pharynx, carcinoma of the cervix, and bladder cancer. This effect is observed both for primary radiation treatment and for postoperative radiotherapy.

More recently, two alternative types of radiation fractionation have been used effectively: accelerated fractionation and hyperfractionation. With *accelerated fractionation*, the fractional doses are given more than once daily, and/or treatment is continued during weekends. This strategy reduces the overall treatment time, thereby providing less opportunity for the repopulation of tumor cells. Unfortunately, these schedules may also increase acute normal tissue toxicity, because there is less time for the repopulation of normal tissue. Accelerated fractionation has improved local control of Burkitt's lymphoma, a hematologic tumor that is known to proliferate rapidly. Accelerated fractionation has been used most extensively for treatment of squamous cell carcinomas of the head and neck, with a small survival benefit and increased loco-regional control. *Hyperfractionation* delivers multiple smaller fractions per day, using conventional overall treatment times, to allow greater normal tissue recovery to occur in each interval between treatments. Accelerated fractionation and hyperfractionation are often combined.

COMBINED RADIOTHERAPY AND CHEMOTHERAPY

The combination of chemotherapy with radiation has improved survival following primary treatment of cancers of the head and neck and uterine cervix, while results are promising for a broader spectrum of cancers, such as lung and bladder cancer. Clinical experience has demonstrated that chemotherapy prior to radiotherapy is not an efficient combination and that chemotherapeutic doses that can be tolerated during radiation are small. The mechanism accountable for the benefit of this combination is not fully elucidated. Chemotherapy might radiosensitize the tumor or have an added antitumor effect. Randomized trials for head and neck cancer have shown that concurrent chemotherapy can overcome the effects of prolonging the overall treatment time when planned treatment gaps are introduced. Although radiation and concurrent chemotherapy is a standard treatment for some types of cancer, toxic reactions prevent many patients from completing their chemotherapy, especially near the end of radiotherapy, when repopulation is most likely to occur. Encouraging results have been reported from phase I and II studies that have evaluated concurrent chemotherapy delivered during the last part of the radiotherapy schedule.

TARGETED THERAPY

Molecular-targeted agents are theoretically the ultimate cancer therapy; as they are designed to destroy cancer cells selectively, sparing the normal tissues of the patient. The "magic bullet" concept of using antibodies to target cancer cells selectively was first proposed by Paul Ehlrich. It took about 100 years for its clinical application. Examples of molecular-targeted agents include small-molecule inhibitors and antibodies against specific proliferation pathway proteins. Some agents are approved for the systemic treatment of cancer, and many others are in clinical trials.

Monoclonal antibodies such as trastuzumab, cetuximab, and rituximab have now successfully made the critical transition from the laboratory to routine clinical protocols for the management of a number of human cancers, such as metastatic breast cancer, limited-volume colorectal cancer, and several types of leukemia. Small-molecule drugs block specific enzymes involved in cancer cell growth. For instance, imatinib is a small-molecule drug that targets abnormal proteins, or enzymes, that form inside cancer cells and stimulate uncontrolled growth. It is approved by the U.S. Food and Drug Administration (FDA) to treat gastrointestinal stromal tumor (a rare cancer of the gastrointestinal tract) and certain types of chronic myeloid leukemia. Gefitinib, which targets the epidermal growth factor receptor (EGFR), which is overproduced by many types of cancer cells, is approved by the FDA to treat advanced non-small-cell lung cancer. Other small-molecule drugs are being studied in clinical trials in the United States.

Most tumors, particularly solid tumors, are usually linked to defects in more than one signaling pathway. Therefore, a dual-targeting or multitargeting therapy might be rational not only to eliminate cancer cells efficiently, but also to limit the emergence of drug resistance. Additionally, many of the recently or currently developed molecular-targeted agents inhibit pathways that when activated stimulate the proliferation of tumor cells, thus arresting growth and not killing cells. Thus, tumor shrinkage is relatively rare, and when it occurs, is usually delayed. In some clinical trials, these agents have been given concurrently and continuously with chemotherapy, and some of the results of most trials have been disappointing. It is quite possible that these negative results are due to a central conceptual flaw in the design of these trials: By giving an agent that arrests proliferation, the agents that kill proliferating cells are rendered inactive. A logical strategy could use a short-acting cytostatic agent between courses of chemotherapy to inhibit the repopulation of tumor cells and to stop it before the next cycle so that cells can resume proliferation and be maximally sensitive to cytotoxic drugs. Alternatively, it could be introduced after the completion of chemotherapy as a long-term effort to avert recurrence. It is thus imperative to design studies based on a robust biological rationale so as not to waste invaluable human scientific and financial resources and condemn a treatment option that if used wisely could improve clinical outcome.

INTRODUCING NEW THERAPEUTIC AGENTS IN THE CLINIC

Drug development is a lengthy, grueling, and costly procedure from design to introduction in the clinic. It takes an average of 15 years to bring an experimental drug out of the lab. The central challenge met at initiation of this process is the choice of candidate drug that will be streamlined. On average, only 1 in a 1000 compounds is chosen. Following the initial basic mechanistic and in vitro studies, an important step in the development that weighs critically on this decision is the application of robust and biologically relevant preclinical models.

Preclinical models have been developed in an effort to recapitulate cancer, yet they are in principle different from human disease. Most of them are generated by introducing cells that are capable of surviving in vitro in mice that are immuno-compromised. The flaws readily identified are that the host is immunodeficient, and additionally, the cancer cells encountered in human disease can survive in vitro only rarely. Other models are based on interfering with gene expression to incur carcinogenesis, while solid tumors are not a single gene disease. So following preclinical testing on a model that is flawed, yet admittedly the best we have, a decision has to be made regarding the fate of the candidate drug. Even though the toxicity and pharmacodynamic data that can be harvested from these models have proven quite reliable, the same does not apply with regard to drug efficiency. A lot of promising compounds were disappointing in the clinic, and we can presume that some of those precluded from the clinic might have proven active in humans.

Once a candidate compound has actually passed 'preclinical testing' it moves onto the *Clinical trial* step. A clinical trial is a research study in volunteering patients with cancer that aims to evaluate and develop new treatments. As some of the drugs have mutagenic effects and acute toxicities, it would be inappropriate to test drugs in early clinical development in normal volunteers, as would be the case with novel drugs in other diseases. Clinical trials determine whether experimental treatments or new ways of using known therapies are safe and effective under controlled environments. The efficient design of a clinical trial is crucial in uncovering the activity of a candidate drug. They are conducted in four different phases (http://www.clinicaltrials.gov/ct/info/). The typical costs of conducting phase I, II, and III clinical trials are $200,000, $1 million, and $10 million, respectively.

Phase I trials test an experimental treatment for the first time in a small group of people (20 to 80) to evaluate its safety, determine a safe dosage range, and identify side effects and study the pharmacokinetics of the agent. Usually, a novel anticancer agent is tested in one to four phase I trials to evaluate distinct schedules. The aim of this phase should be to identify the best initial dose of the new treatment. The maximum dose tolerated has traditionally been the endpoint of phase I studies, as conventional cytotoxic agents are associated with strongly dose-dependent therapeutic effect and toxicity. A narrow therapeutic index is one reason for abandoning a drug after phase I trials.

In view of the new targeted therapies introduced in the clinic, the understanding that more is not always more effective becomes imperative. The main endpoint for phase I trials should be to determine the optimal biological response with the least toxicity; oncopharmacogenomic studies must be performed in tumoral biopsies to assess the target inhibition. Usually, patients recruited for phase I have no other therapeutic option, and treatment starts with a low dose of a drug. If the first group tolerates the dose, the next group receives a higher dose, and this escalation seizes when the toxicity that ensues precludes any further increase. Since almost nothing is known with regard to the clinical aspects of the drug at initiation of these studies, very few patients are expected to benefit clinically. In fact, only around 4% of patients accrued in a single agent and 17% of those participating in combination studies achieve an objective response. Even though patients are informed of the aim of the study and they accept the fact that they may have no therapy effect, the disappointment of a posttreatment scan showing progression of disease is almost always unavoidable. To expedite phase I studies and to minimize the patient population that may be treated suboptimally, alternative trial designs have been used, including a faster dose-escalation strategy or recruiting a single patient in each dose level until toxicity occurs, following which larger numbers entered.

In phase II trials, the experimental study drug or treatment is given to a larger group of people to see if it is clinically effective and to evaluate its safety further. Evaluation of effectiveness is usually achieved by using tumor shrinkage as a surrogate. Phase II trials are typically conducted in five to 10 tumor types. A phase II study may also serve to refine the dose of the treatment tested. For examples patients participating in phase I studies have typically already received multiple myelosuppressive chemotherapy regimens; they may then be more susceptible to the myelosuppressive effects of the investigational agent than patients who are receiving the drug as front-line therapy in a phase II study.

In phase III trials, the experimental study drug or treatment is given to large groups of people (1000 to 3000) to confirm its effectiveness, monitor side effects, compare it to commonly used treatments, and collect information that will allow the experimental drug or treatment to be used safely. *Effectiveness* is defined as definitive evidence regarding the benefit-to-risk profile of the experimental intervention relative to a placebo or an existing standard-of-care treatment.

In phase IV trials, postmarketing studies delineate additional information, including the drug's risks, benefits, and optimal use.

Although improved survival is the "gold standard" for proving clinical benefit of oncologic therapy in phase III studies, the FDA has accepted significant results in clinical trials using surrogate endpoints as the basis for drug approval to expedite a procedure that would otherwise require large long-term and very costly trials. This accelerated approval (AA) process was introduced in 1992 to secure rapid availability of new interventions, particularly for diseases providing risks of death or serious illness. It allowed marketing of interventions shown to have strong effects on measures of biological activity if those measures are potential "surrogates" for true measures of tangible clinical benefit. What appears quite challenging is the definition of a reliable surrogate to avoid compromising what is truly in the best interest of public health: the reliable as well as timely evaluation of an intervention's safety and efficacy. The biological marker chosen for surrogate must not only be correlated with the clinical endpoint but also reflect the net effect of the intervention on the clinical endpoint. The latter, although ideal, is rarely feasible. A biological correlate does not always lie in the causal pathway of the disease progression and clinical outcome. Thus, the candidate therapeutic may be affecting only the surrogate, not the disease. Examples of such correlates are tumor markers such as carcinoembryonic antigen (CEA) for colon cancer and prostate-specific antigen (PSA) for prostate cancer. Their increase is usually the result of increased tumor growth. Since they can be estimates of tumor burden and thus likely morbidity/mortality risk, they can be efficient tools for follow-up. They are not, however, the mechanism through which the disease process induces increased risk of the morbidity mortality, so it is questionable whether treatment-induced changes in these markers could be relied on to predict accurately treatment-induced effects on the clinical endpoints. Furthermore, even if the suggested surrogate is considered causal in cancer morbidity/mortality, the candidate therapeutic may be unlinking it from the clinical outcome, and then the effect of treatment on clinical efficacy endpoints could be over- or underestimated by the effect on the proposed surrogate.

Tumor reduction falls under this category and has been the preferred surrogate in trials. Even though in general this has been a successful surrogate for improved survival, clinical studies of a variety of oncologic agents have not consistently demonstrated a correlation between the two: even more so when we are evaluating cytostatic rather than cytotoxic agents. Results from several clinical studies suggest that patients with solid tumors such as lung cancer may derive clinical benefit from treatment that helps stabilize their disease. In this case the benefit cannot be recognized readily by a trial designed to identify tumor shrinkage. Of course, the reverse could also occur with a tumor shrinkage not necessarily corresponding to a long-term clinical benefit.

To compensate for the lack of ideal surrogates, the AA process expedites marketing for interventions when they have been shown to have compelling effects on biological markers, where these effects are "reasonably likely to predict clinical benefit", on the condition that the sponsor will complete, in a timely manner, one or more clinical trials that will validate that the intervention truly does provide meaningful clinical benefit or tangible measures of clinical benefit. These validation trials should meet all of the usual criteria for quality of trial conduct and reliability of conclusions, including the usual levels for statistical strength of evidence, which would be required for providing full regulatory approval in non-AA settings. The challenge faced should be more or less anticipated: Lack of accrual as the experimental therapy is available in a nonresearch setting.

In fact, clinical trials suffer from limited participation in general. According to the NCI, fewer than 5% of adult cancer patients ever participate in a clinical trial. There are a multitude of reasons for this, including lack of awareness and reluctance of the patient to inquire overtly about trials as well as unreceptive physicians and strict eligibility criteria. If this number increased, new treatments would be evaluated much faster. Ultimately, use of a variety of endpoints as well as different trial designs may provide an adequate basis for expediting the benefit–risk assessment of newer therapies.

PHARMACOGENOMICS IN CANCER TREATMENT

Pharmacogenomics investigate the influence of genetic variation on drug response in patients by correlating gene expression or single-nucleotide polymorphisms with a drug's efficacy or toxicity. Pharmacogenomics aim to develop rational means to optimize drug therapy with respect to the patient's genotype, to ensure maximum efficacy with minimal adverse effects. Pharmacogenetic research has always fascinated the media. It has created a great deal of optimism regarding personalized cancer therapy, as in essence it revolves around the most basic concept of individualized medicine. It is simple and gratifying, as it promises improved outcome and less toxicity, and of course there are economic implications, making it particularly alluring to investors to "get in at the start" of a revolution in drug treatment. Enthusiastic descriptions of the possibility of personal "bar codes" or routine generation of pharmacogenetic profiles prior to treatment with drugs have appeared in the scientific and popular press, driven by the expectation that investigators would move swiftly through the pathway from single-gene studies to predictive profiling.

Understanding the variable response to drugs seems particularly pressing in the field of oncology, in which the stakes are high (failure to cure cancer usually leads to death), drugs commonly have a narrow therapeutic index, and toxicities can be severe (a significant frequency of toxic death is a feature of most acute myeloid leukemia protocols, for example). There are a number of different steps necessary for applying pharmacognenetics toward truly personalized medicine:

1. Identification of significant genes
2. Integration of multiple genes into a profile
3. Demonstration that use of the profile to direct therapy improves outcomes
4. Acceptance of the profile on a population-wide basis, not just in specialized research centers (this is probably the most challenging)

In 25 years of research and despite the original enthusiasm in the scientific community, only two genotypes have been identified. TPMT polymorphism, identified in 1980 by Weinshilboum and Sladek, can predict the toxicity of 6-MP, a drug used to treat some types of leukemia and the consequences of therapy, and UGT1 predicts toxicity for irinotecan, a chemotherapeutic agent used extensively for the treatment of colorectal cancer. Notwithstanding these findings, a recent review of current clinical practice in Europe indicated that only half the clinicians actually thought pharmacogenetic testing to be useful, suggesting comfort with traditional trial-and-error-based drug dosing. Data on improved outcomes will probably need to be compelling to overcome this hesitation in clinical practice.

CHALLENGES OF TREATING METASTATIC
AND MICROMETASTATIC DISEASE

Most cancer patients succumb to the disease because it has spread to other sites. Current approaches to treatment, such as chemotherapy surgery and radiation therapy, are limited in their success by the presence of metastatic disease. With very scarce exceptions, such as testicular cancer, the prognosis of metastatic disease is grim. Treatment with chemotherapy or radiation offers only palliation.

Statistics make it clear that interruption of the metastatic process could be useful for a majority of those with cancer. According to data collected by the Surveillance, Epidemiology, and End Result (SEER) Program of the NCI, of the four most common cancers, fewer than 10% of breast and prostate cancer patients, 20% of colorectal cancer patients, and 40% of lung cancer patients had detectable distant metastases at diagnosis (the period 1988–2001). For patients with breast, colorectal, and lung cancer, another 29 to 37% already had tumor cells in lymph nodes. These people are at the highest risk of metastasis. Invasion has already happened, even though we lack the imaging technology of sufficient sensitivity to verify it and identify at which step of micrometastasis the disease is diagnosed.

The absence of success in treating metastatic disease dictates considerable changes both in preclinical and clinical research involved in the discovery and development of drugs with antimetastatic properties. The challenges faced include the identification of targets strongly linked to tumor metastases, development of biologically relevant and robust preclinical screening models, and the design of clinical development strategies that will maximize the opportunity to demonstrate clinical benefit.

But why do available drugs fail? The steps in metastasis include invasion, survival in the bloodstream, and colonization of the site of metastasis. For colonization, the least efficient of the metastatic steps, to occur successfully, it is imperative that the microenvironment or "soil" interacts favorably with the metastatic cells or "seed." Unfortunately, in humans, only the end stages of the metastatic process are observed, when a metastatic lesion is sufficiently large to be imaged. Thus, compounds that interrupt any of the interactions required prior to establishment of a metastasis may not have conventional efficacy (complete and partial responses) in patients that have an already established metastasis. At this point, the microenvironment has already developed alternative interaction, growth, and survival pathways, making most attempts at controlling disease unsuccessful or at best less successful than at an earlier disease stage.

The concept that the earlier in cancer progression that an effective drug is given, the better, is supported very strongly by the trastuzumab paradigm. Trastuzumab is a monoclonal antibody that acts on the HER2/*neu* (erbB2) receptor. Herceptin's principal use is as an anticancer therapy in breast cancer in patients whose tumors overexpress this receptor. Trastuzumab was originally tested successfully in the metastatic breast cancer and was moved quickly to adjuvant locally advanced disease (lymph node positive, distant metastasis negative).

The magnitude of clinical response data in the metastatic setting, although statistically significant, is dwarfed by that recently reported in the adjuvant locally advanced setting.

Combinations of drugs targeting multiple relevant pathways may be needed to overcome pathway redundancy or resistance. Given the presumed need for chronic dosing, it may also be critical to define a biologically effective dose rather than a maximum tolerated dose, to limit adverse effects of long-term dosing. Preoperative trials that aim at deciphering the mechanism of action and whether the target is actually hit at the tumor level should be performed. Identification of persons whose tumor expresses the target of interest will be critical for success. Increased investment in metastasis targets and logical clinical testing schemas is imperative.

FUTURE PROMISE: TOWARD INDIVIDUALIZED THERAPY

The increased knowledge of mechanisms responsible for carcinogenesis, the development of molecularly targeted therapies in combination with technology improvements that allow us to image, sample, monitor, and destroy previously inaccessible sites selectively, provide the opportunity to develop individualized therapy algorithms. The personalized medicine of the future will depend on the development of cancer classification based on biology rather than anatomy, application of a specific therapy for each person, in anticipation of disease rather than when symptoms of active cancer reported by the patient leads to the diagnosis. Advances in understanding the mechanisms of cancer development at a very basic level are the foundation for this change. For once in the history of human cancer, physicians are armed with sufficient knowledge to make this a realistic possibility for many common cancers.

RECOMMENDED READING

Benson JD, Chen YP, Cornell-Kennon S, et al. 2006. Validating cancer drug targets. *Nature* 441: 451–456.

Chabner BA, Roberts TG. 2005. Chemotherapy and the war on cancer. *Nat Rev Cancer* 5:65–72.

Imai K, Takaoka A. 2006. Comparing antibody and small-molecule therapies for cancer. *Nat Rev Cancer* 6(9):714–727.

Kim JJ, Tannock IF. 2005. Repopulation of cancer cells during therapy: an important cause of treatment failure. *Nat Rev Cancer* 5(7):516–525.

Roberts TG, Chabner BA. 2004. Beyond fast track for drug approvals. *N Engl J Med* 351:501–505.

Roberts TG Jr, Goulart BH, Squitieri L, et al. 2004. Trends in the risks and benefits to patients with cancer participating in phase 1 clinical trials. *JAMA* 292(17):2130–2140.

Takimoto CH. 2003. Anticancer drug development at the US National Cancer Institute. *Cancer Chemother Pharmacol* 52(Suppl 1):S29–S33.

Von Eschenbach AC. 2004. A vision for the National Cancer Program in the United States. *Nat Rev Cancer* 4(10):820–828.

Von Hoff, DD. 1998. There are no bad anticancer agents, only bad clinical trial designs. *Clin Cancer Res* 4:1079–1086.

10

CLINICAL TRIALS
IN ONCOLOGY

Konstantin H. Dragnev and Mark A. Israel

*Norris Cotton Cancer Center, Darthmouth-Hitchcock Medical Center,
Lebanon, New Hampshire*

INTRODUCTION

A major strategy by which progress in oncology is realized is the validation in a clinical trial of a hypothesis generated through laboratory-based scientific investigations. The strong belief and the passionate defense of an attractive idea by cancer experts are not sufficient to establish the efficacy of any new therapy. New cancer treatments are evaluated by the conduct of clinical trials, a robust, stepwise process that begins with the formulation of a testable hypothesis, the design and execution of a definitive clinical evaluation, and the analysis of data that reveal a conclusion about the value of the new therapy (Figure 1). Adherence to strict ethical principles to ensure the safety of all participants and the integrity of each of the steps above is a requirement for all contemporary clinical studies. With the rapid advances in our understanding of the molecular biology of cancer, it is imperative that any cancer therapeutic or preventive agent proposed, as well as novel diagnostic methods, undergo rigorous evaluation in a clinical trial. In this chapter we describe the different types of clinical studies in oncology with an emphasis on

The Biology and Treatment of Cancer: Understanding Cancer
Edited by Arthur B. Pardee and Gary S. Stein   Copyright © 2009 John Wiley & Sons, Inc.

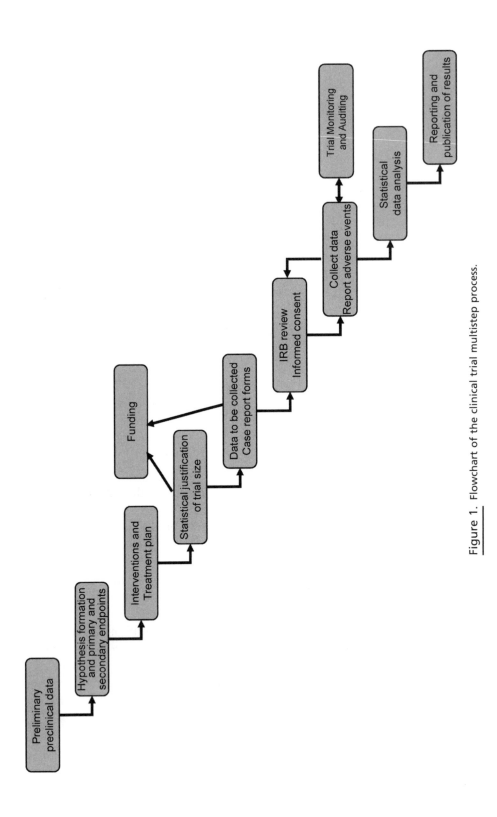

Figure 1. Flowchart of the clinical trial multistep process.

therapeutic trial design. Several excellent reviews on this topic have been published (Pocock, 1996; Hageman and Reeves, 2001; Simon, 2001).

INSTITUTIONAL REVIEW BOARDS AND INFORMED CONSENT

Research involving human subjects invariably presents a wide range of ethical questions. Since the goal of clinical studies is to develop treatments that will benefit future patients, the participants in the trial may not derive any benefit. This may create a conflict between the study participant and those conducting research. A system has to be in place to facilitate the conduct of clinical research without compromising the welfare of individual research subjects. The Institutional Review Board (IRB) is the key to the protection of human research participants (Bohaychuk and Ball, 1999). The IRB is a committee composed of people who understand the concerns of the local community where the studies are conducted. Their mission is to review clinical trial applications and monitor ongoing studies to determine if the conduct of research meets ethical standards. Invariably, to obtain IRB approval, the clinical research protocol should mandate obtaining voluntary and informed consent by potential participants. An IRB also reviews the trial design to be certain that it minimizes the risks to research subjects. There are federal regulations that require all federally funded clinical research to be approved by an IRB. Research participants should be able to understand clearly what will happen to them in the research study, how this will differ from standard care, and what risks are involved as a result of their participation. The process of obtaining informed consent must provide potential clinical trial subjects with sufficient information to make informed choices regarding their participation, especially whether to begin or continue participation in the study. This process includes communication describing the trial and specific discussions detailing the purpose, procedures, risks, and benefits of participating in the trial, as well as the voluntary nature of participation. The informed consent document is a summary of the clinical trial and the rights of the research subject. It can also be used by the study participant as an information resource throughout their participation in the clinical trial. Local IRBs are charged with overseeing the consent documents at their institutions.

PHASE I TRIALS

Once a new drug shows promising activity during preclinical in vitro and in vivo evaluations, it must be studied further to confirm that it is effective in the treatment of patients with specific conditions. Prior to studies designed to determine the efficacy of a treatment, initial studies are conducted to evaluate its adverse effects in human subjects and to determine the dose to be used in subsequent therapeutic investigations. These initial studies to identify toxicities and to find a tolerable dose are referred to as *phase I clinical trials* (Eisenhauer, 1998). Patients with a variety of advanced malignancies for whom no known effective therapy exists are typically the patients enrolled in such studies. The characteristic design of these trials includes the administration of a drug at a starting dose corresponding to a small fraction of the dose that is lethal for the most sensitive laboratory animal species (Simon, 2001). Toxicities that preclude the safe use of a drug are defined as *dose-limiting toxicities* (DLTs). Typically, three patients per dose are treated, and if no DLTs are observed, the next cohort of patients is treated at a higher dose. The most popular dose escalation scheme is the modified Fibonacci series (Simon et al., 1997; Paoletti et al., 2006). Dose levels are increased by 100%, 67%, 50%, 40%, and then 33% until a DLT is encountered. Usually, cohorts of three patients are treated at each dose. When one patient develops a DLT, three additional patients are treated at the same dose. If no other DLT is observed, dose escalation continues. If a second DLT develops in more than 33% of patients (two out of six) at a given dose level, dose escalation stops. Usually, the preceding dose level, a dose level at which fewer than 33% of patients experienced a DLT, is recommended for further study in the next trial, the *phase II evaluation.* Additional patients may be treated at the recommended phase II dose (RPTD) as part of the phase I study to better define the toxicities of the treatment proposed. Detailed description and analyses of all observed toxicities are integral parts of any phase I trial (Eisenhauer, 1998). Since patients with different types of cancer and with different prior treatments are enrolled, phase I studies at best give only suggestions of possible anticancer activity. However, these studies are also frequently designed to study the pharmacokinetics of the drug, and sometimes its pharmacodynamics, by measuring the treatment effect on a marker in blood, in tumor, or in surrogate tissue (Eisenhauer, 1998). Phase I studies provide valuable information about the relationship between dose and toxicities but rarely about dose and anticancer effect.

PHASE II TRIALS

The assessment of activity against specific tumor types is the objective of phase II clinical trials (Wittes et al., 1985). Once an appropriate dose is determined during phase I testing, preclinical data and early signs of benefit seen in phase I studies guide the choice and prioritization of tumor types and the patient populations to be studied. Usually, patients who have not had any prior therapy are studied separately from patients whose disease has become resistant to established treatments. Clinical activity is often measured as the tumor response rate, which is the most common primary endpoint of phase II trials. These studies also provide additional information about safety, and some offer preliminary data on the effect of treatment on survival. Recently, some phase II trials have been designed to evaluate drug activity with respect to delaying disease progression (Ratain and Stadler, 2001). In such studies the primary endpoint becomes the rate of progression at some prespecified time point.

As the goal of phase II studies is to identify the most promising treatments for further testing and to screen out inactive drugs, all studies include precisely defined measures of tumor response (Simon, 1989; Gehan and Tefft, 2000; Curran et al., 2006). Stopping rules are established to discontinue these trials either because the drug's activity is lower than what has been set as the minimal acceptable response rate or because the therapy being tested is definitely more effective than established treatments (Gail, 1982). While stopping rules limit the risk for exposing large numbers of patients to inactive therapies, discontinuing the study early decreases the statistical power to detect differences from other therapies, as there are fewer patients treated. Rarely, additional follow-up after early stopping of a study may change an investigator's interpretation of a study outcome.

It is important to recognize that phase II trials rarely have an appropriate control group of patients, and they do not provide definitive survival results. Comparing results from different phase II trials is inappropriate, as the patient populations in each study are virtually always very different. These trials are valuable because they provide an estimate of the activity of a well-defined treatment intervention for a particular tumor type. Sometimes, randomized phase II clinical trials are conducted (Simon et al., 1985; Simon, 1989; Rosner et al., 2002; Freidlin and Simon, 2005b). This design allows for a determination of which treatment under study performs best according to prespecified parameters. Although randomized phase II trials do not have the statistical power to detect small differences, the information gleaned builds a foundation for selecting the most promising regiment for further evaluation in a definitive phase III trial.

PHASE III TRIALS

Direct comparison of new and established treatments is the objective of *phase III clinical trials.* The choice of a primary endpoint is a critical element in the design of these studies. Typically, investigators evaluate survival, either median survival time or progression-free survival. More recently, other quantifiable measures of benefit to the patient, such as quality of life, have also been studied (Fossella et al., 2003; Gralla and Thatcher, 2004). If a new drug is being evaluated with the intention of seeking regulatory approval for use in a specific disease state, the primary endpoint is determined after discussions with the U.S. Food and Drug Administration (FDA), which must decide whether to approve a treatment based on the clinical trial information (Schneiderman, 1967; Schilsky, 2002). Many studies have shown little correlation between response rates and survival (Weiss et al., 1983; Torri et al., 1992). Consequently, response rates are not used as a primary endpoint in such trials. Statistical input is required while such trials are being designed (Berry, 1986; Simon, 2001; Piantadosi, 2004). To establish that one therapy is better than the other, clinical investigators must determine in advance what degree of difference between the new and the standard treatment regimens is clinically important. Usually, a 30% improvement in survival is considered highly significant. Based on the expected difference, the sample size of the study can be calculated (Freedman, 1982; Donner, 1984; Berry, 1986). The number of patients required to demonstrate convincingly that the prespecified difference between treatments is not due to chance alone is a critical determination, as it helps to define the feasibility of a study, determines the cost of the trial, and allows investigators to determine whether the hypothesis being tested is sufficiently important to justify the expense of conducting a clinical trial.

It is essential that patients whose response to a treatment is being evaluated in a clinical trial of drug efficacy be recognized as having similar prognostic features. This clinical trial design is achieved by stratification, a process of separating patients with known prognostic factors so that they are distributed equally among the types of treatment being evaluated (Piantadosi, 1988). Many other unknown features of a patient's tumor may also influence the treatment outcome. The most important characteristic of phase III studies is randomization, a study design feature that provides an unbiased assignment of patients to one or another treatment that is being examined in a particular trial (Simon, 2001). This process ensures that unknown factors which might affect prognosis are distributed equally between the treatment arms. For randomized trials, any differences in outcomes will probably be due to the different treatments administered. The strength of the conclusions that can be drawn from such studies depends on the degree of the difference and the size of the clinical study (Simon, 1986). Statistical analyses of such trials to evaluate the likelihood that the difference in outcomes observed is not due to chance alone are very important.

PHASE IV TRIALS

Once a drug is approved for use based on the foregoing stepwise process, its safety and efficacy during routine practice may be evaluated in *phase IV clinical trials* (postmarketing trials). Sometimes these studies are mandated as part of the approval process. The results of such studies rarely may lead to removing a treatment from the market, either for lack of confirmed efficacy or for higher than expected toxicities (Schilsky, 2002). Less common side effects are also frequently detected during these trials, since very large numbers of patients are typically being exposed to the new treatment. Although phase IV trials require less rigorous statistical design than phase III randomized studies, they can often be an important part of the overall drug evaluation program.

CLINICAL TRIAL DESIGN FOR TARGETED THERAPIES

The established stepwise approach to the evaluation of new cancer treatments described above has been developed and refined using cytotoxic chemotherapy agents. These drugs rarely act specifically on a single cell type, and treatment with them is usually associated with significant side effects. The dominant drug development paradigm to date has been to determine the maximum dose that can be administered with tolerable toxicities and to use this dose to identify the treatment's therapeutic effectiveness. Whether the desired effects can been achieved at lower doses is usually not studied.

The field of oncology has undergone major changes in the last five years. The progress in molecular and cell biology has led to greater knowledge of the mechanisms of carcinogenesis and the cellular pathways that manifest as cancer-related pathologies such as cellular proliferation and tissue invasion. New drugs are being developed to target specific molecules in pathways that are considered critical for tumor pathology and especially for the survival of the cancer cell. *Targeted therapies* is the collective term used to describe agents that will affect only the malignant cells sparing the normal cells, typically because the molecular target is present only on or in malignant cells. Since the ideal target is likely to vary from tumor type to tumor type and will almost certainly be different in different subgroups of tumors arising in any particular tissue, it is possible that there will be many new drugs in the oncologists' armamentarium going forward. Interestingly, it seems that many different tumor types are characterized by the derangement of a limited number of pathways, and it is possible that some targeted therapies may be useful in subgroups of many different tumors in which that particular target is pathologically modified.

Most of the available targeted agents have fewer toxicities than conventional chemotherapy, since they are typically designed to target specific molecules or pathways that are present or activated only in tumor cells. Interestingly, these agents may also interfere with different pathways, depending on the drug levels achieved in the tumor tissues. For example, at lower doses the desired target may be affected, while at higher doses additional targets may be blocked or induced, and under such conditions might even counteract the beneficial effects or cause more or additional toxicities than were seen at the lower dose (Miller et al., 2005; McNeil, 2006). Clearly, determining the maximum tolerated dose (MTD) as the sole strategy for identifying the dose of a cancer drug that will be evaluated in definitive clinical trials is ill conceived for such targeted agents and also for many biological agents (Eisenhauer, 1998; Korn et al., 2001; Ratain and Stadler, 2001; Fox et al., 2002; Rosner et al., 2002; Simon and Maitournam, 2004; Freidlin and Simon, 2005b). Establishing a biologically effective dose is one alternative approach that has gained some popularity. Instead of monitoring a clinical endpoint such as response rate, investigators seek to evaluate changes in molecular markers that have been determined during preclinical research to change if the pathway desired is affected by the treatment. Some measurements require the examination of biomarkers of response in either body fluids or tissues, although functional imaging in which the activity of specific molecular pathways can be monitored noninvasively are becoming ever more widespread (Gupta et al., 2002; Schechter et al., 2003). The need to establish a dose at which such surrogate markers are repressed or induced has led to the introduction of novel clinical trial designs for the standard phase I and II drug evaluations (Korn et al., 2001; Simon and Maitournam, 2004; Freidlin and Simon, 2005b). Importantly, the relationship of surrogate marker changes and clinical benefit cannot be established through such trials. Rather, classic phase III studies with survival as the primary endpoint are still necessary to prove that a new, targeted treatment is better than standard therapy.

The best cancer treatments available usually benefit only a subset of patients with any particular tumor type. The targeted agents that are being introduced currently will be beneficial only to patients with tumors that carry the appropriate target. Recent advances in molecular medicine have made it ever more possible to evaluate tumors for the presence of the target and/or surrogate markers that will predict which patients are more likely to respond to a particular treatment type. Using advanced technology, it is possible to design trials only for patients who carry the target and biomarker required to monitor response. Simon et al. have proposed a clinical trial design for randomized studies of targeted agents comparing a new treatment to an established treatment (Simon and Maitournam, 2004). These novel designs for targeted agents dramatically reduce the number of patients required to prove that a statistically significant difference exists between treatment groups. For example, responses to small-molecule inhibitors of the epidermal growth factor receptor tyrosine kinase (EGFR-TKI), such as erlotinib and gefitinib, can be predicted if certain mutations in the tyrosine kinase domain of EGFR are present (Lynch et al., 2004). A trial of unselected patients designed to show a 20% improvement in one-year survival of patients treated with a targeted agent will require an estimated 12,806 patients. A trial examining the efficacy of a targeted agent only in patients with mutated EGFR may require as few as 138 total patients (Simon and Maitournam, 2004). Usually, predictive factors are determined by analyses of phase II trials. When targeted therapies are evaluated, every attempt should be made to characterize the responders in phase II studies before large, costly phase III trials are conducted.

Cytotoxic chemotherapy drugs are evaluated for activity in phase II trials with response rates as the endpoint. Response generally is measured as tumor shrinkage; however, many new molecularly targeted agents do not induce such responses, yet they arrest tumor growth. Such treatments are said to be cytostatic rather than cytotoxic. When reliable assays to identify patients who are more likely to respond to cytostatic, targeted drugs are not available, one approach to their evaluation is to assign patients randomly to either the new agent or standard treatment. Alternatively, a randomized discontinuation design can be utilized (Freidlin and Simon, 2005b). In this case, the agent under study is administered to all patients initially, and an evaluation is performed after a predetermined period of time. Patients who progress are removed from the study and receive other treatment; patients who respond continue therapy. Patients with stable disease are randomized to continue treatment with either the agent or a placebo. This phase II trial design may help identify the most promising agent to study further in randomized phase III trials. The randomized discontinuation design is particularly advantageous when only a subset of patients are sensitive to the drug (Freidlin and Simon, 2005). It should be considered in the early development of molecularly targeted therapies when selection for patients expressing the target is not feasible. Traditional randomization is better if slow-growing tumors are targeted and early responses are not expected.

CLINICAL RESEARCH OFFICE AND DATA MANAGEMENT

Even the best trial design will fail if there is not rigorous protocol implementation. Study designs define the type of research data to be collected and often require the creation of specific data management instruments. FDA recommendations and international guidelines specify good clinical practices (GCPs) that must be used in clinical research (Bohaychuk and Ball, 1999). GCPs are invariably guided by the dual focus of protecting study participants and protecting the integrity of the data collected in the course of the study.

Clinical trial data are only a portion of the patient's medical record. To capture the appropriate information relevant to the clinical study, selective data management tools have been developed. Case report forms (CRFs) are guideposts that specify the standard approach to the collection of clinical research data during the course of a clinical trial. These are templates of the data elements that must be captured. Consistency across protocols is reflected in similar generic terms, coding conventions, and the standardized definition of terms. Traditionally, these were hard-copy paper forms, but now electronic CRFs are becoming popular and allow one easily to enter, monitor, and review data. They also facilitate the aggregation of data and the ability to search and share information. The decision to change from paper to electronic CRFs requires a commitment by the research institution to reengineer the data management process. The FDA has adopted guidelines for clinical trial computer systems. When these are adopted, standard operating procedures should be established for system setup, system maintenance, data collection, data backup and recovery, and data security (U.S. Food and Drug Administration, 1999). The widespread adoption of electronic CRFs will be necessary before Internet-based data collection and management can be accomplished. Using a secure web server, the data from large, randomized, multicenter clinical trials can be collected, stored, reviewed, administered, analyzed, and reported. The use of Internet technology will allow participation in such trials of smaller physician groups which are located far from established research centers and which do not have access to an extensive clinical research infrastructure (Santoro et al., 1999).

Computerized data management facilitates the generation of audit trails that allow review of the data history. Viewing the audit trail can establish what was recorded and when, and whether anyone changed data after they were collected.

Ensuring adequate quality control is critical to the conduct of clinical trials. The International Conference on Harmonization, a union of the United States, the European Union, and Japan, has defined *good clinical practice* as "a standard for the design, performance, monitoring, auditing, recording, analyses and reporting of clinical trials to provide assurance that the data and reported results are credible and accurate" (International Conference on Harmonization of Technical Requirements for Registration of Pharmaceuticals for Human Use (ICH) adopts Consolidated Guideline on Good Clinical Practice in the Conduct of Clinical Trials on Medicinal Products for Human Use, 1997). Study performance, monitoring, and auditing are key components of the quality control process (Knatterud et al., 1998). Monitoring is performed by the study monitor, usually a clinical research organization that has the formal responsibility of evaluating the conduct of the trial. Data can be inspected for completeness and adherence to standard operating procedures. Study approvals and reviews and adverse-event reporting activities are typically evaluated during monitoring visits. Auditing is a related but different system for control that assesses the quality of the research process and is carried out by a team independent of the clinical study investigators (Knatterud et al., 1998).

CLINICAL TRIAL RESULT ANALYSES, REPORTING, AND PUBLICATION

The design of clinical trials should include provisions for analyses and reporting of the data collected. A comprehensive publication is an integral part of good research (Bailar and Mosteller, 1988). Methodological guidelines for reporting clinical trials have been developed and adopted by major cancer journals (International Committee of Medical Journal Editors, 1988). The authors should describe adequately the patients enrolled, the data that were collected, and the methods of statistical analyses. The quality control methods ensuring that the data are complete and accurate should be discussed. Major endpoints should include all eligible patients, and a careful distinction should be made between the data that are reported and their interpretation.

FUNDING SOURCES

During the early years of cancer medicine, clinical research was supported almost exclusively through funds provided by the federal government. The National Cancer Institute (NCI) is supporting the development of many new agents and has an extensive clinical trials system. The NCI has its own programs for early drug development and provides grants and contracts to many other institutions to conduct early therapeutic studies. The NCI also supports a large program of clinical trials cooperative groups to conduct later phase trials, including phase III studies. These groups maintain an established mechanism for such studies, including teams of clinical investigators, biostatisticians, and research support staff to design and complete large-scale, multi-institution trials for cancer treatment and prevention. Due to their complexity and size, these studies require extensive infrastructure, such as that supported by the NCI-sponsored clinical trials cooperative groups.

With the improved understanding of the molecular biology of carcinogenesis that has emerged in the past decade, there has been a major increase in the number of clinical trials sponsored by the pharmaceutical industry, either alone or in cooperation with the NCI. The ethical considerations affecting human research subjects are invariant regardless of the sponsor, and the fundamental processes of conducting all clinical trials are similar. A single set of standards exists for the conduct of clinical trials worldwide, including those sponsored by industry, through the International Committee on Harmonization discussed earlier (International Conference on Harmonization of Technical Requirements for Registration of Pharmaceuticals for Human Use (ICH) adopts Consolidated Guideline on Good Clinical Practice in the Conduct of Clinical Trials on Medicinal Products for Human Use, 1997). Almost universally these trials have included independent data and safety monitoring committees to oversee safety-related issues (Gail, 1982). Attempts are being made to develop globally acceptable drug registration metrics, although at the present time every country has its own national drug-approval requirements.

CONCLUSIONS

In adult oncology practice, only 1 to 3% of patients participate in clinical trials. For patients treated at NCI-designated comprehensive cancer centers, trial participation is 5 to 7%. In contrast, more than 70% of pediatric oncology patients are treated in the context of clinical studies. This difference may be one of the reasons for the very effective treatments that are available for some pediatric tumors. The value of a well-designed clinical trial for answering key questions of clinical importance cannot be overstated. Only the joint, integrated efforts of basic cancer researchers, translational scientists, clinical oncologists, biostatisticians, and the entire clinical trials team will improve the outcome for cancer patients in the future.

REFERENCES

Bailar JC, Mosteller F. 1988. Guidelines for statistical reporting in articles for medical journals: amplifications and explanations. *Ann Intern Med* 108:266–273.

Berry G. 1986. Statistical significance and confidence intervals. *Med J Aust* 144:618–619.

Bohaychuk W, Ball G. 1999. *Conducting GCP-Compliant Clinical Research.* New York: Wiley.

Curran SD, Muellner AU, Schwartz LH. 2006. Imaging response assessment in oncology. *Cancer Imaging* 6:S126–S130.

Donner A. 1984. Approaches to sample size estimation in the design of clinical trials: a review. *Stat Med* 3:199–214.

Eisenhauer EA. 1998. Phase I and II trials of novel anti-cancer agents: endpoints, efficacy and existentialism. Presented at the 10th NCI-EORTC Conference on New Drugs in Cancer Therapy, Amsterdam, June 16–19, 1998. *Ann Oncol* 9:1047–1052.

Fossella F, Pereira JR, von Pawel J, Pluzanska A, Gorbounova V, Kaukel E, Mattson KV, Ramlau R, Szczesna A, Fidias P, Millward M, Belani CP. 2003. Randomized, multinational, phase III study of docetaxel plus platinum combinations versus vinorelbine plus cisplatin for advanced non-small-cell lung cancer: the TAX 326 study group. *J Clin Oncol* 21:3016–3024.

Fox E, Curt GA, Balis FM. 2002. Clinical trial design for target-based therapy. *Oncologist* 7:401–409.

Freedman LS. 1982. Tables of the number of patients required in clinical trials using the logrank test. *Stat Med* 1:121–129.

Freidlin B, Simon R. 2005a. Adaptive signature design: an adaptive clinical trial design for generating and prospectively testing a gene expression signature for sensitive patients. *Clin Cancer Res* 11:7872–7878.

Freidlin B, Simon R. 2005b. Evaluation of randomized discontinuation design. *J Clin Oncol* 23:5094–5098.

Gail M. 1982. *Monitoring and Stopping Clinical Trials.* New York: Wiley.

Gehan EA,Tefft MC. 2000. Will there be resistance to the RECIST (response evaluation criteria in solid tumors)? *J Natl Cancer Inst* 92:179–181.

Gralla RJ, Thatcher N. 2004. Quality-of-life assessment in advanced lung cancer: considerations for evaluation in patients receiving chemotherapy. *Lung Cancer* 46(Suppl 2):S41–S47.

Gupta N, Price PM, Aboagye EO. 2002. PET for in vivo pharmacokinetic and pharmacodynamic measurements. *Eur J Cancer* 38:2094–2107.

Hageman D, Reeves D. 2001. Clinical trials in cancer. In: DeVita V, Hellman S, Rosenberg SA, eds. *Cancer: Principles and Practice of Oncology.* Philadelphia: Lippincott Williams & Wilkins, pp. 539–545.

International Committee of Medical Journal Editors. 1988. Uniform requirements for manuscripts submitted to biomedical journals. *Ann Intern Med* 108:258–265.

International Conference on Harmonisation of Technical Requirements for Registration of Pharmaceuticals for Human Use (ICH) adopts Consolidated Guideline on Good Clinical Practice in the Conduct of Clinical Trials on Medicinal Products for Human Use. 1997. *Int Dig Health Legis* 48:231–234.

Knatterud GL, Rockhold FW, George SL, Barton FB, Davis CE, Fairweather WR, Honohan T, Mowery R, O'Neill R. 1998. Guidelines for quality assurance in multicenter trials: a position paper. *Control Clin Trials* 19:477–493.

Korn EL, Arbuck SG, Pluda JM, Simon R, Kaplan RS, Christian MC. 2001. Clinical trial designs for cytostatic agents: Are new approaches needed? *J Clin Oncol* 19:265–272.

Lynch TJ, Bell DW, Sordella R, Gurubhagavatula S, Okimoto RA, Brannigan BW, Harris PL, Haserlat SM, Supko JG, Haluska FG, Louis DN, Christiani DC, et al. 2004. Activating mutations in the epidermal growth factor receptor underlying responsiveness of non-small-cell lung cancer to gefitinib. *N Engl J Med* 350:2129–2139.

McNeil C. 2006. Two targets, one drug for new EGFR inhibitors. *J Natl Cancer Inst* 98: 1102–1103.

Miller KD, Trigo JM, Wheeler C, Barge A, Rowbottom J, Sledge G, Baselga J. 2005. A multicenter phase II trial of ZD6474, a vascular endothelial growth factor receptor-2 and epidermal growth factor receptor tyrosine kinase inhibitor, in patients with previously treated metastatic breast cancer. *Clin Cancer Res* 11:3369–3376.

Paoletti X, Baron B, Schoffski P, Fumoleau P, Lacombe D, Marreaud S, Sylvester R. 2006. Using the continual reassessment method: lessons learned from an EORTC phase I dose finding study. *Eur J Cancer* 42:1362–1368.

Piantadosi S. 1988. Principles of clinical trial design. *Semin Oncol* 15:423–433.

Piantadosi S. 2004. Biostatistics for clinical trials. In: Abeloff, JS, Armitage JE, Niederhuber MB, Kastan I, McKenna WG, eds. *Clinical Oncology*. Philadelphia: Elsevier Churchill Livingstone. pp. 365–382.

Pocock S. 1996. *Clinical Trials: A Practical Approach.* New York: Wiley.

Ratain MJ, Stadler WM. 2001. Clinical trial designs for cytostatic agents. *J Clin Oncol* 19: 3154–3155.

Rosner GL, Stadler W, Ratain MJ. 2002. Randomized discontinuation design: application to cytostatic antineoplastic agents. *J Clin Oncol* 20:4478–4484.

Santoro E, Nicolis E, Franzosi MG, Tognoni G. 1999. Internet for clinical trials: past, present, and future. *Control Clin Trials* 20:194–201.

Schechter NR, Yang DJ, Azhdarinia A, Kohanim S, Wendt R 3rd, Oh CS, Hu M, Yu DF, Bryant J, Ang KK, Forster KM, Kim EE, et al. 2003. Assessment of epidermal growth factor receptor with ^{99m}Tc–ethylenedicysteine–C225 monoclonal antibody. *Anticancer Drugs* 14:49–56.

Schilsky RL. 2002. End points in cancer clinical trials and the drug approval process. *Clin Cancer Res* 8:935–938.

Schneiderman M. 1967. Mouse to man: statistical problems in bringing a drug to clinical trial. *Proceedings of the Fifth Berkeley Symposium on Mathematical Statistical Probability*, University of California, Berkeley, CA.

Simon R. 1986. Confidence intervals for reporting results of clinical trials. *Ann Intern Med* 105:429–435.

Simon R. 1989. Optimal two-stage designs for phase II clinical trials. *Control Clin Trials* 10:1–10.

Simon R. 2001. Clinical trials in cancer. In: DeVita V, Hellman S, Rosenberg, SA, eds. *Cancer: Principles and Practice of Oncology*. Philadelphia: Lippincott Williams & Wilkins, pp. 521–538.

Simon R, Maitournam A. 2004. Evaluating the efficiency of targeted designs for randomized clinical trials. *Clin Cancer Res* 10:6759–6763.

Simon R, Wittes RE, Ellenberg SS. 1985. Randomized phase II clinical trials. *Cancer Treat Rep* 69:1375–1381.

Simon R, Freidlin B, Rubinstein L, Arbuck SG, Collins J, Christian MC. 1997. Accelerated titration designs for phase I clinical trials in oncology. *J Natl Cancer Inst* 89:1138–1147.

Torri V, Simon R, Russek-Cohen E, Midthune D, Friedman M. 1992. Relationship between response and survival in patients with advanced ovarian cancer. *J Natl Cancer Inst* 84:899–900.

U.S. Food and Drug Administration. 1999. *Guidance for Industry: Computerized Systems Used in Clinical Trials.* Washington, DC: FDA.

Weiss GB, Bunce H, Hokanson JA. 1983. Comparing survival of responders and nonresponders after treatment: a potential source of confusion in interpreting cancer clinical trials. *Control Clin Trials* 4:43–52.

Wittes RE, Marsoni S, Simon R, Leyland-Jones B. 1985. The phase II trial. *Cancer Treat Rep* 69:1235–1239.

11

THE DEVELOPMENT OF DRUGS: CURRENT CONCEPTS AND ISSUES

Barry S. Komm

Wyeth Research, Collegeville, Pennsylvania

Christopher P. Miller

Radius Health, Cambridge, Massachusetts

INTRODUCTION

The development of new drugs is an evolving process that has accelerated dramatically over the last several years. There is an expectation that newer, innovative drugs will continue to become available. However, the drug development process is a complex, multifaceted procedure that is coupled with two important issues: It is time consuming and extraordinarily expensive. So, in fact, the appearance of new pharmaceutical entities of any significance does not occur at a very rapid rate. It is probably accurate to state that most end users of pharmaceuticals, whether the prescribing physician or the consumer, don't have a clear understanding of what needs to be accomplished to get a drug to the point where it is available commercially. In this chapter we describe the general process for the development of small-molecule pharmaceuticals. A number of the major points of emphasis also apply to other types of therapy, such as proteins or monoclonal antibodies.

The Biology and Treatment of Cancer: Understanding Cancer
Edited by Arthur B. Pardee and Gary S. Stein   Copyright © 2009 John Wiley & Sons, Inc.

THE COMPLEXITY OF DRUG DEVELOPMENT

The process associated with the development of a drug is tightly associated with the therapeutic area and specific target. Thus, the "rules" are not exact and all encompassing. Different regulatory requirements exist for the many therapeutic areas of research and development. For example, developing a drug for osteoporosis encounters a set of issues completely unrelated to developing a drug for the treatment of breast cancer. Of course, there are overlaps. Although questions are posed from the onset and there is constant review to ensure that the risk of failure is minimized as the process proceeds, it can never be totally eliminated.

The first question that needs to be posed is: What is the need for this drug? In fact, is there a need for another drug in the category? A basic tenet in drug development is that there is almost always room for improvement no matter what exists in the armamentarium. Very few drugs are free of side effects and tolerable for all who have it prescribed for them. In addition, we need to consider potency and, more important, efficacy when contemplating potential advantages for a proposed drug. In other words, is the drug proposed going to improve safety and/or efficacy in such a manner that its overall profile will be advantageous to at least some significant portion of the population? Using osteoporosis as an example, can we find something that will increase bone mass more effectively and/or more safely than that which exists? An extensive knowledge base of the potential is critical. But whether developing a compound targeting a new protein or channel versus an established one, there has to be tangible improvement, for even at the earliest step in drug development there is risk. There is a commitment of physical and human resources and, as stated above, that translates into a considerable monetary investment.

Although there are no specified guidelines for developing a drug, a generalized scheme reveals the complexity associated with drug development (small molecule). Developing drugs is an ordered process with many checkpoints set by both the group generating the new molecule and by the regulatory agencies which ultimately decide if that molecule qualifies to be used in humans and marketed. A somewhat abridged list of steps follows:

1. Disease or therapeutic area need
2. Target identification: basic science
3. Exploratory/discovery: pharmacology and medicinal chemistry
4. Pharmaceutical characterization: pharmacokinetics, metabolism, toxicology
5. Pharmaceutical processing: process chemistry, formulations, production
6. Regulatory filing [Initial New Drug Application (IND)]
7. Clinical evaluation: phase I (safety, PK), II (safety, proof of concept, efficacy), III (pivotal efficacy and safety)
8. Regulatory filing [New Drug Application (NDA)]

9. Launch and marketing
10. Postmarketing clinical evaluation (phase IV): new indications, safety surveillance

OBSTACLES IN THE INITIAL STAGES

As a lead molecule moves along the development pathway, hurdles are always in place. If the drug behaves appropriately, it moves along. Of course, this begets the question of what "appropriate" behavior is for the drug candidate in question. In this regard, the drug discovery team involved will often have set a predetermined benchmark to which they aspire. For an established area, they might compare to a drug already on the market. It may have been decided that improvements could be made that would allow a newer generation to displace or replace that which is currently used. It may also have been decided that the market is so large and the need so great that having more than one drug in the same category has appeal from different perspectives. Certainly, any new drug should be bringing something to the field that is not satisfied by what is already available. What does it take? In addition to the major driving factors already discussed, including better efficacy, safety, and/or tolerability, we may include ease of administration and convenience of dosing manner or schedule. James Black [7] is often quoted as saying: "The most fruitful basis for the discovery of a new drug is to start with an old drug." However, when new targets are identified, the process has to start from scratch. The final clinical endpoint may be the same if the therapeutic endpoint is the same (e.g., treatment of osteoporosis by a new mechanism), but the means to achieving that endpoint have changed with the expectation that the new drug will be "better" in some way. What are the reasons for new drugs failing during clinical evaluation? Safety is one important reason and may be the most difficult parameter to predict preclinically. The other common reason is insufficient efficacy, but that is often due to an inadequate pharmacology database and also that the preclinical assays, both in vitro and in vivo are not always capable of providing the necessary information to make the best, most well-informed decisions.

TARGET IDENTIFICATION

Once the need for a new therapeutic for a disease or symptom is rationalized, the first step is target identification. On the surface this may seem obvious, but in fact, it is not always that simple. What is known about the disease? What basic science has already been published? Are there new data illuminating how a particular pathway may be involved? These are just a few of the questions that can arise. Choosing a particular target will influence many steps in the development process.

How targets are defined and how many are out there are somewhat debatable at this time, since there are differing opinions. Recently [1] it was suggested that a target is "a molecular structure (chemically definable by at least a molecular mass) that will undergo a specific interaction with chemicals that we call drugs because they are administered to treat or diagnose a disease. The interaction has a connection with the clinical effect(s)." A list of potential targets can be generated, but the list can vary depending on the source. The following list conforms well to what are considered "drugable" classes of targets:

- Enzymes
- Protein substrates
- Receptors (nuclear and membrane)
- Channels
- Transporters
- Deoxyribonucleic acid (DNA)/ribonucleic acid (RNA)

The number of individual targets falling within the classes of targets represented by this list has been estimated to range from 120 to 14,000. Obviously, the way that an individual target is defined will affect what number is assigned [2–5], and a recent attempt to reconcile this arrived at 324 drug targets for all classes of approved therapeutic drugs, with the caveat that expansion will probably occur [6].

Targets such as nuclear receptors (e.g., estrogen receptor, glucocorticoid receptor) are well represented by drugs that interact and affect their activity, whereas others are not viewed as amenable to pharmacological intervention. Small molecules (typically, having molecular masses ≤ 500 dalton) have been shown to be capable of affecting some targets effectively, while others, such as nonreceptor protein substrates, are more reluctant. For many nonreceptor protein targets, the desired effect is the direct disruption of a protein–protein interaction. In this venue, antibody and protein therapeutics are much more likely than a small molecule to disrupt the targeted protein–protein interactions. Unlike small-molecule receptors that have conservatively evolved to bind small, endogenous ligands, many protein–protein interactions have no endogenous effector, and due to the size and strength of the protein–protein interface, only another protein is capable of interfering with that process. This one example of target choice illustrates how such a decision can ripple all the way through the research and development (R&D) infrastructure because it affects not only the basic discovery (chemistry, assay development, screening), but also formulation, production, toxicology testing, pharmacokinetic evaluation, and in fact, just about every decision downstream of it.

Whether the target is a nuclear receptor such as the estrogen receptor or an enzyme such as a kinase, it is critical not simply to test compound interaction with these proteins only. Rather, the determination of an interaction with the protein is really only the beginning of an evaluation of the potential drug candidate. Not only is compound cross-reactivity a serious concern early in the process, but often the subtle modulatory effects that a compound has on a target can only be appreciated when examining the drug's effects in vivo. For example, while a drug may demonstrate a certain effect on a given target in vitro (e.g., binding, inhibition), that effect may be very different in vivo when the target is in its native environment. Moreover, a given target may signal differently, depending on the tissue that expresses that target. Using the estrogen receptor as an example shows us that this receptor affects key proliferation signaling pathways in a number of tissues, most notably the uterine endometrium, but estrogens also affect osteoclast resorptive activity in the skeleton via a pathway distinct from proliferation. Kinases may phosphorylate a number of substrates, which demonstrates how difficult target selection can be since any one kinase whose activity is to be manipulated may affect many potential targets and, in turn, multiple pathways. Target specificity is a major stumbling block in drug development that is rigorously monitored. Yet it is often difficult to absolutely know where cross-reactivity or off-target effects are occurring, especially with protein kinase targets, which leads to many safety and tolerability issues, which unfortunately cannot be predicted accurately.

For these reasons, the importance of generating a reliable database characterizing the target and establishing a clear biological role in the physiological process that is to be affected by a small molecule, protein, or nucleic acid cannot be overemphasized. The basic science portion of the development process often requires a substantial period of time to obtain enough reliable data to transition forward to the next step. During this target confirmation timeframe, at least one assay has to be developed that will be used to identify compounds that interact with and/or affect the target appropriately. For small molecules (classic pharmaceutical) this step is usually a high-throughput chemical library screen (HTS), but often these can be focused on a specifically identified group of compounds that are predicted to be likely candidates to interact with the target. It is during this phase that chemistry and biology merge. The chemists categorize the compounds or hits from the HTS based on their chemical structure and search for compounds with similar structural characteristics. This step usually aims to identify two or more series of compounds (chemically distinct) based on their chemical attractiveness, predicted metabolism, and so on.

SAR AND ANIMAL TESTING

The "discovery" phase of the process can last for one to two years (sometimes more) where the chemists structurally modify lead compounds based on feedback from the key biological assays to find out what works best and, just as important, what does not. This is structure–activity relationship (SAR) testing and key to the development of as potent and efficacious a small molecule as possible.

As SAR testing proceeds, lead molecules need to be tested in relevant animal models to determine efficacy and potency under real physiological conditions versus in vitro testing, which, in reality, only aids in prioritizing what compounds move on to animal evaluation. It is also at this point where pharmacokinetic evaluation begins. A number of other activities also take place during this stage of lead compound development. Chemical analysis is always occurring to assess stability, solubility, and other relevant chemical characteristics. In vitro metabolic evaluation provides an early signal for potential metabolic toxicology issues, such as unacceptably high cytochrome activation. Severe limitations are placed on these parameters and become important criteria in prioritization (i.e., which compound should be tested in vivo). They also provide vital feedback to chemists as they seek to improve on the chemical and pharmaceutical properties of the lead series of compounds.

There is a definite limitation on the number of compounds that can be evaluated in vivo, and the type of in vivo model is an important factor in determining the testing throughput. For example, a one-day rapid response in vivo assay versus a chronic dosing model will determine not only the quantities of compound that have to be produced but the number of assays that need to be set up and run simultaneously. Initial in vivo evaluation of a compound most often utilizes broad dose–response regimens to identify the appropriate amount of compound required to achieve efficacy. Ultimately, the goal is to determine the lowest efficacious dosage, but especially in the beginning, relatively high doses may be required to reveal any detectable effect. As the potency of a chemical series is improved, lower doses become feasible. What this implies is that at least in the early stages, the chemists may have to generate relatively large amounts of material, which may sound simple enough, but in fact, depending on the synthetic pathway, can be quite demanding from time, ease of production, and cost of goods considerations. Production of grams versus milligrams of a compound can require a huge change in tactics, so appropriate selection of in vivo models as well as the compounds to go into those models must be made with some care.

What happens to the compound once it is administered to an animal, and by what routes can the compound be delivered? In today's world a successful pharmaceutical is generally orally administrable; however, that does not mean alternative routes of administration are unacceptable. There are many cases, especially with cancer therapeutics and antibiotics, where direct intravenous and intraarterial routes are utilized. However, additional questions must still be addressed. For example, what is the metabolic fate of the compound? Is it rapidly excreted; is it biotransformed into other molecules that have biologic activity; does it accumulate in a particular tissue; is it unable to penetrate the central nervous system; does it bind to proteins in the blood? All of these questions impact dosing and formulation decisions. What is absolutely crucial is that sufficient drug be delivered to the target (absolute bioavailability) to elicit the intended response (e.g., efficacious).

On top of these questions, determining if the drug does anything harmful that would not be predicted based on its mechanism of action is critical. How much drug can an animal tolerate before toxicological signals reveal themselves? A safety window has to be determined. An effective dose would have been determined by this time in one or two animal models and then multiples have to be evaluated to determine the margin of safety. It is at this step where many drugs fail. What is not seen in a rat or mouse efficacy model will often present itself in rodent toxicology studies or when testing occurs in a higher species, such as dogs or nonhuman primates. With efficacy models, investigators are usually not looking for adverse effects or they simply don't occur during the treatment timeframe. Chronic dosing with multiples of the efficacious dosage are carefully staged and evaluated because any toxicologic signal can and often does lead to a critical safety review and termination of the project. The final decision has much to do with the therapeutic endpoint associated with the drug. Stringent requirements are in place for all compounds, yet a drug being developed for certain cancers may be less stringently held to certain guidelines than perhaps a drug for osteoporosis. Nevertheless, the crossbar is set high for all new drugs, because safety is paramount.

CLINICAL EVALUATION

If all boxes are checked up to this point, an IND is filed with the U.S. Food and Drug Administration (FDA) and other documents are filed with regulatory agencies globally. This is the first step prior to the initiation of human testing. In most cases, clinical evaluation is divided into three phases. Phase I is done in steps and normally includes a single ascending dose (1 day of drug) and multiple ascending dose studies (>1 day of drug). These studies provide the pharmacokinetic data necessary to determine dosage for future trials. Often, although usually not required, some pharmacodynamic endpoint is also measured to ensure that the drug is interacting with and affecting its intended target and to record at what dose that interaction is occurring (detectable). The endpoint may be a marker or some simple physiological response and not necessarily the full clinical effect. Phase I trials are usually not more than a few weeks, and many drugs have to be taken for longer periods to demonstrate efficacy. Safety and side effect profiles begin to develop during phase I.

Phase II is proof-of-concept testing. The studies utilize the target population (i.e., if an osteoporosis drug, it would be men or women with a low skeletal mass at risk of fracture), whereas in phase I that is often not the case, since efficacy is not the primary goal. Phase II recruits larger numbers of people and assesses multiple dosages. It is during this stage that the effective dosages are identified. It is in phase II that most compounds meet their demise. In fact, this has stimulated a concerted effort in the pharmaceutical industry to address this problem, determine its cause, and provide potential solutions.

The last stage in clinical evaluation is phase III. This is the pivotal trial, examining the effective dosage in a large population. Like the other phases, safety assessment is central, since efficacy has putatively been established in phase II (albeit usually in a smaller population for a shorter period of time). Drugs that reach phase III are less likely to fail than at any other time during the development process, yet failures still occur and at an alarmingly high rate.

Success in phase III leads to filing a New Drug Application (NDA) in the United States along with similar applications in Europe, Canada, and the rest of the world. The documents are often millions of pages in length, and normal review in the United States takes 10 to 12 months. During that time there is constant communication between the drugmaker and the federal regulatory agency to which the application was submitted. At 10 months the FDA will normally issue a nonapprovable, approvable, or approved letter. If approvable, more information or data may be required prior to final approval. With approval, launch of the drug to the market follows shortly thereafter.

In 2006 the average time for a drug to be developed was approximately 15 years [8]. The bulk of that time is usually spent in clinical trials, but that can vary depending on the clinical endpoints being measured. For example, a drug for the treatment of osteoporosis requires a three-year in-life study (regulatory requirement measured against placebo) with a large sample size because of the rarity of events being measured (spontaneous osteoporosis-related fracture), whereas a pivotal hot-flash trial in postmenopausal women would be 12 weeks in duration. Since each woman in the hot-flash trial is symptomatic, the sample size required is relatively low (hundreds versus 1500 to 2000 for the osteoporosis treatment trial). Trials end with the last patient visit, and because patients are recruited over a time period that can be several years in duration, a three-year-in-life study can cover five to eight years when recruiting is calculated into the equation. The simple diagram in Figure 1 illustrates the basic drug development process that has been discussed.

The costs associated with this process average between $1 billion and $1.5 billion, but that estimate can vary depending on the therapeutic endpoint intended. Perhaps it is also important to keep in perspective that there are significantly more failures than successes. Only about 10% of the drugs that reach phase I achieve FDA approval despite much more stringent testing preclinically [9]. Most compounds never exit exploratory/discovery into the later development stages. The frightening 50% failure rate for compounds in phase III has gained the attention of the FDA, which has recently issued action items with the goal of reducing the attrition of new drugs in clinical trials [10].

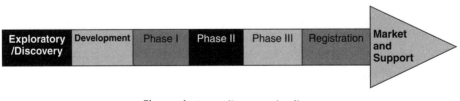

Figure 1. Drug discovery timeline.

Where drug discovery will head in this new century is difficult to predict, especially based on the technologic whirlwind that has already begun and will no doubt continue. High-throughput screening has become an overnight process where, depending on the assay, a million compounds may be assayed rapidly, whereas 10 years ago it could take a year to screen 50,000. Translational medicine is beginning to become a standard component of the drug development process. Although it is too early to measure its impact, conceptually it should improve the success rate of drugs entering clinical trials and streamline the process of efficacy evaluation in the early clinical phases [11]. Many drug discovery gurus suggest that the "low-hanging fruit" has been picked and new drugs are going to become more and more difficult to generate. Potentially, combined pharmaceutical treatment regimes may be the way to address this. Many drugs target similar clinical endpoints, yet achieve efficacy via different mechanisms. A good example of this being used successfully is with combinations of drugs used to treat a variety of cancers [12].

SUMMARY

The drug development process is a protracted, sequential series of steps, culminating in a product that achieves a clinical benefit. The hurdles are high and the regulations are stringent. Importantly, innovations in science and technology coupled with process management should ensure that we continue to see improvements in therapeutics and perhaps cures for some diseases. The clear goal is that application of new technology will address the critical issues of how long it will require to generate these new drugs and the costs associated with their production, because there will always be a need.

REFERENCES

1. Imming P, Sinning C, Meyer A. 2006. Drugs, their targets and the nature and number of drug targets. *Nat Rev Drug Discov* 5:821–834.
2. Drews J. 1996. Genomic sciences and the medicine of tomorrow. *Nat Biotechnol* 14:1516–1518.
3. Drews J, Ryser S. 1997. Classic drug targets. *Nat Biotechnol* 15:1318–1319.
4. Golden JB. 2003. Prioritizing the human genome: knowledge management in drug discovery. *Curr Opin Drug Discov Dev* 6:310–316.
5. Wishart DS, Knox C, Guo AC, Shrivastava S, Hassanali M, Stothard P, Chang Z, Woolsey J. 2006. DrugBank: a comprehensive resource for in silico drug discovery and exploration. *Nucleic Acids Res* 43:D668–D672.
6. Overington JP, Al-Lazikani B, Hopkins AL. 2006. How many drugs targets are there? *Nat Rev Drug Discov* 5:993–996.
7. Raju TN. 2000. The Nobel chronicles. *Lancet* 355:1022.

8. DiMasi JA, Hansen RW, Grabowski HG. 2003. The price of innovation: new estimates of drug development costs. *J Health Econ* 22:151–185.

9. Kola I, Landis J. 2004. Can the pharmaceutical industry reduce attrition rates? *Nat Rev Drug Discov* 3:711–715.

10. Woosley RL, Cossman J. 2007. Drug development and the FDA's critical path initiative. *Clin Pharmacol Ther* 81:129–133.

11. Wagner JA, Williams SA, Webster CJ. 2007. Biomarkers and surrogate end points for fit-for-purpose development and regulatory evaluation of new drugs. *Clin Pharmacol Ther* 81:104–107.

12. Dancey JE, Chen HX. 2006. Strategies for optimizing combinations of molecularly targeted anticancer agents. *Nat Rev Drug Discov* 5:649–659.

12

A NEW GENERATION OF DRUGS IN CANCER TREATMENT: MOLECULARLY TARGETED THERAPIES

Thomas O'Hare and Christopher A. Eide

Howard Hughes Medical Institute, Oregon Health & Science University Cancer Institute, Portland, Oregon

Michael W. Deininger

Oregon Health & Science University, Center for Hematologic Malignancies, Portland, Oregon

INTRODUCTION

Do we know, at the beginning of the twenty-first century, how to cure cancer? Unfortunately, in many cases the answer is no. However, much has changed over the past decade. The discovery and clinical validation of imatinib (Gleevec), a molecularly targeted therapy for chronic myeloid leukemia (CML), has fundamentally redirected drug discovery efforts. In this chapter we focus on kinase inhibitors as molecularly targeted therapeutics, with CML as the paradigm. Targeted therapies taking clinical ground in other cancers are then explored, illustrating the rich potential, as well as obstacles and complexities encountered, in developing new inhibitor treatments.

Whereas the results in CML continue to exceed expectations, experiences in other malignancies have been mixed and sometimes quite sobering. Thus, is CML the exception or the rule, and is the success of targeted therapies limited by the disease or by our incomplete knowledge of disease pathobiochemistry? In the continuing search for improved targeted therapies, deducing a molecular explanation for why some inhibitors have shown limited activity will be as important as understanding why imatinib works in CML. Another important question arising from the CML field is whether imatinib will ever be able to eradicate the disease. Reverse transcriptase–polymerase chain reaction (RT-PCR) data suggest that most patients continue to harbor residual leukemia on therapy, and recurrence is the rule once the drug is discontinued, indicating the persistence of stem cells with full leukemogenic potential. What, then, is the underlying cause of disease persistence, and is it a natural limitation of targeted therapy, implying that life-long therapy is necessary? The answers will have ramifications that reach beyond the laboratory and the doctor's office into the economics of health care.

The field of molecular cancer therapy has expanded so rapidly over the past several years that comprehensive coverage would require an entire book or more. Thus, choices had to be made for this chapter. Significant attention will be given to CML, acknowledging its paradigmatic role for the development of targeted cancer therapies. In the following sections we cover HER2 in breast cancer and EGFR in non-small-cell lung cancer, targets in diseases whose incidence by far exceeds that of CML. The last three sections have been chosen to highlight certain aspects of targeted therapy. BRAF mutations are very frequent in melanoma, yet the limited clinical success of a targeted BRAF inhibitor attests to the complexity of this malignant signaling cascade. JAK2 in the chronic myeloproliferative disorders looks like a perfect target, but the key mutations in this kinase were discovered quite recently, and development of effective inhibitors has just begun. Finally, the activity of a thalidomide analog in myelodysplastic syndromes with a deletion of 5q is a prime example of a drug that is certain to hit a specific target or target pathway, although identifying this pathway is proving to be extremely challenging.

INHIBITING BCR–ABL IN CML: THE GOLD STANDARD OF MOLECULARLY TARGETED THERAPY

Chronic myeloid leukemia is a rare disease, yet has had a profound impact on the development of modern cancer therapy. In 1960, Nowell and Hungerford reported the consistent detection of a shortened chromosome 22, termed the Philadelphia chromosome (Ph), in bone marrow metaphases from CML patients (Figure 1). Thirteen years later, Janet Rowley deduced that this chromosomal anomaly is the product of a reciprocal translocation between chromosomes 9 and 22. The next decade saw the identification of the translocation partners fused by the t(9;22) as *Abl* and *Bcr*, the discovery that the chimeric protein derived from the fusion gene has constitutive tyrosine kinase activity, and confirmation that this activity is

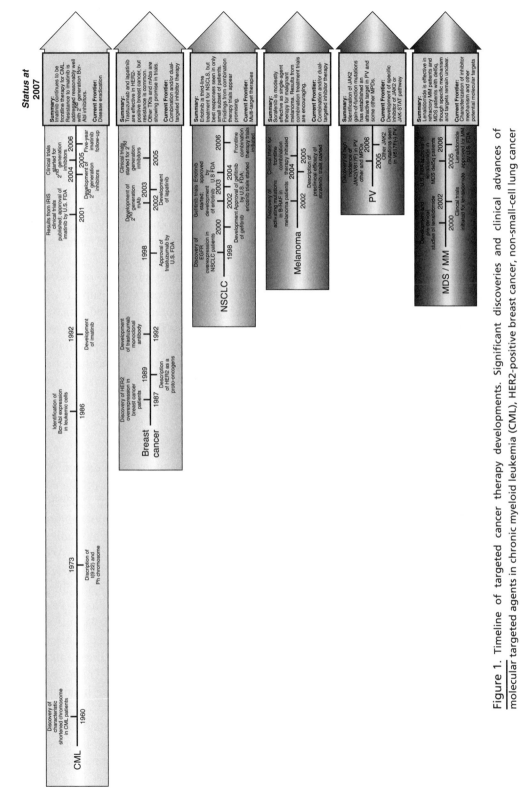

Figure 1. Timeline of targeted cancer therapy developments. Significant discoveries and clinical advances of molecular targeted agents in chronic myeloid leukemia (CML), HER2-positive breast cancer, non-small-cell lung cancer (NSCLC), melanoma, polycythemia vera (PV), and myelodysplastic syndromes (MDS) are displayed chronologically, and progress as of 2007 is summarized for comparison.

absolutely required for malignant transformation. When a murine CML model recapitulated the disease in vivo, the notion took hold that inhibiting Bcr–Abl tyrosine kinase activity could, in principle, be an effective therapy. It took many years of dedicated collaborative effort to convert this concept into reality, but the results were dramatic. Imatinib was granted regulatory approval within four years of its inception in the clinic, an unprecedented pace for a cancer drug. It has become an icon for the potential of targeted cancer therapy, but has also shown some of its limitations.

Imatinib is a selective but not completely specific inhibitor of Bcr–Abl, the deregulated, constitutively activated tyrosine kinase that drives CML. Despite a long-standing recognition of Bcr–Abl as perhaps the most obvious and attractive target in all of oncology, academic researchers and the pharmaceutical industry have, until recently, steered clear of most targets belonging to the kinase class of enzymes. This would appear to be a prudent business decision, given the practical obstacles involved in differentiating individual kinases or even small subsets of kinases. Despite the success of imatinib and several other targeted kinase inhibitors, a frank assessment must admit that we are still not very good at designing highly selective kinase inhibitors. However, the lessons learned from the design and clinical development of imatinib and from the extensive mechanistic research on resistance to imatinib are now being applied to other cancers.

Development of Imatinib

In the late 1980s, scientists at Ciba-Geigy (now Novartis) under the direction of Nick Lydon and Alois Matter, initiated a drug discovery program that produced imatinib (Figure 2A), a micromolar inhibitor of Abl, ARG, Kit, and PDGFR (activity against LCK and FMS was discovered later). Imatinib does not inhibit Src, which is closely related to Abl kinase, which was surprising and not readily explicable. The mystery was solved at least partially when the crystal structure of Abl in complex with a close analog of imatinib [1] and subsequently imatinib itself [2] demonstrated that the inhibitor captured Abl in a unique conformation (Figure 2B), effectively "freezing" the kinase in a catalytically inactive state. Additional key observations from the structural analysis were the extensive downward displacement of the ATP binding loop upon imatinib binding and the extensive surface contact between imatinib and the catalytic groove of the kinase via hydrogen bonds and hydrophobic interactions. Although the structural data were initially more of theoretical interest, they would later prove instrumental for understanding imatinib resistance due to Bcr-Abl point mutations.

In the initial phase I study, patients with chronic-phase CML who had failed interferon-α (IFN-α)–based therapy were treated with imatinib. Nearly all patients treated with at least 300 mg of imatinib daily attained a complete hematologic response (CHR), and 31% attained a major cytogenetic response (MCR) [3]. Based on the efficacy in this population, the trial was expanded to include patients

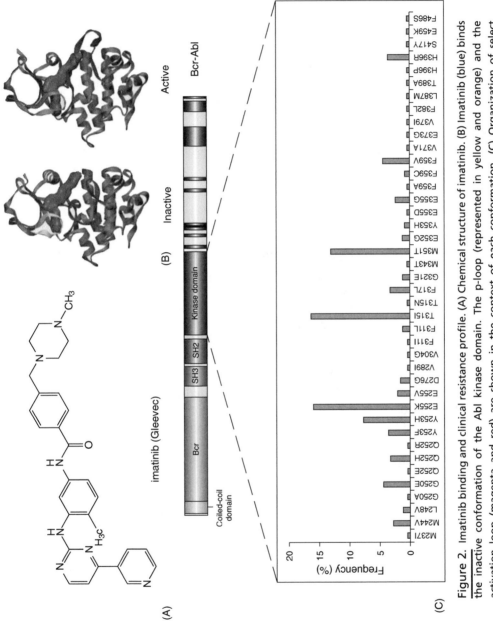

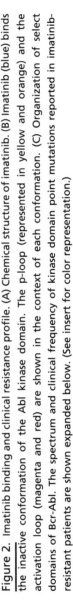

Figure 2. Imatinib binding and clinical resistance profile. (A) Chemical structure of imatinib. (B) Imatinib (blue) binds the inactive conformation of the Abl kinase domain. The p-loop (represented in yellow and orange) and the activation loop (magenta and red) are shown in the context of each conformation. (C) Organization of select domains of Bcr-Abl. The spectrum and clinical frequency of kinase domain point mutations reported in imatinib-resistant patients are shown expanded below. (See insert for color representation.)

with accelerated or blastic phase or with Ph-positive acute lymphoblastic leukemia (ALL). Substantial activity was demonstrated in these cohorts, but unfortunately, many responses were short-lived. A series of phase II trials confirmed the impressive activity seen in the phase I trial, with 41% of patients with chronic-phase CML attaining a complete cytogenetic response (CCR) [3–6]. Based on the phase I/II results, imatinib was approved for the treatment of CML after failure of IFN-α. The superiority of imatinib over the previous standard drug therapy for CML was established in a phase III study in newly diagnosed chronic-phase patients (IRIS trial) [7]. Imatinib produced much higher rates of CHR and CCR as well as superior progression-free survival than those of the previous standard therapy of IFN-α plus cytarabine. A recent update of the IRIS trial at five years of follow-up showed a cumulative CCR rate of 87% and projected overall survival and event-free survival rates of 89% and 83%, respectively, for patients treated initially with imatinib [8].

Imatinib Resistance

Resistance to imatinib is classified as primary if the response target (e.g., CHR) is not achieved upon starting therapy, while secondary (acquired) resistance implies failure after a transient response. Most chronic-phase patients attain profound and durable responses, while primary and secondary resistance is common in patients with blast crisis. The crucial observation from the first study of patients with acquired resistance was that Bcr-Abl signal transduction was suppressed during response but reactivated at the time of relapse. Thus, rather than shifting to a different transforming principle, the leukemia cells continued to be dependent on the activity of Bcr-Abl, consistent with "oncogene addiction" and implying that Bcr-Abl remained an excellent therapeutic target.

Mechanisms of Bcr-Abl–dependent resistance include increased protein expression due to gene amplification or transcriptional activation and point mutations in the kinase domain (KD) of Bcr-Abl that impair drug binding. More than 60 different mutations in the KD of Bcr-Abl have been described in patients with imatinib resistance (Figure 2C), representing the most common resistance mechanism. Mutations cause resistance by (1) altering contact residues and impairing imatinib binding through steric hindrance and/or elimination of important hydrogen bonds or hydrophobic interactions; (2) preventing the kinase from assuming the optimal conformation in regions that undergo extensive conformational adjustments upon drug binding; or (3) favoring the active conformation of the kinase, to which imatinib is unable to bind. Mutational hotspots include the ATP binding loop, threonine 315, methionine 351, and the activation loop. Some mutants, such as E255K and T315I, are completely resistant to imatinib; others, such as M244V and M351T, exhibit a moderate level of resistance, and yet others, such as F311L, are barely distinguishable from native Bcr-Abl. A clinical consequence of the differential imatinib sensitivity is that responses may be recaptured by dose escalation in the case of low-level resistance mutations, while this is ineffective in patients with highly resistant mutations.

Several lines of evidence indicate that many KD mutations pre-date imatinib therapy and are then selected in the presence of drug. In some patients who relapsed with specific KD mutations, the same mutation type was detected in pre-therapeutic specimens using allele-specific PCR [9]. A similar study detected KD mutations in 20% of imatinib-naive patients with advanced CML, but not in patients with chronic phase disease [10]. Surprisingly, not all mutant clones "grew out" upon subsequent imatinib therapy, suggesting that some clones lack other crucial properties required to sustain leukemic hematopoiesis. For example, they may reside in cell clones lacking self-renewal capacity. Data from the IRIS trial also support the notion of the preexistence of mutations [8]. The rate of imatinib failure peaked in the second year of therapy, but decreased in every subsequent year, consistent with the manifestation of a preexisting condition that predisposes to relapse. A strong association between mutations detected and clonal cytogenetic evolution has also been demonstrated in CML, suggesting that the general genetic instability of Bcr-Abl–expressing cells underlies both phenomena. There is increasingly convincing evidence that Bcr-Abl induces self–mutagenesis through generation of reactive oxygen species and that this mechanism is a key to the development of resistance [11,12]. The clinical implications are that (1) complete inhibition of Bcr-Abl should conceivably reduce the mutation risk of an individual cell; (2) a more rapid reduction of the leukemic burden should decrease the number of cells at risk of acquiring mutations; and (3) Abl kinase inhibitors with a broader spectrum of activity should prevent progression in patients who already harbor mutations and are likely to fail on imatinib.

Second-Generation Abl Kinase Inhibitors

The identification of KD mutations as a mechanism of resistance to imatinib therapy prompted the development of additional agents that maintain activity against mutant Bcr-Abl (Table 1). The most important compounds to date are the dual Abl/Src inhibitor dasatinib (Sprycel) [13,14], the only second-line inhibitor that has already been granted regulatory approval for imatinib-resistant and imatinib-intolerant CML and nilotinib (Tasigna) [15,16], which is derived from the 2-phenylaminopyrimidine backbone of imatinib. Nilotinib has been approved in Switzerland and is likely to be approved by the U.S. Food and Drug Administration (FDA) in the near future.

Crystal structure analysis has revealed that dasatinib, unlike imatinib, binds an active conformation of Abl, makes less surface contact, and causes less dramatic structural rearrangements of the ATP binding loop [17]. As a result of these less stringent requirements for binding, dasatinib inhibits native Bcr-Abl but also most KD mutants in the low-nanomolar range. Conversely, the binding mode of nilotinib is nearly identical to that of imatinib, but an improved topological fit within its

TABLE 1. Summary of Clinical and Investigational-Targeted Agents in Various Cancers

Malignancy	Targeted Agent	Chemical Structure	Type of Agent	Main Kinase Targets	Stage of Development	Other Malignancies Possibly Targeted by this Agent
CML	imatinib (Gleevec)		TKI	Abl, Kit, PDGFR	Phase I/II/III, FDA approval	Ph+ ALL, GIST, HES
	nilotinib (Tasigna)		TKI	Abl, Kit, PDGFR	Phase I/II	Ph+ ALL, GIST, HES
	dasatinib (Sprycel)		TKI	Abl, Src	Phase I/II, FDA approval	Ph+ ALL,
HER2-Positive Breast Cancer	trastuzumab (Herceptin)	(Cho et al. 2003, *Nature*)	mAb	HER2	Phase I/II/III, FDA approval	
	pertuzumab (Omnitarg)	(Franklin et al. 2004, *Cancer Cell*)	mAb	HER2	Phase I/II	

NSCLC	lapatinib (Tykerb)	TKI	EGFR, HER2	Phase I/II/III, FDA approval	
	gefitinib (Iressa)	TKI	EGFR	Phase I/II	Colorectal cancer
	erlotinib (Tarceva)	TKI	EGFR	Phase I/II/III, FDA approval	Colorectal cancer
	EKB-569	TKI	EGFR	Phase I/II	Colorectal cancer
	HKI-272	TKI	EGFR, HER2	Phase I/II	

(continued)

TABLE 1. (Continued)

Malignancy	Targeted Agent	Chemical Structure	Type of Agent	Main Kinase Targets	Stage of Development	Other Malignancies Possibly Targeted by this Agent
Melanoma	sorafenib (Nexavar)		TKI	BRAF	Phase I/II	
	SB-590885		TKI	BRAF		
	RAF265		TKI	BRAF, VEGF		
PV	TG101209		TKI	JAK2	Pre-clinical	ET, IMF, CMML
MDS / MM	lenalidomide (Revlimid)		Thalidomide analog		Unknown	Phase I/II

binding site on Abl results in a 30-fold increase in potency compared to imatinib, bringing most KD mutants within the reach of nilotinib (achievable plasma concentration about 1.7 μM). Neither nilotinib nor dasatinib have activity against the T315I mutant.

Dasatinib and nilotinib have shown significant activity in imatinib-resistant or imatinib-intolerant patients in phase I and II studies [14,15,18]. Most patients treated in the chronic phase achieved or maintained a CHR. CCRs were observed in approximately 30% of patients, and although the follow-up is still short, most chronic-phase responses appear durable. Significant activity was also seen in accelerated phase and blast crisis, in particular with dasatinib [19–21], where the rates of CCR exceeded those seen in the early imatinib studies. Unfortunately, in blast-crisis patients there is a considerable rate of primary resistance and a high rate of relapse. Analysis of patients who relapsed after a transient response to dasatinib revealed that acquired resistance is due almost exclusively to a few types of KD mutations, most importantly, T315I.

Predicting Drug Resistance

Several assays have been developed to predict resistance profiles for inhibitors in vitro. The common principle is selection of cells expressing KD mutant Bcr-Abl in the presence of inhibitors, with or without a preceding mutagenesis step to increase the frequency of KD mutations. Demonstrating the ability to recapitulate the spectrum of clinical mutations conferring resistance to imatinib has validated this approach. Compared to imatinib, the spectrum of mutations predicted to confer resistance to Abl/Src inhibitors such as dasatinib was much smaller and limited essentially to mutations of direct contact points [22,23]. This is being confirmed by the emerging clinical data [14]. In vitro, at high concentrations of dasatinib, only T315I was recovered. Combinations of dasatinib and nilotinib were able to eliminate non-T315I resistance at lower concentrations of either agent [22]. These data suggest that addition of a targeted T315I inhibitor may be able to block resistance completely due to KD mutations. Short of eradicating the disease, this may be the natural limit of any therapy directed against Bcr-Abl kinase activity.

Is CML Eradication Possible Using Abl Inhibitors?

Given the excellent results of imatinib in patients with chronic-phase CML, it will be difficult to demonstrate superiority of an alternative drug in endpoints such as overall and event-free survival. The generally good tolerability of imatinib will also hold any new agent to high standards in terms of side effects. An advance that remains on the horizon, however, would be the ability to stop therapy altogether. Experience with imatinib suggests that almost all patients who stop therapy will have a recurrence of disease, even if they had achieved negativity by RT-PCR. Thus, although undetectable with the most sensitive techniques, fully leukemogenic Bcr-Abl–positive cells persist, ready to reconstitute the leukemic cell clone as soon as Bcr-Abl is reactivated. Ex vivo studies on primitive hematopoietic progenitors suggest that noncycling Bcr-Abl–positive cells survive or are even enriched and maintain significant kinase activity in the presence of imatinib and, to a lesser extent, dasatinib [24]. This raises a question as to whether drug transporters may be causative to disease persistence via eliminating imatinib from the target cells, although the data are conflicting. Studies from several labs have shown that high levels of hOCT-1, a transporter that mediates imatinib influx, correlate with cytogenetic response (reviewed by Jiang et al. [25]). Whether this mechanism operates at the stem cell level is presently unknown.

The other possibility is that CML stem cells do not require Bcr-Abl kinase activity for their survival, and inhibiting Bcr-Abl may convert them into phenotypically normal cells that depend on exogenous signals such as GM-CSF signaling with STAT5 and MAP kinase activation. In the case of Bcr-Abl–independent disease persistence, disease eradication with imatinib and in fact all other Bcr-Abl inhibitors would be impossible unless the leukemia stem cell pool were gradually to be depleted by continuous long-term therapy. The fact that the mean Bcr-Abl transcript levels continue to decrease in the IRIS cohorts lends some support to this hypothesis, and one might expect that a more potent inhibitor will expedite the process. If this is not the case, eradicating CML will require therapies that target properties of CML stem cells other than Bcr-Abl kinase. At this point we can only speculate what such properties might be. It also remains to be determined whether disease persistence will be a general phenomenon of kinase-targeted therapies in other diseases. Given that CML has so often established the paradigm, there seems a real possibility that this will be the case. It is important to remember that discussing disease eradication with a well-tolerated oral agent is a luxury that would have been unthinkable less than a decade ago.

The case for targeting certain tyrosine kinases in human cancer is based on their central roles in regulating multiple cellular processes that contribute to tumor development and progression. If a cancer can be shown to be driven by an activated kinase, it should in principle be possible to inhibit or reverse malignant progression. The ongoing clinical validation of imatinib as a targeted drug that inhibits the action of a pathogenic tyrosine kinase has shone light on several key issues. A molecular understanding of CML facilitates the treatment of appropriately selected patients, and new compounds that circumvent acquired resistance have been developed. We now know that tyrosine kinase inhibitors have the potential to be safe, active drugs in selected patient populations. We also know that the therapeutic approach must be tailored to the molecular roots of disease. So, can the paradigm of imatinib be extended? We are still learning, but the following examples highlight the progress and challenges that this approach has yielded in other cancers.

Targeting HER2-Positive Breast Cancer

Unlike CML, breast cancer encompasses several malignancies, and the specific molecular characteristics of disease influence treatment decisions significantly. Expression of the receptor tyrosine kinase HER2 above an empirically derived threshold classifies a tumor as HER2-positive and is an indicator of poor prognosis. On a more positive note, HER2 status has proven to be an excellent molecular marker for selecting proper patient populations for clinical trials [26]. This is in contrast to EGFR overexpression in NSLC (discussed below), which is not a sufficient criterion for linking patient selection and response to inhibitor therapy. Approximately 25% of primary breast cancers are classified as HER2-positive.

HER2 belongs to the human epidermal growth factor receptor (HER) family of transmembrane receptor tyrosine kinases, which also includes EGFR (HER1), HER3, and HER4, all of which play prominent but incompletely understood roles in cancer. HER family members interact in homo- and heterodimeric kinase-active complexes. HER2 is unique in that its extracellular domain is truncated and does not interact directly with receptor ligands. Instead, HER2 is the preferred dimerization partner for all other HER receptors. The extracellular domain of HER2 exhibits a constitutive dimerization-competent conformation resembling the ligand-activated state of EGFR and HER3. Coupling with HER2 potently enhances signaling by HER2-containing heterodimers and increases binding affinity of receptor ligands to EGFR and HER3/4 [26]. HER2/3 heterodimers comprise the most potent mitogenic and transforming receptor complex within the HER family, and this oncogenic unit is a key driver of breast tumor cell proliferation (Figure 3).

An attractive targeting approach would be to interrupt the ability of HER2 to engage other HER members in heterodimeric complexes. Trastuzumab (Herceptin) is an FDA-approved humanized monoclonal antibody (mAb) against HER2

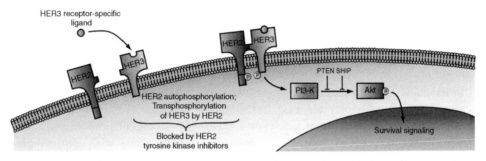

Figure 3. HER2 dimerization and downstream signaling. HER2 readily homo- and heterodimerizes with other HER family members, leading to phosphorylation of the intracellular tyrosine kinase domain. Autophosphorylation of HER2 leads to transphosphorylation of HER3 (which has a receptor-specific ligand but lacks a tyrosine kinase domain), which in turn activates the PI3-K/Akt pathway and promotes survival. Residual signaling through this pathway may serve as an escape mechanism to current HER2-targeted therapies.

that has been in clinical use for some time (Figure 1). The antibody inhibits the growth of HER2-overexpressing cells by binding to the unique extracellular juxtamembrane domain of the HER2 receptor and preventing activation of its intracellular tyrosine kinase. Laboratory data and evidence from clinical trials support several mechanisms to explain its specific route to decreasing subsequent cascade signaling [26].

Early clinical trials of trastuzumab demonstrated modest overall response rates in patients with previously treated HER2-positive metastatic breast cancer, ranging from 11 to 26%, but established a proof of principle for its potential efficacy in a subset of patients. The most pivotal results to date, however, support the clinical use of trastuzumab in combination with paclitaxel or docetaxel chemotherapy, where improved rates of response, overall survival, and progression-free survival have been observed compared to chemotherapy alone [27]. Despite the encouraging nature of these results, the majority of patients who show an initial benefit from regimens containing trastuzumab become resistant within one year of starting therapy. Unfortunately, the mechanisms of resistance to trastuzumab are not currently well understood. The second-generation HER2-targeted mAb pertuzumab (Omnitarg) was developed as a dimerization inhibitor mAb targeting EGFR/HER2 and HER2/3 receptor heterodimerization (Table 1). Several phase II clinical trials are currently under way, including an investigation into the effect of combining trastuzumab and pertuzumab in HER2-positive metastatic breast cancer that had progressed during trastuzumab therapy.

A more recent approach to addressing trastuzumab resistance in HER2-positive patients has been through the development of small-molecule tyrosine kinase inhibitors of HER receptors. Among the compounds in development are lapatinib (Tykerb), a dual EGFR/HER2 inhibitor, and CI-1033, which inhibits all members of the HER receptor family (Table 1). Lapatinib has been approved (March 2007) by the FDA for use in patients with HER2-positive metastatic breast cancer who have failed conventional chemotherapy combined with trastuzumab. Lapatinib acts by potently and reversibly inhibiting the intracellular tyrosine kinase activity of both EGFR and HER2 (IC_{50} for purified enzymes: 10.2 and 8.9 nM, respectively), and it has been demonstrated to have a slower off-rate than similar agents, allowing for prolonged inhibition of HER receptor tyrosine phosphorylation in tumor cells [28]. Results from early single-agent clinical trials in metastatic breast cancer patients showed low overall response rates, although lapatinib was well tolerated and a substantial fraction of the HER2-positive patients had stable disease at four months. However, a recent randomized phase III trial carried out to evaluate lapatinib in combination with capecitabine (a prodrug of 5-FU) in advanced or metastatic HER2-positive patients that had progressed following trastuzumab-containing regimens found a highly significant improvement in the median time to disease progression in the combination arm versus the cohort receiving capecitabine alone (8.4 months versus 4.4 months, respectively) [28].

What are the next steps? Although monoclonal antibodies such as trastuzumab and small-molecule tyrosine kinase inhibitors such as lapatinib are tailored to the same overexpressed target, in vitro studies with breast cancer cell lines suggest synergism [27,28]. Clinical studies are under way to test this concept in HER2-positive metastatic breast cancer patients who have had no prior chemotherapy treatment.

HER2-driven signaling is strongly implicated in several cancers, and drug discovery efforts have produced inhibitors with impressive preclinical profiles. Furthermore, drugs such as lapatinib are well tolerated and appear to effectively diminish HER2 signaling activity. What, then, are the possible reasons for the limited clinical activity of these reagents? It has been suggested that HER2 activation does not play a fundamental role in the pathogenesis of HER2-positive breast cancer, and this may be the case for some patients and/or disease stages. However, an intriguing explanation involving the kinase-inactive HER3 receptor is beginning to gain momentum. Use of HER2 autophosphorylation as a biological readout indicates that HER2 kinase activity is durably inhibited by lapatinib. Surprisingly, blockage of Akt activity is transient rather than sustained. Recent findings demonstrating that inhibition of HER3 transphosphorylation is also transient provide a potential explanation, since constitutive pro-survival, oncogenic signaling via the PI3-K/Akt pathway is driven primarily by transphosphorylation of HER3 [29] (Figure 3). Although still controversial, there is evidence that inhibiting HER2 and/or EGFR leads to compensatory, Akt-mediated feedback signaling that promotes increased expression of membrane-bound HER3, thereby pushing the phosphorylation–dephosphorylation equilibrium of HER3 in the direction of phosphorylation. Re-phosphorylation of HER3 is attributable to residual HER2-based signaling. The finding that in some cases, even residual kinase activity can support a compensatory signaling pathway underscores another design challenge for kinase inhibitors.

It appears that HER3-based signaling must be neutralized for lapatinib and other HER2 inhibitors to reach maximal effectiveness, but how does one inhibit a kinase-inactive HER family member? Since the transphosphorylation of HER3 within HER2/3 heterodimers is ligand dependent with respect to HER3, exploring ways to disrupt engagement by high-affinity ligands such as heregulin may be required. Another possibility is to develop higher-potency HER2 inhibitors. Finally, combining HER inhibitors with inhibitors of downstream pathways such as Akt and PI3-K may be necessary.

Findings implicating HER3 in an escape mechanism to the targeting of HER2-positive breast cancer suggest that evaluating transphosphorylation of HER3 in addition to or instead of HER2 autophosphorylation as a biological marker of response to HER2 inhibitors is warranted. However, given the complexity of the disease, optimism is guarded as to the potential of HER2/3 inhibitors as a curative solution. On the other hand, similar to combinations of Abl kinase inhibitors that may be capable of completely blocking Bcr-Abl-based resistance in CML, it may become possible to intercept HER2/3-based signaling irrevocably, perhaps the first of several punches needed to knock out the disease completely.

EGFR IN NON-SMALL-CELL LUNG CANCER

Smoking-related lung cancer is at once the most deadly and the most preventable cancer. Advanced non-small-cell lung cancer (NSCLC) is the leading cause of cancer death worldwide and accounts for about 80% of all lung cancers. NSCLC originates in lung epithelial cells and encompasses diverse histological subtypes: adenocarcinoma, bronchioaveolar, squamous, anaplastic, and large-cell carcinomas. Notably, the specific histological subtype has turned out to be one important clinical indicator of favorable response to EGFR-inhibitor-based treatment. Ironically, another important finding is that "never smokers" are disproportionately represented in the patient subset with favorable responses to EGFR inhibitors [30].

Advanced lung cancer patients typically present with metastatic disease, and the median survival from diagnosis is four to five months if left untreated. Despite unrelenting research efforts, the results of the various therapies are far from satisfactory. Surgical intervention followed by combination cytotoxic chemotherapy and radiation can bring a modest increase in survival, but this is frequently associated with serious toxicity and quality of life is compromised. Notably, approximately 62% of NSCLC cases demonstrate overexpression of EGFR [30]. However, unlike HER2-positive breast cancer, an increased level of EGFR gene expression is not in itself sufficient to infer a dependency or oncogene addiction. In addition to lung cancer, EGFR overexpression is also observed in cancers of the head and neck, ovary, cervix, bladder, esophagus, stomach, brain, breast, endometrium, and colon.

In the wake of the imatinib/CML story, the search for other suitable kinase targets intensified. Since EGFR is often overexpressed in NSCLC cells, a belief emerged that inhibition of this target would reduce lung cancer cell proliferation. Early studies employing the structurally related tyrosine kinase inhibitors gefitinib or erlotinib (Table 1) in the treatment of chemorefractory NSCLC produced modest objective tumor response rates of 10 to 18% in phase II trials, but in some cases the extent of response was dramatic (Figure 4). Given the lack of significant progress in extending the survival of patients with NSCLC over the course of three decades and the potential market size, it is understandable that these initial findings were met with extreme optimism. However, an important detail is that for cases in which gefitinib or erlotinib was effective, there was little understanding as to why. In several additional phase II trials, a low but appreciable percentage of patients achieved rapid and seemingly sustained responses. These findings were sufficient to secure permission for trials evaluating the benefit of combining gefitinib with the current best-care chemotherapy regimen. Accrual for the trial, for which patient enrollment was unselected and for which no biomarker

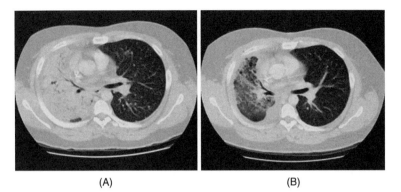

(A)   (B)

Figure 4. Response to gefitinib in a patient with refractory NSCLC. Computerized tomography scans from a 32-year-old male with a large mass in the right lung (A) before beginning gefitinib treatment and (B) after 6 weeks of gefitinib therapy at 250 mg/day. (Images were graciously provided with permission from Daniel Haber [31].)

for gefitinib sensitivity was utilized, was complete in months and expectations were very high. However, the results demonstrated conclusively that inclusion of gefitinib provided no benefit over standard therapy with respect to progression-free or overall survival. Gefitinib was still approved based on low but consistent response rates (in 2002 in Japan; in 2003 in the United States) for patients with chemotherapy-refractive NSCLC and on the basis of its favorable safety profile (Figure 1).

At the time of approval, there was still little understanding of predictive markers. As in the earlier trials but with lower frequency, a small subset of patients had exhibited dramatic responses. Therefore, retrospective studies focused on responders to identify biomarkers correlated with gefitinib sensitivity [31,32]. Unlike the case of HER2-positive breast cancer, there was no correlation between intensity of immunohistochemical staining and response, indicating that EGFR overexpression alone is an insufficient predictor of response. The key finding, however, was that dramatic responders harbor mutations in the intracellular tyrosine kinase domain of EGFR that result in a hyperactivated receptor: a four-residue deletion (ΔE746–A750; accounts for 45% of EGFR-based resistance), L858R (45%), and a scattered few other mutations (10%). Thus, patients that respond to gefitinib display features of oncogene addiction, and addiction is most commonly traced to activating KD mutations. However, the limitations in efficacy of the clinical EGFR inhibitors became readily apparent shortly thereafter. As in CML, but at a much higher frequency and on the time scale of months rather than years, relapses involving acquired KD mutations that confer drug resistance were reported in the majority of responders. The most prevalent mutation associated with resistance to gefitinib and erlotinib involves the gatekeeper residue, T790M, in the catalytic domain of the EGFR kinase.

One possible way to deal with resistance is through the use of irreversible inhibitors. The irreversible inhibitor HKI-272 has shown some promise in early clinical evaluation (Table 1), but this compound cannot completely inhibit EGFR carrying the T790M mutation. The combination of HKI-272 and rapamycin induced dramatic tumor regression in an erlotinib-resistant mouse model of lung cancer [33]. Thus, although an objective criterion has been established to identify patients who are likely to benefit from clinical EGFR inhibitors, further studies addressing the frequent problem of acquired drug resistance, as well as identifying novel targets in patients who lack activating EGFR mutations, will be essential to forward progress in NSCLC therapy.

BRAF V600E MUTATION IN MELANOMA

Melanoma, by far the deadliest form of skin cancer, originates in pigmented cells called melanocytes, which are found primarily in the skin. In concert with a close-lying network of epidermal keratinocytes that secrete factors responsible for regulating melanocyte function, melanocytes respond to exposure to ultraviolet light by producing melanin and bring about the tanning phenomenon [34].

Melanocytes originate from highly motile cells and have unusually low susceptibility to pro-apoptotic cytotoxic agents. Most cases of melanoma (80%) are detected and treated by surgical resection at a relatively early disease stage, and the prognosis is good for these patients. With 25,000 cases annually world-wide, metastatic melanoma is relatively rare but poses a great clinical challenge. Median survival from diagnosis is less than one year and the five-year survival rate is less than 5%.

One smoking gun in the melanoma story is BRAF, a serine/threonine-specific kinase that transduces signals downstream of receptor tyrosine kinases and other signaling cascades via the RAS/RAF/MEK/ERK pathway (Figure 5). BRAF is mutated in at least 70% of melanoma cases, and a single mutation, V600E, accounts for 90% of these occurrences (reviewed in by Gray-Schopfer et al. [34]). Thus, BRAF V600E is detected in about 63% of all melanoma specimens surveyed. Furthermore, this gain-of-function mutation confers a RAS-independent, 500-fold increase in kinase activity and potentiates increased proliferation, survival, and transformation. The structural basis for this dramatic activation has been dissected elegantly and involves disruption of interaction between the glycine-rich loop and the activation segment in the kinase domain of BRAF [35].

There is considerable interest in developing potent BRAF inhibitors. However, the plot is more complicated than was appreciated initially. For example, careful investigation of rare inactivating BRAF mutations that preclude activation of downstream MEK lead to the realization that BRAF can activate CRAF in normal and malignant cells and that CRAF can then activate MEK as well as other signal transduction pathways (Figure 5). Thus, it is difficult to gauge the signaling flow to MEK through these two RAF isoforms. Interestingly, CRAF mutations are exceedingly rare. Although prevalent, the BRAF V600E mutation is not sufficient

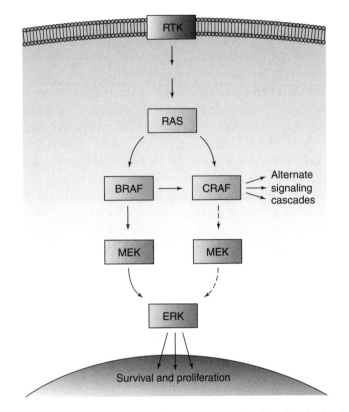

Figure 5. RAS/RAF signaling pathway in melanoma. Normally, signaling in the RAS/RAF/MEK/ERK pathway channels primarily through BRAF, although BRAF can activate CRAF in a RAS-dependent manner. The BRAF V600E mutant causes constitutive activation of the kinase and subsequent increased signaling through the BRAF arm of the pathway. Additionally, activation of CRAF by BRAF becomes RAS independent.

to cause cancer and must cooperate with other processes that are not yet well understood.

Another strong indication that the RAS/RAF/MEK/ERK pathway is central to melanoma biology is that 15 to 30% of melanomas carry an NRAS mutation, most commonly Q61L (reviewed by Gray-Schopfer et al. [34]). Given the observation that RAS and RAF mutations are mutually exclusive, this implies that 85 to 100% of melanoma sufferers carry a RAS or RAF mutation, and the direct consequence in most scenarios is constitutive ERK signaling. What is the best target in this cascade? The first attempts to derail BRAF V600E utilized the multikinase inhibitor sorafenib [36] (Table 1), whose targets include BRAF (IC_{50}: 25 nM), BRAF V600E (IC_{50}: 38 nM), CRAF (IC_{50}: 6 nM), VEGFR1 and VEGFR2 (IC_{50}: 26 and 90 nM, respectively), and PDGFRβ (IC_{50}: 57 nM) [36,37]. Single-agent sorafenib therapy has not been successful in clinical trials for advanced melanoma [38], but phase II trials in which sorafenib is combined with paclitaxel and carboplatin are showing more promise [39] (Figure 1). More recently, impressive preclinical findings regarding the RAF kinase and angiogenesis inhibitor RAF265 (formerly CHIR-265), and a potent and specific BRAF inhibitor, SB-590885 [40], have been reported [34] (Table 1).

Why does sorafenib, a relatively potent BRAF inhibitor, fail as a single-agent therapy for melanoma? One possibility is that the unusual properties of melanocytes come into play. For example, rather than functioning in apoptosis induction, TNF-α signaling appears to confer a survival advantage on melanoma cells in which the activity of BRAF is inhibited [41]. Is BRAF even the right target? It is now generally held that a pan-RAF specific inhibitor might be a better choice than a BRAF-specific inhibitor, and that, at a minimum, an improved potency BRAF inhibitor is needed. Another possibility is that the RAS and RAF mutations provide a signpost as to which cascade or cascades to target, but that MEK is a better target. One problem in targeting MEK is that this kinase also impinges on immune signaling pathways, and long-term inhibition could negatively affect innate immune function.

Despite identification of key dysregulated signaling molecules, the pathway to utilizing this information clinically remains veiled. The benefits of targeting multiple pathways, including angiogenic factors and the PI-3 kinase pathway, as well as combining targeted therapies with HSP90 inhibitors, agents that destabilize multiple client proteins, are under investigation (Table 1). Additionally, the characteristic constitutive activation of MEK-ERK signaling in melanoma has recently been linked to JNK signaling [42]. Cooperation between these two pathways constitutes a rewiring of key signal transduction pathways in melanoma. Once a more complete understanding of the consequences of upregulation of JNK in melanoma has been established, additional therapeutic targets may become clear. We have identified important pieces of the puzzle, but a multipronged approach appears necessary. BRAF mutations, predominantly V600E, also occur with high frequency in ovarian (30%), thyroid (30%), and colorectal cancer (15%). One hope is that the lessons learned in the beautiful detective work pertaining to melanoma biology will have therapeutic implications for these diseases as well.

JAK2 IN POLYCYTHEMIA VERA

Classified as one of the myeloproliferative disorders (MPDs), polycythemia vera (PV) is an acquired disorder of the bone marrow that results in characteristic erythrocytosis, accompanied by moderate leukocytosis and thrombocytosis. Currently, recommended treatment typically involves frequent phlebotomy to control heightened hematocrit levels, in addition to administering low-dose aspirin to reduce the risk of thromboembolic complications [43]. For patients with evidence of a high risk of thrombosis or progressive myeloproliferation, hydroxyurea, an antimetabolite inhibitor of DNA synthesis, is first-line cytoreductive treatment.

In 2005, several research groups identified a single point mutation in the JAK2 tyrosine kinase in the vast majority of PV patients as well as in subsets of patients with various other MPDs, in particular essential thrombocytosis and idiopathic myelofibrosis (reviewed by Levine and Gilliland [44]; Figure 1). This somatic mutation, a phenylalanine substituted for valine at residue 617 (termed V617F), occurs in the catalytically inactive pseudokinase domain of JAK2 and is detected in approximately 95% of patients with PV. Functionally, this amino acid exchange renders the kinase constitutively activated and leads to increased cellular growth and proliferation via overactivation of the JAK-STAT signaling pathway [45]. The pseudokinase domain is believed to serve an autoregulatory function, maintaining the JH1 kinase domain in a conformation that precludes phosphorylation of a specific tyrosine residue required for full activation of the kinase. The crystal structures of the kinase domains of JAK2 [46] and JAK3 [47] have been solved and are strikingly similar (Figure 6). Molecular modeling and functional studies

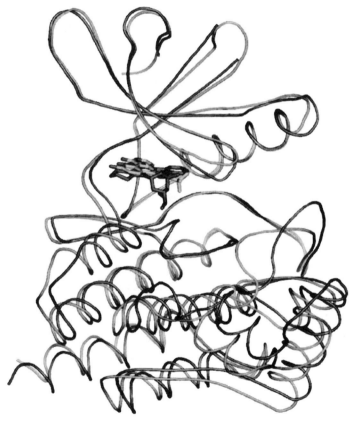

Figure 6. Crystallographic comparison of JAK2 and JAK3. The tyrosine kinase domains of JAK2 (blue) and JAK3 (green) bound to the specific small-molecule pan-JAK inhibitor CMP6 (yellow) and staurosporine analog AFN941 (magenta), respectively, feature a high degree of homology and are shown superimposed above. (Image graciously provided with permission from J. Rossjohn [46].) (See insert for color representation.)

examining the interaction of the pseudokinase and kinase domains of JAK2 predict that three specific regions within the pseudokinase domain form an interface with the kinase domain, and that phosphorylation of Tyr 1007 within the kinase domain disrupts this interaction and thereby activates JAK2 in an EPO-receptor-independent fashion [48]. These studies do not reveal an obvious role for the clinically prevalent JAK2 V617F mutation in disrupting regulatory control, and further structural studies are clearly warranted.

Is JAK2 V617F as central to PV as the Bcr-Abl tyrosine kinase is to CML pathogenesis? It has been shown that hematopoietic stem cells expressing JAK2 V617F produce a PV-like phenotype in a murine model, and exposure of patient primary cells to JAK2 siRNA prevents EPO-independent colony formation, a hallmark of PV [49]. Taken together, these results add to the building evidence supporting a critical role for JAK2 V617F in the development of PV. Also, novel activating mutations were reported recently in exon 12 of JAK2 in 10 of 10 patients with a diagnosis of V617F-negative PV. These mutations demonstrated effects similar to those of JAK2 V617F in functional assays, including EPO-independent in vitro erythroid colony formation [50]. However, there is also evidence to suggest that, while important, mutating JAK2 may not be the primary event in disease development. For example, the V617F mutation can be detected at low levels in a small percentage of normal subjects who do not have PV.

As a relatively new arrival to the molecularly targeted cancer therapy scene, the excitement surrounding the discovery of JAK2 mutations in PV and other MPDs has prompted a rapid move to develop a clinical inhibitor of JAK2. Several pan-JAK inhibitors have been reported, but these are not clinically viable, due to formulation and toxicity issues. It is difficult to predict whether a pan-JAK kinase inhibitor could be acceptable in the treatment of JAK2 V617F-positive MPDs, but it is unlikely, since the JAKs play important, nonredundant roles in hematopoiesis. At the same time, due to the fact that members of the JAK family all bear a high degree of homology to one another (Figure 6), the design of a clinical JAK2-specific small-molecule inhibitor may prove quite challenging. One compound that has shown some promise in preclinical studies, TG101209 [51] (Table 1), is likely to enter clinical trials in the near future. However, if JAK2 specificity remains a high hurdle to clear in the clinic, it could perhaps dictate a shift in development focus to productive interference with another downstream component of the JAK-STAT pathway [45,49]. Another consideration is health care economics. Current PV therapies, although strictly speaking mostly only symptomatic (with the possible exception of IFN-α), are quite effective in reducing complications of the disease; and they are cheap. It is difficult to see how an agent with therapy costs of $24,000 a year (the costs of standard-dose imatinib therapy for CML) could compete with hydrea and aspirin in economic terms. Thus, large-scale comparative studies will be required to establish whether a specific JAK2 inhibitor demonstrates significant clinical benefit in the treatment of PV and other JAK2 V617F-positive MPDs.

THERAPEUTIC STRATEGIES FOR MYELODYSPLASTIC SYNDROMES

Myelodysplastic syndromes (MDS) span a range of clinical and biological manifestations [52]. The affected patient population encompasses older persons, and outcomes vary widely for patients allocated to the same risk groups based on the International Prognostic Staging System (IPSS). In this and other cases (e.g., NSCLC), disease heterogeneity presents a formidable challenge with respect to designing targeted therapy.

The occurrence of symptomatic anemia is the most common indicator of early-stage MDS. Erythropoietin therapy is beneficial in selected patients, although efficacy often diminishes over time and red blood cell transfusions are then required [53]. Aside from continued fatigue, the major long-term concern with chronic transfusion therapy is iron overload with resulting cardiac or hepatic impairment. Allogeneic transplantation is the only curative treatment for MDS, but this procedure is associated with considerable morbidity and mortality. Therefore, transplantation is generally reserved for patients at high risk. Unfortunately, even upon successful transplantation, there is still significant risk of relapse if the disease is advanced [53].

The nucleoside analogs 5-azacytidine (Vidaza) and decitabine (Dacogen) (reviewed by Corey et al. [52]), have been investigated over the past decade for their potential in treating MDS, and although they have been approved for all patient risk groups, their DNA demethylation mode of action inherently limits their specificity. Although significant responses have been seen in MDS patients at intermediate and high IPSS risk, multiple courses of treatment are required and the median response duration is less than one year. More recently, lenalidomide (Revlimid), an orally administered analog of thalidomide, has been approved by the FDA after producing dramatic responses in patients with the 5q-syndrome, a specific subtype of MDS clinically characterized by anemia, a normal platelet count, low bone marrow blasts, and at the cytogenetic level, isolated interstitial deletion of the long arm of chromosome 5, including bands q31 to q33 [54] (Figure 1 and Table 1). Responses included significant improvements or normalization of hemoglobin and suppression of the abnormal clone in approximately two-thirds of patients [55]. The duration of responses is not yet known, and insufficient data are currently available for patients with more advanced MDS [56].

How does lenalidomide work against MDS, and does lenalidomide therapy represent a targeted therapy? One would surmise that a gene contained in the commonly deleted region of chromosome 5 must be involved in a pathway that is targeted by lenalidomide, and hence in disease pathogenesis. As decades of research into the genes in this region failed to identify inactivating mutations of the remaining allele in any of the candidates, this must be a haploinsufficient tumor suppressor gene. Thus, the prediction is that the drug may suppress a pathway that is overactive in cells that are haplodeficient for the presumed tumor suppressor. Several candidates have been identified by gene expression profiling comparing the lenalidomide response of normal versus 5q- erythroblasts [57,58]. However, it has not yet been established how these transcriptional changes relate to the hypothetical disease-initiating gene(s) in patients with 5q-syndrome. Interestingly, the 5q-abnormality has a dominant effect on responses, as evidenced by the fact that patients with a complex karyotype that includes 5q- also achieve responses to lenalidomide. On the other hand, responses are much less frequent in MDS patients without deletions of 5q- [59].

Overall, we currently do not fully understand why and how lenalidomide works, and it seems that deciphering the script will be more difficult than in the case of NSCLC. However, as lenalidomide has also been observed to exhibit activity in patients with refractory multiple myeloma (reviewed by Strobeck [60]), it appears that the importance of characterizing lenalidomide's specific targets and mode of action may extend beyond MDS to benefit therapeutic progress in other malignancies as well.

CLOSING THOUGHTS

The success of imatinib in CML created a surge to find and target the Achilles' heel in other malignancies. To date, the unearthing of highly prevalent, activating mutations has been reasonably successful, including the discovery of JAK2 V617F in PV and other MPDs and BRAF V600E in melanoma. However, it has also become increasingly clear that the business of interrupting malignant signaling cascades is filled with unexpected twists and turns. Even in cases for which an oncogenic kinase is unequivocally identified and effectively inhibited, there is no guarantee of results mirroring the imatinib/CML paradigm. We also now recognize that overexpression of a given kinase (e.g., EGFR in NSCLC) does not in itself provide target validation and may in fact be misleading. Indeed, it seems that our ability to identify appropriate targets in other malignancies remains contingent upon a gradual dissecting of molecular anomalies and pathways that are essential in a subset of patients from those that are merely common.

Imatinib has revealed the potential of small-molecule kinase inhibitors as effective and well-tolerated therapies in selected patients with diseases that have a relatively simple molecular design. In other cancers, however, avenues to progress have been very slow to materialize, as deciphering the molecular details of oncogenic targets does not mean that we can necessarily design small-molecule inhibitors with narrow specificity. Engineering candidate compounds still requires sifting through substantial chemical libraries looking for hits while being mindful of toxicity and off-target effects. Regardless, even when such inhibitors are developed and validated in vitro and in preclinical models, the reality remains that effective translation of these results into the clinic has proven a challenging task.

How can we apply the imatinib paradigm to these more complex situations? It is important not to lose sight of the need for a molecular understanding of why we expect a targeted-therapy approach to accomplish its goal. This may require consideration of rational approaches to targeting more than one pathway and/or cutting off workarounds when one pathway is targeted successfully. For HER2 overexpression in breast cancer and BRAF V600E in melanoma, adequate inhibition of target tyrosine kinase activity is achieved, although there is insufficient interruption of downstream signaling (Akt pathway via HER3 or MEK-ERK pathway via CRAF, respectively). In general, it appears that progress will require simultaneous oversimplification (to design intervention strategies) and recognition of complexity (to be vigilant in anticipating and responding to problems such as unanticipated escape pathways and acquired drug resistance).

Assuming that the imatinib paradigm in CML is extendable to other cancers, what are the roots of success? A partial list includes matching patient subsets to the appropriate drug, improvements in genetic screening, detection diagnostics and technology for monitoring degree of remission, anticipating and minimizing resistance, and continuing to streamline the drug development process. Using NSCLC as an example, "perceived failures" are often, in fact, attributable to the difficulty of identifying and stratifying receptive patient populations at the outset of a trial. Therefore, it is important not only to design trials as effectively as possible but also to sift through the results meticulously to identify reasons for rare responses, as was done elegantly subsequent to the large NSCLC trials. Unfortunately, this necessarily comes very late in an expensive process for large, unselected trials.

Our current understanding of cancer is fundamentally different from that a decade ago, and this has greatly informed current treatment strategies. There is now less focus on where a particular cancer occurs in the body and more emphasis on pinpointing the molecular dependencies that allow the tumor to expand. There is a push to develop novel targeted therapies, but also mounting evidence that even under best-case scenarios, kinase inhibitors, although effective for debulking malignancies, may not be curative. Imatinib, the exemplar of successful targeted therapy, dramatically changed the prognosis for patients with CML, but it probably does not cure the disease. Whether a combination of Abl inhibitors will be capable of achieving this aim remains to be answered in clinical trials. Nonetheless, the past decade has seen enormous progress in understanding and treating cancer, and just as each advance that is rebuked illuminates further complexities, it also enhances our knowledge. Much remains to be done, but we continue to move closer to our goal of understanding a disease, knowing how to treat it effectively from the ground up, and striving toward a cure.

REFERENCES

1. Schindler T, Bornmann W, Pellicena P, Miller WT, Clarkson B, Kuriyan J. 2000. Structural mechanism for STI-571 inhibition of Abelson tyrosine kinase. *Science* 289(5486):1938–1942.
2. Nagar B, Bornmann WG, Pellicena P, Schindler T, Veach DR, Miller WT, et al. 2002. Crystal structures of the kinase domain of c-Abl in complex with the small molecule inhibitors PD173955 and imatinib (STI-571). *Cancer Res* 62(15):4236–4243.

3. Druker BJ, Talpaz M, Resta DJ, Peng B, Buchdunger E, Ford JM, et al. 2001. Efficacy and safety of a specific inhibitor of the Bcr-Abl tyrosine kinase in chronic myeloid leukemia. *N Engl J Med* 344 (14):1031–1037.

4. O'Brien SG, Guilhot F, Larson RA, Gathmann I, Baccarani M, Cervantes F, et al. 2003. Imatinib compared with interferon and low-dose cytarabine for newly diagnosed chronic-phase chronic myeloid leukemia. *N Engl J Med* 348(11):994–1004.

5. Sawyers CL, Hochhaus A, Feldman E, Goldman JM, Miller CB, Ottmann OG, et al. 2002. Imatinib induces hematologic and cytogenetic responses in patients with chronic myelogenous leukemia in myeloid blast crisis: results of a phase II study. *Blood* 99(10):3530–3539.

6. Talpaz M, Silver RT, Druker BJ, Goldman JM, Gambacorti-Passerini C, Guilhot F, et al. 2002. Imatinib induces durable hematologic and cytogenetic responses in patients with accelerated phase chronic myeloid leukemia: results of a phase 2 study. *Blood* 99(6):1928–1937.

7. Hughes TP, Kaeda J, Branford S, Rudzki Z, Hochhaus A, Hensley ML, et al. 2003. Frequency of major molecular responses to imatinib or interferon a plus cytarabine in newly diagnosed chronic myeloid leukemia. *N Engl J Med* 349(15):1423–1432.

8. Druker BJ, Guilhot F, O'Brien SG, Gathmann I, Kantarjian H, Gattermann N, et al. 2006. Five-year follow-up of patients receiving imatinib for chronic myeloid leukemia. *N Engl J Med* 355 (23):2408–2417.

9. Willis SG, Lange T, Demehri S, Otto S, Crossman L, Niederwieser D, et al. 2005. High-sensitivity detection of Bcr-Abl kinase domain mutations in imatinib-naive patients: correlation with clonal cytogenetic evolution but not response to therapy. *Blood* 106(6):2128–2137.

10. Chu S, Xu H, Shah NP, Snyder DS, Forman SJ, Sawyers CL, et al. 2005. Detection of Bcr-Abl kinase mutations in $CD34^+$ cells from chronic myelogenous leukemia patients in complete cytogenetic remission on imatinib mesylate treatment. *Blood* 105(5):2093–2098.

11. Koptyra M, Falinski R, Nowicki MO, Stoklosa T, Majsterek I, Nieborowska-Skorska M, et al. 2006. Bcr/Abl kinase induces self-mutagenesis via reactive oxygen species to encode imatinib resistance. *Blood* 108(1):319–327.

12. Skorski T. 2002. Bcr/Abl regulates response to DNA damage: the role in resistance to genotoxic treatment and in genomic instability. *Oncogene* 21(56):8591–8604.

13. Shah NP, Tran C, Lee FY, Chen P, Norris D, Sawyers CL. 2004. Overriding imatinib resistance with a novel ABL kinase inhibitor. *Science* 305(5682):399–401.

14. Talpaz M, Shah NP, Kantarjian H, Donato N, Nicoll J, Paquette R, et al. 2006. Dasatinib in imatinib-resistant Philadelphia chromosome–positive leukemias. *N Engl J Med* 354(24):2531–2541.

15. Kantarjian H, Giles F, Wunderle L, Bhalla K, O'Brien S, Wassmann B, et al. 2006. Nilotinib in imatinib-resistant CML and Philadelphia chromosome–positive ALL. *N Engl J Med* 354 (24):2542–2551.

16. Weisberg E, Manley PW, Breitenstein W, Brüggen J, Ray A, Cowan-Jacob SW, et al. 2005. Characterization of AMN107, a selective inhibitor of wild-type and mutant Bcr-Abl. *Cancer Cell* 7:129–141.

17. Tokarski JS, Newitt JA, Chang CY, Cheng JD, Wittekind M, Kiefer SE, et al. 2006. The structure of dasatinib (BMS-354825) bound to activated Abl kinase domain elucidates its inhibitory activity against imatinib-resistant Abl mutants. *Cancer Res* 66(11):5790–5797.

18. Kantarjian HM, Giles F, Gattermann N, Bhalla K, Alimena G, Palandri F, et al. 2007. Nilotinib (formerly AMN107), a highly selective Bcr-Abl tyrosine kinase inhibitor, is effective in patients with Philadelphia chromosome–positive chronic myelogenous leukemia in chronic phase following imatinib resistance and intolerance. *Blood* 110(10):3540–3546.

19. Quintas-Cardama A, Kantarjian H, Jones D, Nicaise C, O'Brien S, Giles F, et al. 2007. Dasatinib (BMS-354825) is active in Philadelphia chromosome–positive chronic myelogenous leukemia after imatinib and nilotinib (AMN107) therapy failure. *Blood* 109(2):497–499.

20. Cortes J, Rousselot P, Kim DW, Ritchie E, Hamerschlak N, Coutre S, et al. 2007. Dasatinib induces complete hematologic and cytogenetic responses in patients with imatinib-resistant or intolerant chronic myeloid leukemia in blast crisis. *Blood* 109(8):3207–3213.

21. Guilhot F, Apperley J, Kim DW, Bullorsky EO, Baccarani M, Roboz GJ, et al. 2007. Dasatinib induces significant hematologic and cytogenetic responses in patients with imatinib-resistant or -intolerant chronic myeloid leukemia in accelerated phase. *Blood* 109(10):4143–4150.

22. Bradeen HA, Eide CA, O'Hare T, Johnson KJ, Willis SG, Lee FY, et al. 2006. Comparison of imatinib, dasatinib (BMS-354825), and nilotinib (AMN107) in an *N*-ethyl-*N*-nitrosourea (ENU)-based mutagenesis screen: high efficacy of drug combinations. *Blood* 108:2332–2338.

23. Burgess MR, Skaggs BJ, Shah NP, Lee FY, Sawyers CL. 2005. Comparative analysis of two clinically active Bcr-Abl kinase inhibitors reveals the role of conformation-specific binding in resistance. *Proc Natl Acad Sci USA* 102(9):3395–3400.

24. Copland M, Hamilton A, Elrick LJ, Baird JW, Allan EK, Jordanides N, et al. 2006. Dasatinib (BMS-354825) targets an earlier progenitor population than imatinib in primary CML but does not eliminate the quiescent fraction. *Blood* 107(11):4532–4539.

25. Jiang X, Zhao Y, Smith C, Gasparetto M, Turhan A, Eaves A, et al. 2007. Chronic myeloid leukemia stem cells possess multiple unique features of resistance to Bcr-Abl targeted therapies. *Leukemia* 21(5):926–935.

26. Hudis CA. 2007. Trastuzumab: mechanism of action and use in clinical practice. *N Engl J Med* 357(1):39–51.

27. Nahta R, Esteva FJ. 2006. HER2 therapy: molecular mechanisms of trastuzumab resistance. *Breast Cancer Res* 8(6):215.

28. Moy B, Kirkpatrick P, Kar S, Goss P. 2007. Lapatinib. *Nat Rev Drug Discov* 6(6):431–432.

29. Sergina NV, Rausch M, Wang D, Blair J, Hann B, Shokat KM, et al. 2007. Escape from HER-family tyrosine kinase inhibitor therapy by the kinase-inactive HER3. *Nature* 445(7126):437–441.

30. Sun S, Schiller JH, Gazdar AF. 2007. Lung cancer in never smokers: a different disease. *Nat Rev Cancer* 7(10):778–790.

31. Lynch TJ, Bell DW, Sordella R, Gurubhagavatula S, Okimoto RA, Brannigan BW, et al. 2004. Activating mutations in the epidermal growth factor receptor underlying responsiveness of non-small-cell lung cancer to gefitinib. *N Engl J Med* 350(21):2129–2139.

32. Paez JG, Janne PA, Lee JC, Tracy S, Greulich H, Gabriel S, et al. 2004. EGFR mutations in lung cancer: correlation with clinical response to gefitinib therapy. *Science* 304(5676):1497–1500.

33. Li D, Shimamura T, Ji H, Chen L, Haringsma HJ, McNamara K, et al. 2007. Bronchial and peripheral murine lung carcinomas induced by T790M-L858R mutant EGFR respond to HKI-272 and rapamycin combination therapy. *Cancer Cell* 12(1):81–93.

34. Gray-Schopfer V, Wellbrock C, Marais R. 2007. Melanoma biology and new targeted therapy. *Nature* 445(7130):851–857.

35. Garnett MJ, Rana S, Paterson H, Barford D, Marais R. 2005. Wild-type and mutant B-RAF activate C-RAF through distinct mechanisms involving heterodimerization. *Mol Cell* 20(6):963–969.

36. Wilhelm SM, Carter C, Tang L, Wilkie D, McNabola A, Rong H, et al. 2004. BAY 43-9006 exhibits broad spectrum oral antitumor activity and targets the RAF/MEK/ERK pathway and receptor tyrosine kinases involved in tumor progression and angiogenesis. *Cancer Res* 64 (19):7099–7109.

37. Wilhelm S, Carter C, Lynch M, Lowinger T, Dumas J, Smith RA, et al. 2006. Discovery and development of sorafenib: a multikinase inhibitor for treating cancer. *Nat Rev Drug Discov* 5 (10):835–844.

38. Eisen T, Ahmad T, Flaherty KT, Gore M, Kaye S, Marais R, et al. 2006. Sorafenib in advanced melanoma: a phase II randomised discontinuation trial analysis. *Br J Cancer* 95(5):581–586.

39. Flaherty KT. 2006. Chemotherapy and targeted therapy combinations in advanced melanoma. *Clin Cancer Res* 12(7 Pt 2):2366s–2370s.

40. Takle AK, Brown MJ, Davies S, Dean DK, Francis G, Gaiba A, et al. 2006. The identification of potent and selective imidazole-based inhibitors of B-Raf kinase. *Bioorg Med Chem Lett* 16 (2):378–381.

41. Gray-Schopfer VC, Karasarides M, Hayward R, Marais R. 2007. Tumor necrosis factor-alpha blocks apoptosis in melanoma cells when BRAF signaling is inhibited. *Cancer Res* 67(1):122–129.

42. Lopez-Bergami P, Huang C, Goydos JS, Yip D, Bar-Eli M, Herlyn M, et al. 2007. Rewired ERK-JNK signaling pathways in melanoma. *Cancer Cell* 11(5):447–460.

43. Finazzi G, Barbui T. 2007. How I treat patients with polycythemia vera. *Blood* 109(12):5104–5111.

44. Levine RL, Gilliland DG. 2007. JAK-2 mutations and their relevance to myeloproliferative disease. *Curr Opin Hematol* 14(1):43–47.

45. Tefferi A. 2007. JAK2 mutations in polycythemia vera: molecular mechanisms and clinical applications. *N Engl J Med* 356(5):444–445.

46. Lucet IS, Fantino E, Styles M, Bamert R, Patel O, Broughton SE, et al. 2006. The structural basis of Janus kinase 2 inhibition by a potent and specific pan-Janus kinase inhibitor. *Blood* 107 (1):176–183.

47. Boggon TJ, Li Y, Manley PW, Eck MJ. 2005. Crystal structure of the Jak3 kinase domain in complex with a staurosporine analog. *Blood* 106(3):996–1002.

48. Giordanetto F, Kroemer RT. 2002. Prediction of the structure of human Janus kinase 2 (JAK2) comprising JAK homology domains 1 through 7. *Protein Eng* 15(9):727–737.

49. Levine RL, Pardanani A, Tefferi A, Gilliland DG. 2007. Role of JAK2 in the pathogenesis and therapy of myeloproliferative disorders. *Nat Rev Cancer* 7(9):673–683.

50. Scott LM, Tong W, Levine RL, Scott MA, Beer PA, Stratton MR, et al. 2007. JAK2 exon 12 mutations in polycythemia vera and idiopathic erythrocytosis. *N Engl J Med* 356(5):459–468.

51. Pardanani A, Hood J, Lasho T, Levine RL, Martin MB, Noronha G, et al. 2007. TG101209, a small molecule JAK2-selective kinase inhibitor potently inhibits myeloproliferative disorder-associated JAK2V617F and MPLW515L/K mutations. *Leukemia* 21(8):1658–1668.

52. Corey SJ, Minden MD, Barber DL, Kantarjian H, Wang JC, Schimmer AD. 2007. Myelodysplastic syndromes: the complexity of stem-cell diseases. *Nat Rev Cancer* 7(2):118–129.

53. Schiffer CA. 2006. Clinical issues in the management of patients with myelodysplasia. *Hematol Am Soc Hematol Educ Prog* 2006:205–210.

54. Giagounidis AA, Germing U, Wainscoat JS, Boultwood J, Aul C. 2004. The 5q-syndrome. *Hematology* 9(4):271–277.

55. List A, Dewald G, Bennett J, Giagounidis A, Raza A, Feldman E, et al. 2006. Lenalidomide in the myelodysplastic syndrome with chromosome 5q deletion. *N Engl J Med* 355(14):1456–1465.

56. List A, Kurtin S, Roe DJ, Buresh A, Mahadevan D, Fuchs D, et al. 2005. Efficacy of lenalidomide in myelodysplastic syndromes. *N Engl J Med* 352(6):549–557.

57. Pellagatti A, Jadersten M, Forsblom AM, Cattan H, Christensson B, Emanuelsson EK, et al. 2007. Lenalidomide inhibits the malignant clone and up-regulates the SPARC gene mapping to the commonly deleted region in 5q- syndrome patients. *Proc Natl Acad Sci USA* 104(27):11406–11411.

58. Joslin JM, Fernald AA, Tennant TR, Davis EM, Kogan SC, Anastasi J, et al. 2007. Haploinsufficiency of EGR1, a candidate gene in the del(5q), leads to the development of myeloid disorders. *Blood* 110(2):719–726.

59. Raza A, Reeves JA, Feldman EJ, Dewald GW, Bennett JM, Deeg HJ, et al. 2008. Phase II study of lenalidomide in transfusion-dependent, low- and intermediate-1-risk myelodysplastic syndromes with karyotypes other than deletion 5q. *Blood* 111(1):86-93.

60. Strobeck M. 2007. Multiple myeloma therapies. *Nat Rev Drug Discov* 6(3):181–182.

13

EPIDEMIOLOGY: IDENTIFYING CANCER'S CAUSES

James R. Hebert*

Department of Epidemiology and Biostatistics, Arnold School of Public Health, South Carolina Statewide Cancer Prevention and Control Program, University of South Carolina, Columbia, South Carolina

INTRODUCTION

The word *epidemiology* is derived from the Greek roots *epi* (on or among) and *demos* (people). Epidemiology is conventionally defined as the "study of the distribution and determinants of health-related states or events in specified populations and the application of this study to control health problems" [1]. Although laboratory animal, cell culture, and other sorts of experiments conducted in highly controlled environments can deepen our understanding of the pathophysiological bases of disease, what we know definitively about human cancers must come from studies of human beings. This difficult business of establishing "cause" is the province of epidemiology.

As highlighted in other chapters of this book, cancer represents a wide variety of diseases that vary in terms of anatomical site, histology, molecular biology,

*Funding to support Dr. Hebert was provided by the National Cancer Institute, Center for Research and Cancer Health Disparities (Community Networks Program) to the South Carolina Cancer Disparities Community Network (SCCDCN) [1 U01 CA114601-01].

morphology, and a variety of other characteristics. The study of human cancers is complicated by the heterogeneous nature of cancer and by a number of other factors, including generally long, but variable, periods of latency; the multi-factorial nature of "cause"; methodologic challenges inherent in measuring common risk factors; and ethical issues that preclude examining the natural history of cancer in a manner analogous to methods employed in studies of cells in culture and of laboratory animals.

Reflecting the heterogeneity of the disease processes implied in the natural histories of cancers and the complex relationships between and among factors that can cause or prevent disease, many different outcome measures are used in epidemiologic studies of cancer. These include detection of new cancers (inci-dence), the presence of cancer in a population (prevalence), and survival from a cancer after diagnosis (disease-free survival and mortality). In addition, there are various intermediate endpoints, such as precancerous lesions (e.g., colorectal polyps and oral precancerous lesions). Some cancers, such as colorectal, oral, and cervical, can be screened to detect such precancerous lesions, and such screening therefore constitutes real *primary prevention* (i.e., to lower incidence) by removing a lesion before it becomes cancer. Screening for others, such as breast and prostate, are focused on "downstaging" of disease at the time of diagnosis and therefore represent *secondary prevention* (because we can influence survival and thereby prevalence). One consequence of screening is that incidence may actually increase artificially for a time [as was the case for prostate cancer in the early to mid-1990s with the advent of prostate-specific antigen (PSA) for widespread, population-based screening]. There also are attempts to improve quality of life, and some of these types of studies have resulted in apparent survival benefits [2,3].

Despite the many challenges that face cancer epidemiologists in conducting studies, we actually know a lot about how to prevent many cancers, and the best way to treat or control many others that we cannot, or will not, be able to prevent for the foreseeable future. Much of what remains to be done in advancing the field requires moving past the normal boundaries of what we have defined as the domain of conventional epidemiology.

In the following sections we focus on the ways in which we collect information and gain knowledge, the factors that influence the probability of getting or dying of cancer, and brief summaries of what we know about specific cancers. Besides acting as a practical guide toward understanding the current knowledge basis, in the final section we point out challenges and directions for future research.

TYPES OF STUDIES

Virtually all studies of humans are epidemiologic. Typically, these are organized in a hierarchical fashion, with those representing the least stringent types of control being seen as methodologically inferior to those in which tighter control is exercised or at least possible. Of course, there is a trade-off between possible control and both methodologic complexity and risk factor heterogeneity. For example, we sacrifice access to greater generalizability in identifying and quantifying risk factors in order to recruit well-educated, compliant persons into our studies. Indeed, the narrow range of exposures that are often entailed in large-scale epidemiologic studies limits our ability to discern effects that may be seen in more tightly controlled human studies or in laboratory animal experiments in which researchers can drastically alter the amounts of particular substances given "research subjects" [4].

Descriptive Studies

Descriptive studies rely on the use of aggregate data to describe a situation or condition. These sorts of studies are generally exploratory and do not attempt to infer causation to a specific exposure–disease relationship. Often, they are conducted in advance of some other sort of formal study: either a methodologically more rigorous epidemiologic study or a more tightly controlled laboratory experiment. As such, they are often used as ideal places in which to generate hypotheses to be tested using other studies. The advantages of these sorts of studies include:

- *A large range of outcomes.* For cancer rates these might be 100-fold or more different, compared to just a few percentage points different in comparing subpopulations in a particular population (say, African Americans versus European Americans in the United States) [5].
- *A large range of potential predictors.* Dietary factors, for example, may vary 10- or even 100-fold between populations, as opposed to just a few percentage points within populations.

However, they also have disadvantages, including the inability to:

- *Examine relevant subgroups.* Because the data are aggregated, it is not possible to understand how specific groups of people might have been exposed to a particular agent or substance.
- *Control for confounding or to estimate how one factor might influence another.* Because we do not have data on individuals, we cannot rule out factors that would interfere with our seeing clearly how certain risk factors influence cancer or understand how various factors may interact with one another at the level of the individual in order to modify risk.
- *Reproduce/replicate results.* One of the hallmarks of science is to be able to replicate studies and verify results obtained in particular experiments; clearly, this cannot happen in nonexperimental situations where we have limited capability to examine aggregate results.

Cross-Sectional Comparisons

These compare data that are aggregated from smaller sampling frames, or sometimes at the level of individuals, into groups. Although such data may be from repeat surveys conducted over time, for the purposes of these comparisons the focus is on observations made at only one point in time. Completion of this type of study can be conducted relatively inexpensively and quickly compared to virtually any other study design. However, by their very design, cross-sectional studies cannot reveal the temporal sequence of events in relation to one another or establish a causal relationship between the exposure and disease. Furthermore, only disease prevalence, not incidence, can be calculated in this type of study. Cross-sectional studies often simply compare, for example, prevalence rates of particular cancers in one place or geographical region to those in another place or geographical region. As such, they require no special statistical modeling.

Ecological Studies

These studies represent a transition to analytical studies in that they employ aggregate data of cancer rates to compare populations in relation to putative risk factors. Exposure and disease information is collected at a group or population level, not at an individual level, at "virtually the same time." Group mean values or rates of the outcome of interest and the postulated risk factor(s) are calculated. Typically, these are plotted to ascertain if a relationship is evident. Sometimes, analyses may entail statistical modeling. Some of the classical early identification of dietary factors (primarily fat and total energy) in relation to cancer fall into this category [6]. Aggregated measurements, such as the average amount of fat intake, summarize the characteristics within a population and are then compared to an aggregate measure of disease or a disease-related outcome. Measurements also can be made at an environmental level to represent the physical attributes of a geographic location, such as average sunlight exposure, air pollution, and water or soil contamination. A third type of variable used in ecological studies is a measurement representing populations that are not reducible to the individuals within that group, also known as a *global measure*. Examples include the existence of health inequalities, the presence or absence of a certain law, or a type of political, social, or health care system.

There are two general types of ecological studies:

1. Those that compare cancer rates and risk factor exposures at "virtually the same time" but in various places (e.g., the classic cross-national comparisons of diet and cancer mortality rates). These include the earliest ecological studies from which many of the diet–cancer hypotheses arose [6] and have now expanded to the use of sophisticated mathematical modeling [7,8]. Results from these studies tend to be consistent with

findings from laboratory animal experiments showing that diet is a powerful determinant of the incidence of many cancers, especially the hormone-sensitive cancers and other cancers of affluence, such as colorectal.

2. Those that follow the experience of populations that move (i.e., migrate) compared to genetically similar ones that stay in one place. In these comparisons it is possible to control for possible genetic factors (e.g., these would include the classic comparisons of Japanese migrants to Japanese remaining in Japan on aggregate cancer rates in relation to aggregate rates of exposure to factors of interest such as diet) [9].

Analytical Studies

Analytical studies measure both disease-related outcomes and putative risk factors, such as diet, physical activity, and alcohol and tobacco use, at the level of the individual. The vast majority (>99%) of all epidemiologic studies in the medical literature fall into this category. The advantages and disadvantages of these types of studies are the converse of those listed for descriptive studies. The advantages include:

- *The ability to focus on relevant subgroups.* Because we collect data at the level of the individual it is possible to estimate measures of association based on specific sociodemographic subgroups. There may, however, be practical limitations in terms of numbers of people within groups who are enrolled and measured.

- *The capacity to control for confounding and estimate effect modification.* Again, because measurements are made at the level of the individuals it is possible to control for *confounders* (i.e., factors that may be related to outcome only because of a spurious statistical association and not because of a causal relationship) and estimate effect modification (i.e., the degree to which one factor, e.g., tobacco, may affect that of another, e.g., alcohol or dietary fat).

- *Scope for reproducing/replicating results.* Although this may be expensive, it is possible to repeat, reproduce, or replicate such studies.

However, they also have disadvantages, including:

- *Limited variability in disease rates.* Although not an inherent problem with such studies, the practical reality is that these studies are based within populations such that variation in cancer rates is usually much smaller than that observed across populations [7].

- *Narrow range of potential predictors.* Essentially, this problem is similar to the preceding problem: Populations that are convenient to study usually occupy a fairly narrow range of the "exposure spectrum" [4,5,10].

- *Biased exposure estimates.* Unlike ecological studies, we rely in these studies on self-estimates of exposures (e.g., diet, sexual behavior). These are known or suspected to have numerous, often serious biases that can distort the results of epidemiologic analyses and result in faulty inferences [11].

Case–Control Studies

These studies comprise the majority of analytic epidemiologic studies in cancer. In studies of this design, participants are compared according to whether they have disease (i.e., a *case* is defined as a person with cancer or a precancerous lesion) or not [i.e., a *control* is either known not to have the disease under study (typically the case in hospital-based studies) or is assumed to have a low probability of having the disease (typically the case in population-based studies)]. Past exposures to potential risk factors are measured retrospectively. Cases and controls are then compared on the measured exposures and the odds ratio (the odds of being a case versus a control, given exposure) is then calculated. Advantages of this type of design include the ability to estimate associations in a timely and efficient manner because follow-up is not necessary and the number of participants needed to obtain a necessary sample size is smaller (because we can know in advance approximately how many "cases" can be enrolled over a set period of time and no expense is incurred for having to "wait" for people to get disease). However, the possibility of methodological bias may affect case–control studies more readily than cohort or prospective studies. Selection bias can occur if cases and controls are not selected from similar populations. Also, case–control studies are subject to recall bias, for example, in situations in which the study subjects are asked retrospectively to recall an exposure postulated (or assumed by the participant) to be a risk factor.

An interesting variant of the traditional case–control design is the *nested case–control study*, in which cases are identified within a well-established cohort. The cases are persons who have developed the outcome or disease of interest over the cohort follow-up period. Controls are selected among persons at risk (i.e., disease-free) at the time that each case occurs. Cases and controls are selected from the same reference cohort population, so that selection bias tends to be diminished in a nested case–control design. Most large-scale cohorts using biomarkers of exposure are analyzed in this way.

Cohort Studies

In contrast to the case–control study design, in which the study subjects are classified according to whether or not they have cancer (or another endpoint related to cancer, such as a precancerous lesion), here people are defined according to exposure status. A cohort or prospective study is considered the "gold standard" in observational epidemiology in that data obtained in a study of this design, if unbiased, reflect the temporal sequence of cause and effect. The basic components of a cohort study include the identification and follow-up of a group of disease-free people (i.e., a cohort) over a specified period of time in order to ascertain the development of a certain outcome. Once a defined population is identified and all prevalent cases of the outcome are excluded, the cohort subjects are classified according to exposure status. Follow-up over a period of time allows for researchers to ascertain the incidence of the outcome of interest and to compare the outcome between the exposure groups. Because the cohort is healthy at the beginning of the study (and means are available for helping to ensure that this assumption is met), the overall objective of a cohort study is to determine whether the incidence of a cancer is related to postulated exposures. Obviously, a cohort study allows us to follow a population to examine its experience of a variety of disease endpoints and relate the occurrence of these outcomes to as many risk factors as we may have been able to measure.

The main advantage of a cohort study is the ability to investigate causality in an exposure–disease relationship in order to capture temporal sequence (without biases resulting from retrospective assessment). However, the undertaking of such a study is generally very time consuming, costly, and requires many thousands (often, hundreds of thousands) of subjects in order to obtain enough disease or other outcomes. A variant of the traditional prospective cohort design is the nonconcurrent, or historical cohort, in which a cohort is identified retrospectively on the basis of existing data or records and followed up to the time when the study is being conducted. Historical studies, often using occupational records, can be done more quickly and inexpensively than prospective cohort studies. However, researchers must rely on available information, which may not be accurate or adequate to fulfill the study objectives. Nonetheless, nonconcurrent study designs are a useful tool in epidemiologic investigations. This is especially true in regard to the study of cancer. The latency period for most cancers can be decades long. The ability of a researcher to obtain a disease-free population and measure exposures for this amount of time in order to ascertain cancer incidence may not be feasible or preferred. Therefore, the use of a retrospective study design may prove advantageous in these situations.

Interventions

Interventions can take the form of clinical or community trials. Essentially, these are cohort studies in which one (or occasionally, two) factors are manipulated by design (e.g., by random assignment of a study agent).

RISK FACTORS AND CAUSES OF CANCER

Age

Age is the most ubiquitous cancer-related risk factor. Most, but not all, cancers evince a pattern of increasing incidence with age. This is due to the fact that genetic damage leading to cancer accumulates over time, and that the machinery necessary to detect and eradicate cancer (e.g., immune surveillance systems) tends to become more error prone and less efficient with age. Exceptions to the general rule of incidence increasing with age include some of the soft-tissue neoplasms of childhood (several types of leukemias), lymphoma, and testicular cancer. For some cancers, most notably hormone-sensitive cancers such as breast and prostate, virulence is associated inversely with age; the older the age at presentation, the more indolent, or slowing, the cancer tends to be. For both of these reasons, it is recommended that efforts aimed at early detection cease at age 74 years for most cancers for which we commonly screen. When comparing cancer rates across populations, it is very important to age-standardize the data to account for differences that might exist in the age structure of the populations (and therefore would mislead in terms of misestimating the real risk or the public health impact of cancer). In epidemiologic studies, age must be controlled, either by matching, by using statistical methods of adjustment, or both.

Gender

Certain cancers occur exclusively in men (e.g., prostate, testicular) or women (e.g., cervical, ovarian, vaginal, and endometrial). Others are much more common in one gender than the other (e.g., breast in women and esophageal cancer in men). Others are about evenly distributed (e.g., colorectal). In general, men have higher overall cancer incidence and much worse survival than women. Analyses of cancer data require control for gender. Usually, this entails stratifying by gender (i.e., looking at men and women separately) but also can entail use of more sophisticated statistical methods of control.

Lifestyle Factors

Diet

The importance of diet in maintaining health and preventing disease, including cancers of many anatomical sites, has been recognized for millennia. A quarter of a century ago, Richard Doll and Richard Peto estimated that 35% of all human cancers are caused by diet [12], an estimate that is current despite uncertainty and correspondingly wide confidence limits. Early in the scientific study of diet and cancer it was shown that dietary fat increases risk in certain animal models of cancer and subsequent work in humans. Analytical studies have not been supportive.

Over the past several decades there has been greatly increased focus on specific micronutrients (nutrients such as minerals and vitamins that do not contribute calories to the diet) and other constituents of the diet, including compounds in spices and categories of fiber (e.g., some nondigestible components). On balance, patterns of nutrient consumption associated with vegetarian diets and certain traditional foodways (e.g., East Asian, South Asian, Mediterranean cuisines) are associated with lower overall cancer rates. Consistent with this, there is a body of evidence showing that meat (especially processed and red meat) intake is associated with increased cancer risk. The International Agency for Research in Cancer (IARC) concludes that greater consumption of vegetables and fruits is associated with decreased risk of lung, esophageal, stomach, and colorectal cancer. The connections with other cancers are considered "probable." In general, the strongest evidence for diet and cancer comes from free-living populations that choose to eat diets that diverge from the Western norm. Cross-cultural studies designed to measure and test the effect of diets of *individuals* who differ from one another to as great a degree as countries represented in cross-national comparisons have not been undertaken.

In summary, whole-food, vegetarian, or near-vegetarian diets are associated with lower rates of cancer. Usually, supportive findings derive from studies outside the nutritional mainstream in countries such as the United States. Many of the components of these diets appear to be protective. Attempts to study specific dietary components, especially in humans, generally have not met with much success [13].

Physical Activity

Physical activity and the result of energy expenditure influence overall health, including the management of weight, increasing one's psychological well-being, and reducing the risk of obesity, diabetes, high blood pressure, and heart disease. In addition to these health benefits, investigators have found that physical activity is advantageous in reducing the risk of various types of cancer. Various mechanisms through which physical activity can influence the risk of cancer include alterations in the distribution of body fat, production of sex hormones and other metabolic factors, and changes in weight and body mass index. Several studies have indicated a reduced risk of hormone-sensitive cancers among people who are physically active. Changes in body mass and a person's relative weight can alter the metabolism of sex hormones, such as estrogens, thus influencing a woman's risk of breast and ovarian cancer. Researchers have also found that people who are physically active reduce their risk of colon cancer by as much as 50%. This may be due to regular activity aiding in regulating bowel movements, thus reducing the exposure time of possible carcinogens to the colon, and may alter other influences on colon cancer risk, such as inflammatory or immune factors. Physical activity, or the lack thereof, later in life has been shown to greatly affect breast cancer. Weight change and physical activity influence a woman's risk of breast cancer more dramatically after menopause than before, due primarily to the association of central or upper body fat and changes in hormone production. In summary, energy balance, body mass, immune and inflammatory functions, and other factors influenced by regular physical activity may help reduce a person's risk of cancer by preventing tumor development and growth.

Use of Tobacco

Tobacco use is the single most important modifiable cause of cancer in most populations. It accounts for about 40% of total cancer incidence in the United States. In some countries, where use is higher than in this country, the percentage is even higher. Some cancers are so strongly related to tobacco use that they would be very rare diseases in the absence of tobacco. In the United States and other populations where cigarette smoking is the most common form of use, lung is the most prominent of these. However, other sites that are strongly linked to tobacco include those of the upper aerodigestive tract and the urinary bladder. For some of these sites, most prominently those of the upper aerodigestive tract, alcohol is an important cocarcinogen. In the United States, tobacco use in men has decreased over time. In a time-lagged pattern, incidence and mortality in lung cancer have decreased following a drop in prevalence of this risk factor. In many Western countries, especially the United States, women have continued to increase their use of tobacco after the rate in men has decreased. The pattern evident in men is just now emerging in women, and it appears that the concomitant fall in incidence and mortality will follow the same pattern as that seen for men. Reinforcing the idea that tobacco is a primary cause of many cancers is the sharp rise evident in populations, especially in Asia, in which many males choose to smoke. In the 2006 Surgeon General's Report [14], secondhand smoke is also a concern among persons who are regularly exposed and is classified as a carcinogen, with no safe nonzero level of exposure.

While the smoking of tobacco is the most common form of exposure in many parts of the world (e.g., Europe, North America, and China), there are many other places (e.g., India, other parts of South Asia) where tobacco is often chewed. Such exposures are much less strongly associated with lung cancer but tend to be strongly related to oropharyngeal cancer.

Use of Alcohol

Alcohol's primary role is as a cocarcinogen, along with other strongly carcinogenic compounds such as those found in tobacco. Indeed, its most important role in cancer results from its strong synergistic relationship with tobacco. For some sites, such as the esophagus, the effect of alcohol is to strongly amplify the effect of tobacco, by a factor of 10 or more. Work conducted in the 1980s on the role of mouthwash (which is usually around 26.5% ethanol) showed that alcohol, by itself, is not a cause of cancer of the oral cavity or other sites of the upper aerodigestive tract. There is a literature showing a modest increase in breast cancer at lower levels of exposure (i.e., up to about one drink per day) and a possible weak relationship with cancers of other sites, such as prostate. Unlike tobacco, for which there is no redeeming value from a public health perspective, consumption of specific alcoholic beverages (e.g., red wine) may confer other health benefits.

Sexual Behavior

It has long been recognized that sexual promiscuity and poor sexual hygiene are related to several urogenital cancers, especially penile and cervical. It is now known that the real, underlying cause of these cancers is human papilloma virus (HPV), especially the high-risk or oncogenic types 16 and 18. Furthermore, HPV appears to be responsible for some oral cancers. Vaccines for some of the common types that cause cancer or venereal warts (type 6 and 11) came on the U.S. market in 2006.

Meditation and Other Stress Reduction and Relaxation Practices

Many years ago it was observed that persons with acquiescent personality types were more likely to get cancer and to do poorly after a diagnosis. Although the concept of a type C (i.e., cancer-prone) personality type has been largely discredited, there are elements of this hypothesis that have been, and currently remain, under study. Some of the most fruitful work has been conducted through studies of persons enrolled in programs focused on stress reduction, group support, or some combination of these modalities [2,3,15].

Psychosocial Factors

There is an overlap between practices related to "personal improvement" and psychosocial factors that represent more closely people's "traits" (i.e., long-term, stable psychological characteristics or predispositions). It is known that psychological orientation toward potentially stressful life experiences has a strong influence on immune responses [16]. These, in turn, can influence the probability of getting cancer or succumbing to the disease [17]. The observation of most people who deal with cancer treatment and care on a frequent basis is that some people with very poor-prognosis disease do well, and conversely, some with good-prognosis disease do poorly. This observation is consistent with a literature showing that attitude and orientation to life are important determinants of subsequent disease course [18]. This is also consistent with an interesting literature on caregiver stress (e.g., a person who cares for a spouse with life-threatening illness), showing that such caregivers are at increased risk of being diagnosed with cancer. This line of work emphasizes the importance of social support, which is known to affect disease course in those diagnosed with cancer.

Socioeconomic Status and Social Deprivation

It is well known that cancer rates move predictably across well-known socio-economic gradients. The most reliable predictor of outcome is education [19], which may be related to a variety of other health-related behaviors [20] as well as to the role of status in health per se [21]. Although some cancers in the United States (e.g., breast) are more common in the affluent, most tend to be more common in those who are poor. Almost without exception, cancer mortality rates per unit incidence are higher, usually much higher, among the poor. For example, blacks in South Carolina, which is one of the poorest states in the United States, have the highest mortality : incidence rates in the country for almost all cancers [22]. In general, people under economic duress also experience stress in the form of disturbed sleep, increased rate of shift work, worries about unemployment and loss of income, and less wherewithal to practice healthful behaviors. Of all the socioeconomic "predictors" of cancer, education is the most important. This may be due to factors ranging from life choices (e.g., lower rates of tobacco use and better diet) to improved access to medical care.

Chronobiological Factors

Chronobiological factors, including circadian-related phenomena, are an impor-tant, although normally neglected, factor in most biological processes. Their influence extends from the development of specific cancers to their treatment. Cancer rates are known to vary by season and by timing within the biological rhythms of individuals (e.g., menstrual cycles) [23], including the role of clock genes in determining cancer risk [24]. Timing of treatment, including chemother-apy and surgery, may also produce drastically better results if they are optimally timed within circadian, menstrual, and annual cycles to maximize their efficacy and minimize their side effects [25,26].

Occupational Exposures

Probably only a small proportion of overall cancer risk is attributable to on-the-job exposures. This is not to say that occupationally determined exposures are not important for specific cancers and for particular types of exposures. Often, the work environment entails heavy exposure to chemicals and other substances that are rarely encountered in other settings. These may be carcinogens or precarcinogens that require activation to active forms. Classic examples of such exposures include heavy metals such as lead, mercury, and hexavalent chromium; and organic solvents and other chemicals, such as polycyclic aromatic hydrocarbons, aromatic amines, polychlorinated biphenyls; and asbestos and synthetic fibers. In addition to classical exposure to chemical and physical agents, the work environment can influence risk by increasing psychological factors related to stress, restricting access to healthy behavioral choices, and simply by forcing workers to work at odd hours (i.e., shift work), which entails disruption of circadian rhythms.

Studies of occupational exposures and cancer suffer from the fact that careful descriptions of exposure are usually not readily available and cannot easily be reconstructed from historical records. Complicating studies on occupation and cancer is the *healthy worker effect*. Simply stated, people who work tend to be healthier than demographically similar people who do not work. So the study of occupational cancers is confounded by the fact that people who work are generally healthy enough to do so.

Physical Environment/Spatial Variations

Although cancer is a genetic disease, even simple comparisons of genetically similar populations living in different environments (e.g., West Africans vs. African Americans and Japanese living in Japan vs. those residing in the United States) emphasize the importance of environment in carcinogenesis. If studies of occupational exposures and cancer are difficult, those focusing on ambient exposures are even more difficult. For example, exposure estimates from residential histories and subjects' recalls are notoriously imprecise. Classical examples of difficulties in this arena include studies attempting to study the effect of electromagnetic fields in breast and other cancers. Ecological approaches, however, have proven to be successful in identifying gross patterns of disease occurrence that have led to generating hypotheses that have been tested in both laboratory animal studies and analytic epidemiologic studies. A good example of this is the observation of a latitude gradient for breast and prostate cancers and generation of the vitamin D hypotheses relating to these cancers.

Genetic Factors

Although cancer is assuredly a set of genetic diseases, the literature clearly indicates that the factors responsible for the dramatic rate differences observed internationally and with migration are environmental, primarily lifestyle-related [6,27]. Rate differences across populations are up to 500-fold for some cancers, 100-fold or so for many, and virtually all respond to changes in migration very quickly (i.e., usually within a couple of generations) [28]. So even though cancers are diseases of genetic alterations, only a relatively small proportion of all cancers are due to major inherited susceptibility (e.g., disease-conferring mutations in *BRCA1* and *BRCA2*). A much larger proportion of the interindividual differences in susceptibility to environmental factors may be determined by low-penetrance, common genetic variants related to detoxification, and activation of carcinogen exposures and deoxyribonucleic acid (DNA) repair.

Gene–Environment Interactions

Given the lack of clearly dominant genetic factors in explaining much of the overall variation in cancer rates between populations, one of the most important challenges to cancer epidemiology includes identifying predisposing genetic factors (e.g., polymorphisms in common genes) that interact with putative life-style factors (including diet, physical activity, and tobacco smoke) to modify risk. A huge literature on this topic has emerged. Indeed, research in this arena has spawned two new subdisciplines: bioinformatics (to deal with the staggering number of permutations of genes and possible gene–environment interactions) and molecular epidemiology (with its focus on making sense of all of the data, i.e., drawing reasonable inferences).

Time Trends

Of the six criteria for judging causality that were defined by Bradford Hill [29] and popularized in the 1964 Surgeon General's Report linking tobacco to lung cancer [30], only one criterion is a *sine qua non*: temporality. A cause must precede its effect. Therefore, examination of time trends either in terms of cancer rates or the relationship between changes in cancer rates and putative risk factors can provide important clues for study. Examples of fruitful exploration in this arena include the protective relationship between refrigeration and stomach cancer and the suggestion that transition to a higher-fat diet is related to increases in rates of certain cancers, including breast and prostate, in Japan [31–33]. The issue of *temporal relatedness* is an underpinning of the conclusion we draw from migrant studies, from which we deduce that environmental factors, changes in which can evince their effects quickly, are much more important than genetic factors, which change much more slowly.

Mortality to Incidence (M : I) Ratio

Overall, about 43% of people diagnosed with cancer will die of the cancer with which they have been diagnosed (i.e., M : I = 0.43). Some cancers, such as breast

(21%) and prostate (19%), are much less deadly; while others, such as pancreatic and esophageal, are much more deadly (i.e., $M:I > 0.90$). An important determinant of mortality is the stage at diagnosis. Therefore, an important strategy of most screening programs is to downstage disease at the time of diagnosis. Even a cursory examination of cancer registry data shows very clearly that mortality increases markedly by stage. As mentioned previously, some cancers, such as those of the upper aerodigestive tract, evince a pattern of increasing virulence with age; others, including those that are hormone related, evince an inverse pattern. There are also differences in virulence by race; for example, African-Americans tend to have very high mortality rates for most cancers relative to their European-American counterparts. Age relatedness tends to be preserved in such comparisons. That is, African-American men and women tend to have *both* more virulent prostate and breast cancers *and* they tend to occur at younger ages.

There are a few cancers for which screening is not only effective in downstaging disease, but can actually prevent the cancer from recurring entirely by identifying and removing a precancerous lesion. For three common cancers, screening can function as a primary preventive: oral cavity, cervical, and colorectal.

CANCERS BY SITE

Oral Cavity and Pharynx

Oropharyngeal cancers account for about 5% of all cancers in men worldwide and 2.5% in women. Histologically, all oral and pharyngeal cancers are squamous. As with the other sites of the aerodigestive tract, these cancers are highly age dependent and tend to be very strongly related to tobacco exposure. Rates vary markedly across regions, with the highest rates in Asian populations that traditionally chew tobacco. In India, for example, these cancers comprise about 13% of all cancers, as opposed to 3% or so in the United States. Familial factors are suspected in these diseases. Cancers of the oral cavity are one of the sites for which screening can be used as a primary preventive rather than simply as a method of early detection [34]. About 200 precancerous lesions are detected for each frank cancer found [35]. DNA repair genes such as p53 appear to be important, as do low-penetrance genes such as these that encode enzymes involved in metabolism of tobacco, alcohol, and other environmental agents. Glutathione S-transferase enzymes appear to have an important role, as does the CYP1 family, which metabolizes products of combustion such as benzo[a] pyrene. Other detoxifying enzymes, such as alcohol dehydrogenase, may figure prominently. N-Acetyltransferases involved in the metabolism of compounds from cooked meats may have a role. Besides tobacco and alcohol, other possible factors include fruits and vegetables; iron and zinc; a number of micronutrients, such as copper, iron, and zinc; and vitamins C and E and β-carotene. Also, there may be a role for human papilloma virus (HPV) and herpes simplex virus in the etiology of these cancers [35].

Larynx

As for oropharyngeal cancers, these cancers are exclusively squamous. Cancers of this site are very rare, and rates have been very stable for a long time. Known risk factors include tobacco, especially chewing and smoking of dark tobacco. HPV is also implicated in this cancer. Protective factors appear to include a diet rich in fruits and vegetables [36].

Esophagus

Esophageal cancers are relatively uncommon. However, they tend to be fatal (M : I ratio = 0.92). Rates are much higher in men than in women (about three- to ninefold, depending on the population), across all races. Esophageal cancers fall into two histologic categories. Squamous cell carcinomas, which are conventionally thought to be more strongly associated with tobacco and alcohol, tend to arise from the body of the proximal esophagus [37–39]. Adenocarcinomas generally arise from the distal esophagus, near its junction with the stomach, and are strongly associated with gastroesophageal reflux disease (GERD).

Esophageal cancer incidence and mortality rates among blacks were over three times those of whites in the late 1980s [40,41]. This large differential emerged between 1950 and 1977, when the age-adjusted esophageal cancer incidence rate approximately doubled in blacks. Thereafter, the incidence increased slightly until leveling off in the mid 1980s [40,41]. During the same period, the rates of squamous cell cancers remained virtually unchanged in whites, and rates of adenocarcinomas remained relatively constant in both races [42,43]. Since the early 1980s, rates of squamous cell carcinomas have remained approximately constant in both races. However, blacks remain at a distinct disadvantage in relation to whites, owing to the large increases in incidence prior to the mid-1980s. In contrast to squamous cell cancer, adenocarcinoma rates began increasing markedly from the late 1980s, rising about 3 to 4% per year, with the increase being confined almost entirely to whites, and primarily men [42,43].

Across countries of the world there is marked geographic variability in the incidence of, and mortality from, squamous cell esophageal cancer, amounting to about a 500-fold difference. Within the United States, Washington, DC and coastal South Carolina have the highest incidence in the United States, more than twice the national average [44–46]. The racial disparity in this disease is among the most pronounced of any illness in the United States and is especially evident in South Carolina, where the incidence among black men is 7.63 times that observed in white men [46].

Rates of adenocarcinoma of the esophagus are higher in whites than in blacks. Men's rates are about four to eight times higher than those of women, a gender difference about as extreme as that observed for squamous cell cancers. Esophageal adenocarcinomas are thought to be less strongly associated with tobacco than is squamous cell carcinoma [42,43,47,48]. In the United States, increasing obesity is a possible contributing factor to the rising incidence of adenocarcinoma [49]. However, white men are no more obese than other population subgroups. One of the strongest risk factors for adenocarcinoma is GERD [50], the backflow of acid from the stomach into the esophagus, which irritates and sometimes damages the delicate lining on the inside of the esophagus. If this condition remains untreated, it can lead to Barrett's esophagus, which is defined as an abnormal change in the growth of cells of the esophagus. It is generally accepted that this condition is a precursor to adenocarcinoma [50,51]. The role of infectious agents, most notably *Helicobacter pylori*, is much less certain and more complicated.

Stomach

Coinciding with the replacement of other means of preservation by refrigeration, there has been a large global decline in the rate of this type of cancer [52]. The decrease has been mainly for adenocarcinoma of the intestinal type. As often is the case, rates in men are much higher (about twice) than in women. Stomach cancer is strongly age related; except in Japan, it is rarely diagnosed in persons younger than 50. There is some familial aggregation (e.g., the family of Napoleon Bonaparte).

H. pylori infection, in particular, is an important risk factor for the disease. Salt induces superficial and atrophic gastritis, and ecological studies support the salt hypothesis, as do several prospective or cohort studies. Consistent with the refrigeration hypothesis, pickled food, nitrate, nitrite, and nitrosamines are associated with increased risk. Tobacco use also increases the risk, whereas consumption of fruits, vegetables, antioxidants, and green tea appear to be protective. Despite considerable controversy in this area, there appears to be no effect of coffee or caffeine on the risk of stomach cancer. Similarly, alcohol appears to be unrelated [53].

Despite the obvious gender imbalance, hormonal factors have not been studied. The inverse relationship with body height may reflect the effect of early nutritional status. Consistent with the inflammatory hypotheses of cancer, there is a possible inverse relationship with nonsteroidal anti-inflammatory drugs (NSAIDs), including aspirin [53].

Colon and Rectum

As with other cancers, age is a major colorectal cancer (CRCA) risk factor. Around 90% of incident colorectal cancer occurs in people over 50. Certain populations are at greater risk for CRCA, due to genetics and heredity. A family history of CRCA accounts for approximately 25% of cases, which suggests a role for an inherited genetic trait, common exposures among family members, or a combination of these factors. Even after controlling for the effects of stage at diagnosis, comorbidities, and socioeconomic status, blacks are more likely than whites to die from this cancer. Genetic differences may at least partially explain these observations. Differences in mismatch repair genes among African American populations have been observed in comparison with European Americans [54].

Contrasts among rates of disease in different countries may provide clues as to nongenetic causes of CRCA and point towards effective prevention strategies. As for other cancers associated with affluence, such as breast and prostate, there are marked international variations in the incidence and mortality rates of colorectal cancer [6]. These geographical differences suggest that environmental factors probably play an important role in CRCA etiology. Ecological studies have revealed associations between CRCA rates and per capita consumption of meat, fat (positive correlations), and dietary fiber (negative correlation) [55]. The incidence in certain low-risk areas is now rising as these areas become more industrialized and adopt more Western-type diets. Furthermore, the rates of colorectal cancer in migrants from low- to high-incidence countries tend to increase toward the rates of host countries. These results further support an environmental component to CRCA risk and also indicate that CRCA rates are responsive to changes in lifestyle, which can be used to inform potential intervention and prevention strategies. Epidemiologic evidence therefore supports a role for nongenetic factors, especially lifestyle (e.g., dietary) factors, in the pathogenesis of CRCA.

The modifiable risk factors for CRCA include too little physical activity (including the lack of intentional or occupational physical exercise); nonsteroidal anti-inflammatory drugs (NSAIDs); calcium; a diet high in saturated fat and low in fiber from a variety of fruit, vegetable, and grain sources; obesity; and smoking cigarettes. Several studies suggest that occupational physical inactivity is a risk factor for colon cancer but not for rectal cancer [56]. Cigarette smokers are 30 to 40% more likely to die of colorectal cancer than are nonsmokers. It should be noted, however, that tobacco use often clusters with a variety of other known risk factors thought to be related to disease risk [57].

Colorectal tumors may arise from sites of chronic, asymptomatic inflammation, the body's natural response to infection. In general, diet is a powerful determinant of inflammation, and diets in the West tend to be pro-inflammatory, whereas those in parts of the world that have higher concentrations of phytochemicals and lower levels of fat, particularly the ω-6 polyunsaturated and saturated fatty acids, which would be expected to exert anti-inflammatory effects [55]. Consistent with the inflammation hypotheses, chronic inflammatory and symptomatic conditions, such as ulcerative colitis, are strongly associated with increased carcinogenesis of the colon. At the population level, ulcerative colitis and Crohn's disease, collectively known as *inflammatory bowel disease* (IBD), are chronic inflammatory conditions that are associated with increased risk for colorectal cancer [58]. Similarities in the biological and molecular mechanisms between IBD-associated and sporadic colorectal cancers have led to speculation that sporadic cancers in non-IBD patients may be a result of constant low-level inflammation of the bowel and that this may arise from interactions between the bacterial flora and the colonic mucosa [59]. It is important to note that CRCA is one of the cancers that can be screened for primary prevention. With widespread age- and race-appropriate screening, mortality from colorectal cancer can be reduced by about 90 to 95%.

Liver and Biliary Tract

Liver and biliary tract cancers represent one of the most common types of malignancies in the world. However, these cancers [consisting of mainly hepato-cellular carcinoma (HCC), cholangiocarcinoma, and angiosarcoma] are relatively rare in the United States and northern Europe. There tends to be a male predominance of disease, especially in countries of high incidence [60].

The epidemiology of liver cancer, which clearly implicates infectious agents hepatitis B virus (HBV) and hepatitis C virus (HCV), reflects the consistency and importance of both descriptive and analytical studies. Aflatoxin is another known risk factor, the exposure to which is much more common in developing countries. Alcohol is an important exposure, but mainly as a cofactor, highlighted by the fact that in countries with high rates of alcoholic beverage consumption and alcohol-ism, HCC is very rare. Occupationally, vinyl chloride and inorganic arsenic exposure appear to increase risk. Most clustering within families reflects shared risk factors, including chronic HBV infection. Tobacco is a relatively minor factor in HCC. Little research has been done on biliary tract cancer because it is so rare and so fatal. However, we do know that obesity and high-fat diets are associated with increased risk.

Pancreas

Like liver and esophageal cancers, pancreatic cancer is very fatal. About 95% of all pancreatic cancers develop in the exocrine pancreas, about two-thirds of these in the head of the pancreas. This is mainly a disease of the elderly [61]. Because it is a very rare cancer, our work is pretty much relegated to case–control approaches. We do know that there are instances of family clusters, including the family of former U.S. President Jimmy Carter. In terms of prevention, there is a modest effect of tobacco; the fact that risk reduces rapidly after smoking cessation suggests that tobacco smoke is a late-stage component in the carcinogenic process. Diets high in vegetables or fruits seem to be protective. Nutrients associated with such diets, such as vitamin C and various antioxidants, appear to be protective. Both ecological studies and laboratory animal experiments have implicated high-fat intake as a factor that increases risk.

Lung and Bronchus

Cancers of the lung and bronchus are the leading cause of cancer death in both men and women in the United States. The predominant cause of lung cancer is cigarette smoking, which accounts for approximately 85% of the lung cancer burden [62]. On average, a patient's risk of lung cancer is determined largely by smoking history and age, which in turn is a major determinant of duration of exposure because most people begin smoking early in life [62]. Compared to those who quit smoking, the risk of lung cancer decreases after smoking cessation and continues to decrease further with longer duration of sustained cessation [63]. Compared to never-smokers, though, the residual risk of lung cancer in quitters lasts many decades, indicating that the powerful carcinogenic effects of cigarette smoke also have an effect in the early stages of lung carcinogenesis. Although the effect of primary exposure has been known for decades, the effect of secondhand smoke has now been implicated and has led to a variety of antismoking ordinances around the United States [14].

The substantial contribution of lung cancer to the overall mortality burden is due to the combined effects of a disease that has a high incidence rate and a poor overall five-year relative survival rate, 16% [64]. Nationally, lung cancer incidence and mortality rates are much higher in men than women, but the gap is narrowing, as the rates in men have decreased during the past 15 years, whereas the rates in women have risen steadily during the past five decades [65]. There appear to be inter-individual differences in susceptibility, including by race. Biomarkers of tobacco carcinogens have been observed to be present in higher concentrations in African-American male smokers than in white male smokers per unit exposure [66].

In addition to tobacco smoke exposure, many other factors are established causes of lung cancer, although they account for only a small fraction of the total lung cancer burden. These include occupational agents such as chromium, nickel, arsenic, asbestos, and radon. Outdoor air pollution also contributes to lung cancer risk, and may be responsible for 1 to 2% of the overall lung cancer burden.

Diet and physical activity may modify risk. Although protective associations have been observed with increased fruit and vegetable consumption, the specific constituents of fruits and vegetables that might confer protection are unknown. The results of large-scale randomized primary prevention trials now clearly indicate that regular use of dietary supplements containing β-carotene or vitamin E does not protect against lung cancer. Several studies have reported that more physically active individuals have a lower risk of lung cancer than those who are more sedentary, even after adjustment for cigarette smoking.

Skin

Skin cancer falls into three main categories: basal cell carcinoma (BCC), squamous cell carcinoma (SCC), and melanoma. Incidence of all types is much more common in light-skinned persons and is much more common at lower latitudes. SCC of the lip is related to tobacco smoke. The most important risk factor for melanoma is ultraviolet light exposure. Risk is particularly high in light-skinned persons. As such, the most important primary preventive is avoidance of excessive exposure to sunlight, especially sporadic severe sunburning. There is evidence that regular sun exposure that does not result in sunburn may actually be protective. There is no evidence that any aspect of diet is related to BCC or SCC. However, there is a suggestion that antioxidant vitamins, especially those that are oil soluble, may be protective against melanoma [67].

Breast

Breast cancer (BrCA) is the most commonly diagnosed cancer among women, and risk increases substantially with age [44]. It is the second-leading cause of cancer death among women in United States. BrCA is one of the cancers for which virulence is inversely related to age. Although BrCA can occur in men, women are at a much ($\approx$ 100-fold) higher risk of developing the disease.

It is clear from cross-country comparisons [6,68] and migrant studies [69] that nongenetic (i.e., primarily lifestyle-related) causes of breast cancer dominate as plausible explanations of interpopulation rate differences in incidence as well as rates of change over time. Although somewhat controversial, some studies have found that conventional risk factors (including those related to reproduction, family history, and socioeconomic status) explain less than 50% of breast cancer incidence [70]. Lifestyle-related factors such as obesity, decreased physical activity, and hormone therapy use may explain a larger proportion of breast cancer incidence. However, these documented factors do not easily explain the BrCA differences between populations, including the ethnic disparities observed.

Long-term exposure of breast tissue to estrogen plays a major role in breast tumor formation. Consequently, reproductive factors such as total numbers of pregnancies, age at first pregnancy, breastfeeding, age at first menstruation, age at menopause and hormone replacement therapy, which affect a woman's lifetime exposure to estrogen, have been shown to be strongly associated with breast cancer risk. Consistent with the increase in incidence with age, most breast cancers occur among postmenopausal women, and several large prospective studies have identified an association between elevated postmenopausal estrogen levels and BrCA risk. The relationship between premenopausal estrogen levels and subsequent breast cancer development is more difficult to ascertain, but is supported by some studies. Substantial adult weight gain is associated with a decreased risk of breast cancer premenopausally and increased risk postmenopausally. Various mechanisms can explain the effect of overweight, including increased extra-ovarian conversion of androstenedione to estrone in adipose tissue, the potential for carcinogen storage in adipose tissue, and the contribution of hyperinsulinemia. Physical activity, which tends to be related to dietary behavior, also can influence risk, and its impact is independent of diet and body weight. Other important and potentially modifiable risk factors for BrCA are alcohol consumption and smoking.

Ethnic differences in cancer incidence and mortality within the United States can also provide important etiologic clues that may not be apparent when focusing on studies conducted within homogeneous populations. Breast tumors in African-American women tend to be more aggressive even within the same size category, leading to poorer stage specific prognoses than in their white counterparts. Two distinct hypotheses have been proposed for these differences: (1) that socio-economic disparities in the African-American community adversely affect access to care and disease screening; or (2) that the biological nature of breast cancer and its disease manifestation are inherently worse for African-American women. Although a body of literature has addressed these hypotheses over the last few years, no clear answer has emerged [71].

Cervix

Within the past 20 years, oncogenic (i.e., high-risk) genital HPV infection has been identified as the main etiological factor in the development of cervical cancer [72]. There are over 100 known types of HPV, of which 40 infect the genital tract; however, only 15 types are currently considered oncogenic (high-risk). Infection with one of 13 types of oncogenic HPV DNA can be detected by a U.S. Food and Drug Administration (FDA)-approved method, Hybrid Capture II (Digene Corporation, Gaithersburg, Maryland). The HPV DNA test is approved for triage of women with equivocal Pap test results (i.e., atypical squamous cells of undetermined significance) and for primary screening in conjunction with Pap tests for women 30 years and older.

Genital HPV infection is transmitted by skin-to-skin contact in the genital area. Most HPV infections are transient, not persistent, and are resolved within nine months to a year. Only persistent oncogenic HPV infection is a risk factor for cervical cancer. HPV infection is very common among women and their partners. According to the Centers for Disease Control and Prevention, approximately 20 million people are currently infected with HPV in the United States. At least 50% of sexually active men and women acquire genital HPV infection at some point in their lives. By 50 years of age, at least 80% of women will have acquired genital HPV infection. About 6.2 million Americans get a new genital HPV infection each year, whereas cervical cancer is very rare (<10,000 women per year) [57]. Thus, HPV infection is necessary, but not sufficient, to cause invasive cervical cancer. Currently, the most effective preventive measure that a woman can adopt to protect herself from cervical cancer is to have regular Pap tests, with HPV DNA testing as appropriate. Condoms have been shown to decrease the risk of cervical dysplasia and cervical cancer; however, until recently, the effectiveness of condoms in preventing transmission of HPV has been debated. It is now known that condoms are effective in preventing transmission of HPV.

Additional cofactors that contribute to cervical cancer are smoking, other sexually transmitted infections (especially *Chlamydia*), immunosuppression (e.g., HIV infection, other chronic comorbid conditions, pregnancy, autoimmune disorders), and dietary factors. Smoking may contribute because it leads to the concentration of carcinogenic substances in the cervical mucus. Also, antioxidant vitamins such as β-carotene and vitamin C that may counteract the effect of smoke-borne carcinogens may reduce the risk of cervical cancers. The hormones in oral contraceptives may act by modulating HPV gene expression in cervical cells. In addition, socioeconomic factors have been identified as correlates of cervical cancer mortality, in particular.

Endometrium

Endometrial cancer is a common malignancy in the West that occurs late in life (i.e., postmenopausally) and tends to have an excellent prognosis. This cancer is very sensitive to hormone signaling and is therefore affected by the range of factors that affect exposure to hormones, including past oral contraceptive use, reproductive history, obesity, smoking, energy imbalance, and physical activity [73].

Ovaries

Ovarian cancer does not have established precursor lesions and women generally present at a very late stage [74]. As with most hormone-sensitive cancers, incidence is generally much higher in developed countries than in less-developed regions of the world. The most strongly associated factors are those related to reproduction. Reduced risk is observed with increasing parity (reduced risk with increasing parity and with higher age at first parity; this effect diminishes with time) and breast-feeding. Risk increases with increased lifetime ovulatory cycles, including due to oral contraceptive (OC) use and postmenopausal hormone replacement therapy (HRT) [75]. Although only a small proportion of ovarian cancers are associated with a positive family history, such history does confer a 2- to 10-fold increase in risk. Dietary factors are suggested as important based on international comparison studies. For example, intake of total fat is highly correlated ($r = 0.79$) with ovarian cancer mortality [6].

Prostate

Prostate cancer (PrCA) is the most commonly diagnosed cancer among men in the United States, accounting for 30% of all male cancer diagnoses. About one out of five American men will have a diagnosable PrCA sometime during his life [44]. Based primarily on autopsy results, PrCA appears to be much more common than published incidence data would indicate [76]. In fact, were screening to continue past age 74 years, virtually all men in the United States would be found to have pathological or histological evidence of the disease. Despite the relative indolence of the disease, especially in older men, PrCA is a major cause of cancer-related deaths, second only to lung cancer among men in the United States as a whole [44].

Although PrCA tends to be a relatively indolent disease (M : I ratio = 0.19), studies also have shown that African-American men are at significantly higher risk than white men for being diagnosed with advanced-stage prostate cancer. They also tend to be diagnosed with more aggressive disease at younger ages. Racial disparities are larger for PrCA than for any other common cancer in the United States. For example, the incidence rate is 55% higher in blacks than in whites and the mortality is about 1.5 times higher; both rates are about 50% higher in South Carolina (where the African gene pool is more strongly preserved) than for the nation as a whole [77].

Given the higher rates of PrCA, the migration toward lower ages and the related tendency to be diagnosed with later-stage disease, it has been suggested that efforts aimed at early detection may be a better strategy in black men than in their white counterparts. Since the inception of widespread prostate-specific antigen (PSA) screening in the early to mid-1990s, mortality in white men has dropped by about 12%. However, in the same period it has risen in black men by around 20%. This highlights the fact that screening for PrCA and issues related to informed decision making are more controversial for this cancer than for any other. Essentially, the debate revolves around issues of disease aggressiveness and its relationship to age: essentially the tension between overtreatment of indolent disease and undertreatment of aggressive disease. In the early 1990s the American Cancer Society and the American Urological Association advocated that all men over 50 years of age receive PSA tests annually [78]. This recommendation was opposed by specialty groups of primary care physicians: the American College of Physicians, the American Academy of Family Physicians, and the United States Preventive Service Task Force [79]. The majority of physician organizations oppose routine prostate cancer screening, whereas most community-based organizations such as the Prostate Cancer Foundation and the American Foundation for Urologic Disease have recommendations for screening that include modifications for differences in age, race/ethnicity, and family history.

The reasons for the large racial disparities in PrCA incidence and mortality are not yet understood, but point to important clues. Dramatic international variations in age-adjusted incidence and mortality rates provide hints to the etiology of prostate cancer [7]. Japanese men have much lower PrCA incidence and mortality rates than those for Americans. However, upon migration to the United States their rates increase four- to ninefold within one generation and approximate American rates by the second generation [80]. The clear dominance of environmental (i.e., nongenetic) factors in "explaining" rapid changes in incidence should not, however, lead one to underestimate the role of genetic factors in determining risk profiles, either individually or across races (or other identifiable population subgroups). There may very well be subsets of the population that are particularly sensitive to the influences of environmental factors because of their genetic constitution.

Epidemiologic studies that have used different study designs suggest that among environmental influences, dietary factors constitute the most important of modifiable risk factors. Total fat and meat consumption is associated with overall increased incidence of prostate cancer as well as with incidence of more aggressive tumors. Saturated fat, primarily from meat and dairy intake, is the most strongly associated fat subtype [81]. Conversely, intake of whole grains and soy products is associated with decreased mortality [7]. In cross-national comparison studies of both prostate and breast cancers, we can use "disappearance data" (i.e., the difference between population-level estimates of production + imports − experts − estimates of food wastage) to estimate population-level estimates of food intake. Using these data, which are available from United Nations sources, we have been able to explain up to 90% of variability in mortality with dietary factors accounting the vast majority of the variation [7]. Results from laboratory animal experiments are consistent with the findings of the international studies: Fat restriction has been shown to inhibit growth of transplanted prostate cancer cells in rodents [82]. Preliminary evidence also suggests that PrCA may continue to be sensitive to dietary factors even after development of metastases. Substantive dietary changes, marked by adoption of plant-based diets, have been associated with prolonged survival and instances of remission of bone metastases in men with advanced disease.

Unlike dietary factors, there is no repository of physical activity "disappearance" data that can be used to exploit the huge variations in cancer rates observed across countries of the world. Recent reviews of the physical activity (PA) and PrCA association have therefore had to rely exclusively on results of studies conducted at the level of the individual. Using criteria previously used to assess diet–cancer relationships, the association was "probable," based on findings that 15 of 26 published studies demonstrated that higher levels of activity are associated with reduced risk and that 9 of 19 reported a dose–response effect [83]. In a review of studies that have assessed obesity with PrCA mortality, higher-grade and advanced-stage disease have consistently produced results showing that obesity may not increase the risk of PrCA, but rather, promote growth of the tumor once established. Biologically active polypeptides called adipokines have been linked to a number of carcinogenic mechanisms, such as cell proliferation, metastasis, and alterations in sex-steroid hormone levels [84].

Testicles

Testicular cancer, which should not be confused with scrotal cancer, consists of two main histological types, seminomas and nonseminomas. The disease usually presents as a painless mass on the testicle. Unlike many cancers, testicular cancer incidence peaks at around age 30 years and then declines to about zero by age 60 years. For this reason, it is thought that exposures early in life are most important. The early age of onset among familial cases as well as the high proportion of bilateral cancer indicates a genetic component. Work is being conducted to sort out the molecular epidemiology of the disease. Currently, only age, region of residence, ethnic group (Western Europeans and European-Americans have the highest rates of disease), time, and "age cohort" effects (the disease is evincing of strong tendency to increase over time) and cryptochordism (RR ≈ 5 for undescended testicles) are established risk factors [85].

Urinary Bladder

Urinary bladder cancer is much (three- to nine-fold) more common among men than women. It is one of the cancers most strongly associated with occupational exposures. The occupations that are strongly linked with bladder cancer include painting, machining, mechanical work in the metal industry, textiles, leatherwork, dry-cleaning, and transportation. The agents that appear to be the most strongly related to bladder cancer are aromatic amines, polyaromatic hydrocarbons, and hair dyes. In Western countries such as the United States, transitional cell carcinomas constitute about 95% of all cancers of the site. The remaining 5% or so include squamous cell carcinomas, adenocarcinomas, and other minor histological types. Incidence is highest in Western Europe and North America and tends to be much lower in Asia (probably in Africa as well; however, incidence registration is so poor there it is difficult to know with much certainty). Tobacco, particularly in the form of cigarette smoking, is the most important established risk factor for bladder cancer. In terms of dietary exposures, the only consistent findings are for the protective effects of vegetables [86].

Kidneys

Kidney cancer is one of the first cancers for which obesity was observed to be an important risk factor [87]. Cigarette smoking is responsible for up to 40% of kidney cancers in high-risk countries. Asbestos is the only established occupational exposure. Physical activity is probably important both in terms of direct effects and the indirect effect on body weight. Intake of fruits and vegetables is probably protective.

Brain and Nervous System

Brain and nervous system cancers represent a set of diseases of diverse histological type. Primarily from work in atomic bomb survivors and other nonintentional exposures [88], we know that ionizing radiation is one of the few known causes of these cancers. In general, exposures in childhood seem to be more important than those later in life. Occupational exposures, including parental exposures to solvents such as vinyl chloride and electromagnetic fields may be important for childhood cancers [89]. Other modifiable risk factors have not been identified. One clue, however, is the secular trend toward higher rates in cohorts of people born after the early decades of the twentieth century. Currently, there is little evidence to suggest that the increased incidence in older people is explained by improved access to medical care, including better methods of diagnosis [90].

Thyroid

Most (i.e., 90%) thyroid cancers are epithelial (of these 50 to 80% are papillary; 15 to 20% are follicular). In addition, there is a small minority of medullary and anaplastic tumors. Although variable, survival is excellent in general, with a 90% five-year survival rate. Unlike most sites, the incidence is highest in younger people (especially those under 40 years old). The disease is more common in women, especially those in the reproductive ages. There is a weak suggestion of familial aggregation. Dietary and supplemental iodine may be a risk factor. An extensive literature on the subject shows that ionizing radiation is the *only known cause* [91].

Lymphomas and Leukemias

Hodgkin's lymphoma accounts for about 8% of all lymphomas. It is one of the most curable types of cancer. Rates have been very stable over time. There are variations in age (with a young adult peak, then a rise again at about 60 years of age), gender (10 to 45% higher in men), and a socioeconomic gradient indicating a strong environmental role. Epstein–Barr virus may be important at young ages. Incidence also has been associated with occupation in the wood industry [92].

Non-Hodgkin's lymphoma represents a very heterogeneous group of diseases. Rates are increasing very rapidly in many parts of the world and are highest in United States. Incidence is 40 to 70% higher in males and in whites than in blacks. Incidence increases progressively with age, in a pattern more typical of most cancers. Regarding occupation, there is nothing conclusive. Well-established risk factors such as immunosuppression, autoimmunity, and HIV explain only a small proportion of cases; therefore, the rapid worldwide rise in incidence is perplexing [92].

Leukemias represent a variety of soft-tissue cancers. As is the case for Hodgkin's disease, there is not a monotonic increase in incidence with age. There are two childhood peaks and another peak again in late adulthood. Currently, most (>70%)

childhood leukemias are treated effectively. By contrast, we know almost nothing about preventing these cancers. Growth hormone seems to be important, however. Benzene appears to increase risk in adults [93].

FUTURE DIRECTIONS

The Problem of Type III Error

Type III error results from a faulty conception of how the world works, or selection of a study design that produces an answer (even if correct) to the *wrong question.* Unlike type I error (denoted by the *p*-value of a statistical test on the effect of a putative "risk factor" in relation to a disease outcome and defined as accepting the alternative hypothesis of an effect on the assumption that the null hypothesis of no effect is true) and type II error [also known as statistical power $(1 - \beta)$ and defined as accepting the null hypothesis of no effect on the assumption that the alternative hypothesis is true], no statistical tests exist for type III error. Type III errors are therefore not tested, but are probably very common. Future research will have to overcome this ubiquitous problem that has plagued analytic epidemiologic studies.

Health Disparities: Population Difference

As noted, many of the clues that guide our understanding of cancer causation come from comparisons of populations and subgroups within populations that have divergent rates of cancer. Unfortunately, observations made in descriptive studies rarely are tested adequately in analytical epidemiological studies. Subjects recruited for study represent those who are easiest to enroll, from a number of sociodemographic perspectives, rather than those who might be more likely to provide explanations for large rate differences. Challenges of the future will entail getting off the "epidemiologic beaten path" in order to understand why some populations suffer cancer rates far in excess of what their exposure levels would suggest [5].

Community-Based Participatory Research (CBPR)

CBPR holds great promise for engaging those individuals and groups at especially high risk of certain diseases. Unless we do this, we will continue being in the dark regarding the true underlying causes of most cancers. CBPR is a process wherein the community is actively engaged in the actual design of the research [94]. Because community members are partners in the process, the likelihood of asking the right questions is enhanced and recruitment will surpass the usual low rates experienced in epidemiologic studies.

Gene–Environment Interactions

Although cancer is assuredly a set of genetic diseases, we know that the factors responsible for the dramatic rate differences observed internationally and with migration are environmental, primarily lifestyle-related [6,27]. One of the most important challenges to the field of cancer epidemiology is to identify predisposing genetic factors (e.g., polymorphisms in common genes) that interact with putative lifestyle factors (including diet, physical activity, and tobacco smoke) to modify risk. This is a challenging field, especially daunting in terms of the number of permutations possible for interactions among genetic and environmental factors. This will necessitate undertaking large studies in the future, and developing and using state-of-the-art statistical methods to manage the data in order to answer important questions about gene–environment interactions in relation to cancer causation.

REFERENCES

1. Last JM, ed. 2001. *A Dictionary of Epidemiology*, 4th ed. New York: Oxford University Press.
2. Spiegel D, Bloom J, Kraemer H, Gotheil E. 1989. Effect of psychosocial treatment on survival of patients with metastatic breast cancer. *Lancet* 2:888–891.
3. Fawzy FI, Fawzy NW, Arndt LA, Pasnau RO. 1995. Critical review of psychosocial interventions in cancer care. *Arch Gen Psychiatry* 52:100–113.
4. Hebert JR, Kabat GC. 1991. Distribution of smoking and its association with lung cancer: implication for fat–cancer studies. *J Natl Cancer Inst* 83:872–874.
5. Hebert JR. 2005. Epidemiologic studies of diet and cancer: the case for international collaboration. *Austro-Asian J Cancer* 4(3):125–134.
6. Armstrong B, Doll R. 1975. Environmental factors and cancer incidence and mortality in different countries with special references to dietary practices. *Int J Cancer* 15:617–631.
7. Hebert JR, Hurley TG, Olendzki B, Ma Y, Teas J, Hampl JS. 1998. Nutritional and socioeconomic factors in relation to prostate cancer mortality: a cross-national study. *J Natl Cancer Inst* 90:1637–1647.
8. Wynder EL, Hebert JR, Kabat GC. 1987. Association of dietary fat and lung cancer. *J Natl Cancer Inst* 79:631–637.
9. Haenszel W, Kurihara M. 1968. Studies of Japanese migrants: I. Mortality from cancer and other diseases among Japanese in the United States. *J Natl Cancer Inst* 40:43–68.
10. Hebert JR, Miller DR. 1988. Methodologic considerations for investigating the diet–cancer link. *Am J Clin Nutr* 47:1068–1077.
11. Hebert JR, Ebbeling CB, Matthews CE, Ma Y, Clemow L, Hurley TG, Druker S. 2002. Systematic errors in middle-aged women's estimates of energy intake: comparing three self-report measures to total energy expenditure from doubly labeled water. *Ann Epidemiol* 12:577–586.

12. Doll R, Peto R. 1981. Avoidable risks of cancer in the U.S. *J Natl Cancer Inst* 66(6):1191–1308.

13. American Institute for Cancer Research. 1997. *Food, Nutrition and the Prevention of Cancer: A Global Perspective.* Washington, DC: AICR.

14. U.S. Department of Health and Human Services. 2006. *The Health Consequences of Involuntary Exposure to Tobacco Smoke: A Report of the Surgeon General–Executive Secretary.* Atlanta, GA: USDHHS.

15. Saxe GA, Hebert JR, Carmody JF, Kabat-Zinn J, Rosenzweig PH, Jarzobski D, Reed GW, Blute RD. 2001. Can diet, in conjunction with stress reduction, affect the rate of increase in prostate specific antigen after biochemical recurrence of prostate cancer? *J Urol* 166:2202–2207.

16. Cohen S, Rabin BS. 1998. Psychologic stress, immunity, and cancer. *J Natl Cancer Inst* 1:314.

17. Bovbjerg DH. 1991. Psychoneuroimmunology and psycho-oncology. Presented at Current Concepts in Psycho-Oncology IV, Oct. 10–12, 1991, Memorial Sloan-Kettering Cancer Center, New York.

18. Cooper CL, Faragher EB. 1993. Psychosocial stress and breast cancer: the inter-relationship between stress events, coping strategies and personality. *Psychol Med* 23(3):653–662.

19. Schwartz KL, Crossley-May H, Vigneau FD, Brown K, Banerjee M. 2003. Race, socioeconomic status and stage at diagnosis for five common malignancies. *Cancer Causes Control* 14(8): 761–766.

20. Schoenborn CA, Adams PF, Barnes PM, Vickerie JL, Schiller JS. 2004. Health behaviors of adults: United States, 1999–2001. *Vital Health Stat* 10(219):1–79.

21. Marmot MG. 2006. Status syndrome: a challenge to medicine. *JAMA* 295(11):1304–1307.

22. Hebert JR, Elder K, Ureda JR. 2006. Meeting the challenges of cancer prevention and control in South Carolina: focus on seven cancer sites, engaging partners. *J SC Med Assoc* 102:177–182.

23. Hrushesky WJ. 2000. The temporal organization of life: the impact of multi-frequency non-linear biologic time structure upon the host–cancer balance. *Jpn J Clin Oncol* 30(12):529–533.

24. You S, Wood PA, Xiong Y, Kobayashi M, Du-Quiton J, Hrushesky WJ. 2005. Daily coordination of cancer growth and circadian clock gene expression. *Breast Cancer Res Treat* 91(1):47–60.

25. Hrushesky WJ, Bjarnason GA. 1993. Circadian cancer therapy. *J Clin Oncol* 11(7):1403–1417.

26. Wood PA, Hrushesky WJ. 1996. Circadian rhythms and cancer chemotherapy. *Crit Rev Eukaryot Gene Expr* 6(4):299–343.

27. Jones LA, Chilton JA, Hajek RA, Iammarino NK, Laufman L. 2006. Between and within: international perspectives on cancer and health disparities. *J Clin Oncol* 24(14):2204–2208.

28. Parkin DM. 1989. Cancers of the breast, endometrium and ovary: geographic correlations. *Eur J Cancer Clin Oncol* 25(12):1917–1925.

29. Hill AB. 1953. Observation and experiment. *N Engl J Med* 248:3–9.

30. U.S. Department of Health Education and Welfare. 1964. *Smoking and Health: Report of the Advisory Committee to the Surgeon General of the Public Health Services.* P.H.S. Publ. 1103. Washington, DC: USDHEW.

31. Boyle P, Kevi R, Lucchini F, LaVecchia C. 1993. Trends in diet-related cancers in Japan: a conundrum? *Lancet* 349:752.

32. Wynder E, Fujita Y, Harris R, Hirayama T, Hiyama T. 1991. Comparative epidemiology of cancer between the United States and Japan: a second look. *Cancer* 67:746–763.

33. Tajima D, Tominaga S. 1985. Dietary habits and gastro-intestinal cancers: a comparative case–control study of stomach and large intestinal cancers in Nagoya, Japan. *Jpn J Cancer Res (Gann)* 76:705–716.

34. Sankaranarayanan R, Ramadas K, Thomas G, Muwonge R, Thara S, Mathew B, et al. 2005. Effect of screening on oral cancer mortality in Kerala, India: a cluster-randomized controlled trial. *Lancet* 365(9475):1927–1933.

35. Yen KL, Horner MJD, Reed SG, Daguise VG, Johnson MG, Day TA, Wood PA, Hebert JR. 2006. Head and neck cancer disparities in South Carolina: descriptive epidemiology, early detection, and special programs. *J SC Med Assoc* 102:192–200.

36. Cattaruzza MS, Maisonneuve P, Boyle P. 1996. Epidemiology of laryngeal cancer. *Eur J Cancer Part B Oral Oncol* 32B(5):293–305.

37. Macfarlane GJ, Zheng T, Marshall JR, Boffetta P, Niu S, Brasure J, Merletti F, Boyle P. 1995. Alcohol, tobacco, diet and the risk of oral cancer: a pooled analysis of three case–control studies. *Eur J Cancer Part B Oral Oncol* 31B(3):181–187.

38. Blot WJ, McLaughlin JK, Winn DM, Austin DF, Greenberg RS, Preston-Martin S, Bernstein L, Schoenberg JB, Stemhagen A, Fraumeni JF, Jr. 1998. Smoking and drinking in relation to oral and pharyngeal cancer. *Cancer Res* 48(11):3282–3287.

39. Franceschi S, Talamini R, Barra S, Baron AE, Negri E, Bidoli E, Serraino D, La Vecchia C. 1990. Smoking and drinking in relation to cancers of the oral cavity, pharynx, larynx, and esophagus in northern Italy. *Cancer Res* 50(20):6502–6507.

40. Hebert JR, Kabat GC. 1988. Menthol cigarette smoking and esophageal cancer. *Am J Public Health* 78:986–987.

41. Hebert JR, Kabat GC. 1989. Menthol cigarette smoking and oesophageal cancer: results of a case–control study. *Int J Epidemiol* 18:37–44.

42. Chalasani N, Wo JM, Waring JP. 1998. Racial differences in the histology, location, and risk factors of esophageal cancer. *J Clin Gastroenterol* 26(1):11–13.

43. Nguyen AM, Luke CG, Roder D. 2003. Comparative epidemiological characteristics of oesophageal adenocarcinoma and other cancers of the oesophagus and gastric cardia. *Asian Pac J Cancer Prev* 4(3):225–231.

44. U.S. Cancer Statistics Working Group. 2005. *United States Cancer Statistics: 2002 Incidence and Mortality.* Atlanta, GA: US DHHS/CDC/NIH-NCI.

45. National Cancer Institute. 2004. SEER Cancer Statistics Review, 1975–2001. Bethesda, MD: NCI. (Accessed January 4, 2005, at http://seer.cancer.gov/csr/1975_2001/.)

46. South Carolina Central Cancer Registry Incidence (finalmast2005-statfile) and Mortality (cancermortality9404-statfile). 2006. Office of Public Health Statistics and Information Services, Department of Health and Environmental Control.

47. Stoner GD, Gupta A. 2001. Etiology and chemoprevention of esophageal squamous cell carcinoma. *Carcinogenesis* 22(11):1737–1746.

48. Ahsan H, Neugut AI, Gammon MD. 1997. Association of adenocarcinoma and squamous cell carcinoma of the esophagus with tobacco-related and other malignancies. *Cancer Epidemiol Biomark Prev* 6(10):779–782.

49. Lagergren J, Bergstrom R, Nyren O. 1999. Association between body mass and adenocarcinoma of the esophagus and gastric cardia. *Ann Intern Med* 130(11):883–890.

50. Pera M. 2001. Recent changes in the epidemiology of esophageal cancer. *Surg Oncol* 10(3): 81–90.

51. Shaheen NJ. 2005. Advances in Barrett's esophagus and esophageal adenocarcinoma. *Gastroenterology* 128(6):1554–1566.

52. Coggon D, Barker DJ, Cole RB, Nelson M. 1989. Stomach cancer and food storage. *J Natl Cancer Inst* 81(15):1178–1182.

53. Crew KD, Neugut AI. 2006. Epidemiology of gastric cancer. *World J Gastroenterol* 12(3):354–362.

54. Ashktorab H, Smoot DT, Farzanmehr H, Fidelia-Lambert M, Momen B, Hylind L, Iacosozio-Dononue C, Carethers JM, Goel A, Boland CR, Giardiello FM. 2005. Clinicopathological features and microsatellite instability (MSI) in colorectal cancers from African Americans. *Int J Cancer* 116(6):914–919.

55. Krzystyniak KL. 2002. Current strategies for anticancer chemoprevention and chemoprotection. *Acta Pol Pharm* 59(6):473–478.

56. Vena JE, Graham S, Zielezny M, Swanson MK, Barnes RE, Nolan J. 1985. Lifetime occupational exercise and colon cancer. *Am J Epidemiol* 122(3):357–365.

57. American Cancer Society. 2006. *Cancer Facts and Figures 2005.* Atlanta, GA: ACS.

58. Levin B. 1992. Inflammatory bowel disease and colon cancer. *Cancer* 70(5 Suppl):1313–1316.

59. Rhodes JM, Campbell BJ. 2002. Inflammation and colorectal cancer: IBD-associated and sporadic cancer compared. *Trends Mol Med* 8(1):10–16.

60. Sherman M. 2005. Hepatocellular carcinoma: epidemiology, risk factors, and screening. *Semin Liver Dis.* 25(2):143–154.

61. Lowenfels AB, Maisonneuve P. 2006. Epidemiology and risk factors for pancreatic cancer. *Best Pract Re Clin Gastroenterol* 20(2):197–209.

62. U.S. Department of Health and Human Services. 2004. *The Health Benefits of Smoking Cessation: A Report of the Surgeon General.* Atlanta, GA: Public Health Service, Centers for Disease Control, Center for Chronic Disease Prevention and Health Promotion, Office on Smoking and Health.

63. U.S. Department of Health and Human Services. 1990. CH2, Assessing smoking cessation and its health consequences. *The Health Benefits of Smoking Cessation: A report of the Surgeon General.* DHHS Publication (CDC) 90-8416. Atlanta, GA: Centers for Disease Control, Office on Smoking and Health.

64. Ries LAG, Eisner MP, Kosary CL, Hankey BF, Miller BA, Clegg L, Edwards BK. 2005. *Cancer Statistics Review* 1975–2002. Bethesda, MD: National Cancer Institute.

65. Alberg AJ, Samet JM. 2003. Epidemiology of lung cancer. *Chest* 123(1 Suppl):21S–49S.

66. Muscat JE, Djordjevic MV, Colosimo S, Stellman SD, Richie JP. 2005. Racial differences in exposure and glucuronidation of the tobacco-specific carcinogen 4-(methylnitrosamino)-1-(3-pyridyl)-1-butanone (NNK). *Cancer* 103(7):1420–1426.

67. Geller AC, Annas GD. 2003. Epidemiology of melanoma and nonmelanoma skin cancer. *Sem Oncol Nurs* 19(1):2–11.

68. Hebert JR, Rosen A. 1996. Nutritional, socioeconomic, and reproductive factors in relation to female breast cancer mortality: findings from a cross-national study. *Cancer Detect Prevent* 20:234–244.

69. Buell P. 1973. Changing incidence of breast cancer in Japanese–American women. *J Natl Cancer Inst* 51:1479–1483.

70. Madigan MP, Ziegler RG, Benichou J, Byrne C, Hoover RN. 1995. Proportion of breast cancer cases in the United States explained by well-established risk factors. *J Natl Cancer Inst* 87(22):1681–1685.

71. Adams SA, Hebert JR, Bolick-Aldrich S, Daguise VG, Mosley CM, Modayil MV, Berger SH, Teas J, Mitas M, Cunningham JE, Steck SE, Burch J, Butler WM, Horner MJD, Brandt HM. 2006. Breast cancer disparities in South Carolina: early detection, special programs, and descriptive epidemiology. *JSC Med Assoc* 102:231–239.

72. Cox JT. 2006. The development of cervical cancer and its precursors: What is the role of human papillomavirus infection? *Curr Opin Obstet Gynecol* 18 (Suppl 1):s5–s13.

73. Purdie DM, Green AC. 2001. Epidemiology of endometrial cancer. *Best Pract Res Clin Obstet Gynaecol* 15(3):341–354.

74. Morrison J. 2005. Advances in the understanding and treatment of ovarian cancer. *J Br Menopause Soc* 11(2):66–71.

75. Lukanova, Kaaks R. 2005. Endogenous hormones and ovarian cancer: epidemiology and current hypotheses. *Cancer Epidemiol Biomark Prev* 14(1):98–107.

76. Yatani R, Chigusa I, Akazaki K, Stemmermann GN, Welsh RA, Correa P. 1982. Geographic pathology of latent prostatic carcinoma. *Int J Cancer* 29(6):611–616.

77. Drake BF, Keane TE, Mosley CM, Adams SA, Elder KT, Modayil MV, Ureda JR, Hebert JR. 2006. Prostate cancer disparities in South Carolina: early detection, special programs, and descriptive epidemiology. *JSC Med Assoc* 102:241–249.

78. Schmid H-P, Riesen W, Prikler L. 2004. Update on screening for prostate cancer with prostate-specific antigen. *Crit Rev Oncol Hematol* 50(1):71–78.

79. Sorun PC, Shim J, Chasseigne G, Bonnin-Scaon S, Cogneau J, Mullet E. 2003. Why do primary care physicians in the United States and France order prostate-specific antigen tests for asymptomatic patients? *Med Decision Making* 23:301–313.

80. Shimuzu H, Ross RK, Bernstein L, Yatani R, Henderson BE, Mack TM. 1991. Cancers of the prostate and breast among Japanese and white immigrants to Los Angeles County. *Br J Cancer* 63:963–966.

81. Mettlin C, Selenskas S, Natarajan N, Huben R. 1989. Beta-carotene and animal fats and their relationship to prostate cancer risk: a case–control study. *Cancer* 64:605–612.

82. Carroll KK, Noble RC. 1987. Dietary fat in relation to hormonal induction of mammary and prostate carcinoma in Nb rats. *Carcinogenesis* 81:851–853.

83. Friedenreich CM. 2001. Physical activity and cancer prevention: from observational to intervention research. *Cancer Epidemiol Biomark Prev* 10:287–301.

84. Baillargeon J, Rose DP. 2006. Obesity, adipokines, and prostate cancer. *Int J Oncol* 28(3): 737–745.

85. Garner MJ, Turner MC, Ghadirian P, Krewski D. 2005. Epidemiology of testicular cancer: an overview. *Int J Cancer* 116(3):331–339.

86. Pelucchi C, Bosetti C, Negri E, Malvezzi M, La Vecchia C. 2006. Mechanisms of disease: the epidemiology of bladder cancer. *Nat Clin Pract Urol* 3(6):327–340.

87. Albanes D. 1987. Caloric intake, body weight, and cancer: a review. *Nutr Cancer* 9(4):199–217.

88. Preston DL, Ron E, Yonehara S, Kobuke T, Fujii H, Kishikawa M, Tokunaga M, Tokuoka S, Mabuchi K. 2002. Tumors of the nervous system and pituitary gland associated with atomic bomb radiation exposure. *J Natl Cancer Inst* 94(20):1555–1563.

89. Johnson CC, Spitz MR. 1989. Childhood nervous system tumours: an assessment of risk associated with paternal occupations involving use, repair or manufacture of electrical and electronic equipment. *Int J Epidemiol* 18(4):756–762.

90. Muir CS, Storm HH, Polednak A. 1994. Brain and other nervous system tumours. *Cancer Surveys* 19–20:369–392.

91. Nagataki S, Nystrom E. 2002. Epidemiology and primary prevention of thyroid cancer. *Thyroid* 12(10):889–896.

92. Swerdlow AJ. 2003. Epidemiology of Hodgkin's disease and non-Hodgkin's lymphoma. *Eur J Nuclear Med Mol Imag* 30 (Suppl 1):S3–12.

93. Rinsky RA, Smith AB, Hornung R, Filloon TG, Young RJ, Okun AH, Landrigan PJ. 1987. Benzene and leukemia: an epidemiologic risk assessment. *N Engl J Med* 316(17):1044–1050.

94. Viswanathan M, Ammerman A, Eng E, Gartlehner G, Lohr KN, Griffith D, Rhodes S, Samuel-Hodge C, Matry S, Lux L, Webb L, Sutton SF, Swinson T, Jackman A, Whitener L. 2004. *Community-Based Participatory Research: Assessing the Evidence.* AHRQ Publication 04-E022-1. Rockville, MD: Agency for Healthcare Research and Quality.

14

CONSUMER HEALTH INFORMATION

David Shepro

Biology Department, Boston University, Boston, Massachusetts
Marine Biological Laboratory, Woods Hole, Massachusetts

Catherine N. Norton

MBLWHOI Library, Marine Biological Laboratory,
Woods Hole, Massachusetts

OVERVIEW

In this chapter we immodestly take on the challenge to create a layperson's medical road map with explicit directions for searching and finding databases that provide clear information on cancer prevention, detection, and diagnosis. How to access the most extensive listing of past, present, and future cancer clinical trials is also provided. Since the reader is the starting point, success in selecting an accurate route to the desired information destination will depend in no small measure on your involvement as a "smart traveler."

However, locating an information source alone does not make you a smart traveler. How does the consumer know that the information can be trusted? Some guidelines from the Medical Library Association are provided to help you evaluate a relevant site and to ensure that the information is not a product sales pitch—or worse, that the information is wrong and may be harmful.

The Biology and Treatment of Cancer: Understanding Cancer
Edited by Arthur B. Pardee and Gary S. Stein   Copyright © 2009 John Wiley & Sons, Inc.

1. *Sponsorship.* Can you easily identify who publishes a site? The web address may be helpful: *.gov* tells you that a government agency has responsibility for a site's information; *.edu*, an educational institution; and *.org*, a professional scientific or research entity. Commercial sites have *.com* in the address, and although some of these sell products, many do have credible information. You need to determine who funds a *.com* site.

2. *Currency.* Check to make sure that the site is updated with the newest information about the disease. The dates and the latest revisions are clearly posted, usually at the bottom of the page.

3. *Factual information.* The statements should be factual and not opinions, and easily verifiable from primary information sources such as the professional literature.

4. *Audience.* Look to see if the site is for a health professional or an information consumer. Many sites have materials for both, so be sure to check so as to make a selection with which you are comfortable.

5. *Ethical commitment.* The Health on the Internet Foundation Code of Conduct (HONcode) for medical and health websites (http://www.hon.ch/HONcode/) specifies eight principles intended to hold website developers to basic ethical standards and to make sure that consumers always know the source and purpose of the data they arc reading. Participation is voluntary throughout the world, but sites displaying the foundation's symbol are generally considered credible sources of information. Unfortunately, the number of sites participating is small.

In the presentation, we attempt to adhere to Albert Einstein's admonishment: "Everything should be made as simple as possible, but not simpler."

CONSUMER INFORMATION RETRIEVAL

In the annals of medical practice, never has there been such an extensive direct linkage of patients (*consumers*) to medical information as exists at present. Newspapers, magazines, and television advertise drug information, almost indiscriminately, direct to consumers. In addition there is on line prescription shopping. The frequently used headline, "Ask Your Doctor" is followed by an A-to-Z list: Alzheimer's, breast cancer, elevated cholesterol, erectile dysfunction, migraine, rheumatism. But even these commercial ventures are but the proverbial drop in the bucket compared to the information on *patient-centered health care* available free on the Internet. Now that patients are regarded as active consumers, they also take on the responsibility of decision making for their own and their family's health care. This requires new health literacy and new skills to access the literature. And therein lays a problem.

"Information" [gathering, storing, retrieving, evaluating] is the second-largest industry worldwide, surpassed only by the manufacture of machinery for waging wars. In medicine, the global growth is at the speed of light (there are over 26,000 clinical journals alone). Where does all this information come from? Major sources beyond commercial publications are books, libraries, librarians, physician records, patient records, government documents, websites, and for most diseases there are national organizations that communicate tailored, updated medical information. For nonprofessionals who seek information, insight, and help with a disease, navigating the paper and electronic literature, vast beyond imagination and frequently highly technical, can be a major hurdle. The largest percentage of persons seeking information are those who, randomly and intermittently, wish to learn about minor issues such as headaches, weight gain or loss, and skin care. Those with chronic ailments are the most regular seekers of health information. The beginners are usually persons newly diagnosed with a serious health condition. Regardless of which group you fall into, the steps for self-teaching, self-improvement, and continuing education, beyond "googlelization," are similar.

The cornerstone to becoming a wise and active health consumer is motivation. Once you jump-start an initiative *to know*, you will find many avenues to target information. By far the most heavily used resource today is the Internet. [Currently there are between 15 and 30 billion web pages and over 1 billion Internet users. On one Sunday alone (2/25/07), 100 million users were clocked on Pandia Search Engine News.] You can zero-in on a specific drug that will list benefits, use, and cautions; listen and see professionals discuss diagnosis and treatments; join support groups and hear stories from others who have similar health problems; and learn strategies for choosing proper providers and hospitals. The bottom line is that all this information will help you to (1) learn valuable details about a disease, (2) understand how quality care is measured, and (3) assess the quality of health care you are receiving so that you can make informed decisions.

Be wary—market research has shown that very attractive websites are used more often than ones that do not have flash and dazzle that attract attention. A sensible first place to start your search, if you have been diagnosed or someone in your family has been diagnosed, is to ask your doctor where to look. Many studies are available that describe how physicians handle patients who come armed with Internet information. Two examples are:

- Potts HWW, Wyatt JC. Survey of doctors' experience of patients using the Internet. *J Med Internet Res* 2002;4(1):e5; http://www.jmir.org/2002/1/e5/.
- Ahmad F, Hudak PL, Bercovitz K, Hollenberg E, Levinson W. Are physicians ready for patients with Internet-based health information? *J Med Internet Res* 2006:8(3):e22; http://www.jmir.org/2006/3/e22/.

Interaction between the informed patient and the physician will be more "helpful" and less challenging if the patient and his or her advocates use trusted

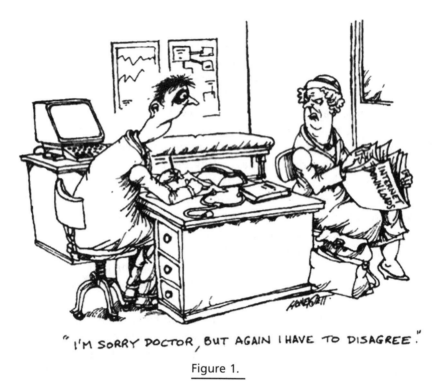

"I'M SORRY DOCTOR, BUT AGAIN I HAVE TO DISAGREE."

Figure 1.

information sources on the Internet (Figure 14.1). In the last analysis, the consensus by health providers is that the benefits of searching for information outweigh the problems that physicians voice about Internet information.

The very large hospitals all have websites with plentiful information. Many have separate pages for the beginning search on all varieties of cancer: bone marrow transplant, breast cancer, cutaneous cancer, gastrointestinal cancer, genitourinary cancer, gynecologic cancer, head and neck cancer, metabolic oncology, hematology, neurological cancer, pain and palliative care, pathology, psychosocial oncology, radiology, radiation oncology, sarcoma, and thoracic cancer. "Surviving cancer" types of sites will provide a patient with a place to start to collect information before moving on to more detailed information.

What is detailed or full information? Some of the components that make up a full complement of information about the disease that is affecting the patient are stored in a variety of places. For example, patient data collected in a health care setting include diagnosis, lab tests, and treatment regimen. All of these bits of information are helpful. Increasingly many hospitals are making all information available through a patient record system that allows patients to view their own health records, such as the Beth Israel/Deaconess Hospital in Boston (http://bidmc.harvard.edu). These personal patient sites (https://www.patientsite.org/) provide appointment schedules, doctors involved, financial accounts, referrals, test results, and complete medical records. The patient can learn about her or his current condition; the etiology, diagnosis, prognosis, and therapies that are available; and risk factors. There are also links to learning centers about diseases, drug information, exercise and fitness programs, and medical dictionaries to decipher the medical jargon.

Information Sources and Retrieval

Patient records, hospital records, insurance records, scientific articles, books, and bedside practice reports by caregivers are major suppliers of information. Although we are in the "Google" generation of access, a serious problem is that the availability of high-quality information is not always in the open-access arena. Many journal articles in the scientific literature are only accessible through institutional subscriptions in hospital libraries, clinical research settings, and universities. Moreover, the prices of these subscriptions have increased well beyond inflation and certainly beyond the financial value to the lay consumer. Not all institutions provide access to this literature or patient's records. Nevertheless, your health care professional can help you to find open-access publications that are available for unrestricted use, distribution, and reproduction (provided that the original work is cited properly). The "Public Library of Science Medicine" is an example of a publication by authors who place their article in an open-access journal so that it is freely available over the Internet. These publications are also able to be archived in institutions repositories, such as PubMed-Central.gov, whose mission is to archive this information and make it freely available over the Internet for generations to come. There are many players in the open-access movement apart from physicians, such as librarians, scientists, publishers, funding agencies, legislators, and consumer groups. In the last analysis, the consensus by health providers is that the benefits of searching for information outweigh the problems.

Many websites stay active for very short periods of time. A report aired by the Kansas Public Radio in October 2006 notes that in two years, the average life of a website diminishes drastically: One-half of the *.com* sites are lost, one-third of the *.edu* sites are gone, and one-tenth of the *.gov.* sites disappear, so you must keep a critical eye on the websites and their longevity. Listed below are 14 sites that have longevity and credibility.

1. http://medlineplus.gov is the most-trusted authoritative source for quality and accuracy of content for health information most suitable for the nonprofessional. This site is a service of the U.S. National Library of Medicine (NLM), National Institutes of Health (NIH). The primary purpose is educational, and the information is current and consistently available. There are many special features on this site, such as diagrams, a glossary, health news, links to videos, tutorials and e-mail updates, and Really Simple Syndication (RSS) feeds to keep you up to date on the latest information on

your particular clinical interest. This site also features the local resources for health-related issues, libraries, organizations, and international sites from Canada and Australia. Also provided is information on care giving and advocacy from the National Rehabilitation Information Center.

2. The NLM also provides a database on clinical trials (http://www.clinical-trials.gov). This site provides information about federally funded and privately supported clinical research with human volunteers. You can find information on whether a clinical trial is still open for volunteers, how to participate, the different types of cancer trials, explanations of informed consent, placebo groups, past trial results, and future trials. For the latter, the site provides contact information, dates, location, eligibility, and other pertinent information. The Cancer Trials from the National Cancer Institute (NCI) are the U.S government's focal point for clinical trials on cancers: http://www.cancer.gov/clinicaltrials/.

3. NCI Clinical Trials Education Series provides publications, such as self-paced workbooks, slide programs on CD-ROM, booklets, and videos, for individuals and health care professionals to understand clinical trials: http://www.nci.nih.gov/clinicaltrials/resources/clinical-trials-education-series.

4. The Veterans Administration and NCI provide information on their inter-agency partnership agreement in clinical trials for cancer especially valuable to veterans: http://www.va.gov/cancer/.

5. The U.S. Food and Drug Administration (FDA) Cancer Liaison Program, Office of Special Health Issues with NCI, answers questions directed to FDA by participants, their families, and participant advocates about therapies for life-threatening diseases: http://www.fda.gov/oashi/cancer/cancer.html.

6. National Cancer Institute, Office of Liaison Activities, "Understanding NCI: Toll-Free Teleconference Series": http://ola.cancer.gov/activities/teleconferences.

7. The other area of research that is important to these trails is the Information of Bioethics sites from the Office of Extramural Research (OER), NIH. OER provides information on policies and regulations, Institutional Review Board resources, guidance for clinical investigators, research resources, and courses and tutorials on bioethical issues in human studies: http://www.nih.gov/sigs/bioethics/.

8. The NLM compiled a comprehensive bibliography from 1989 through November 1998, "Ethical Issues in Research Involving Human Partici-pants": http://www.nlm.nih.gov/archive/20061214/pubs/cbm/hum_exp.html.

9. U.S. Department of Health and Human Services (HHS) Office of Human Research Protection (OHRP). OHRP provides a guide and training materi-als on regulations and procedures governing research with human subjects and includes a guidance document on financial relationships in clinical research: http://www.hhs.gov/ohrp/.

10. Worthy of repetition are two valuable and important websites for non-health professionals: MedlinePlus.gov and Clinical Trials: http://www.nlm.nih.gov/medlineplus/clinicaltrials.html. An other site that lists clinical trials is the Thompson Site Center Watch, a Clinical Trials Listing Service that includes more than 41,000 active industry- and government-sponsored clinical trials, as well as new drug therapies in research. Center Watch covers clinical research worldwide and is an open site: http://www.centerwatch.com/.

11. Genetic Home Reference (http://ghr.nlm.nih.gov/) is a consumer-friendly web resource about the effects of genetic variations and information about the genes associated with those conditions. If you search for breast cancer on this site, it explains how these cancers could be caused by mutation in particular genes, such as *BRCA1* or *BRCA2* and variations of the *ATM*, *BRCA1*, *BRCA2*, *CHEK2*, and *RAD51* genes, which increase the risk of developing breast cancer. This web resource is a great help in understanding basic genetic principles.

12. Cancercare (http://www.cancercare.org) is dedicated to helping advanced cancer patients and their families and friends. Many of the publications are in Spanish and Russian and deal with a wide range of cancer topics. This site provides free professional support services to anyone affected by cancer and has a number of publications and telephone workshops on medical, emotional, and practical concerns, along with some online counseling.

13. Many universities have a website that deals with the treatment of cancer, one example being, ONCOLINK from the University of Pennsylvania: http://www.oncolink.upenn.edu. This site has information on types of cancer, treatment, coping, care plans, and so on.

14. Memorial Sloan Kettering Cancer Center (http://www.mskcc.org) is one of the most extensive websites, with menus for each type of cancers that gives an overview, risk factors, screening, diagnosis, surgery, systemic therapy, radiation therapy, clinical trials, and survivorship and support information.

Top Cancer Websites Recommended by the Medical Library Association

Not withstanding the redundancy, the reader may be interested in another evaluation, a list by librarians from the Medical Library Association (MLA). The MLA has issued a guide that helps identify health information on the web that is credible, timely, and safe: http://www.mlanet.org/resources/userguide.html. Anyone searching for information using their favorite search engine (e.g., Google, Yahoo) knows that a simple search on "cancer" will bring up an overwhelming number of "hits." By simply learning to use their advance search capabilities and combining terms such as "breast cancer" and "drug therapy" will return a more precise list of hits. Librarians also recommend that you look at the general health information–finding tools, such as MEDLINEPLUSMEDLINEPLUS (http://www.medlineplus.gov), produced by the National Library of Medicine, or Healthfinder (http://www.healthfinder.gov) from the HSS, which can get you started by pointing you to good, credible health information quickly. These librarians search the web everyday for good-quality information that is safe and reliable, so their list of sites is a "trusted information source."

Since most of the health-related information that you do find from credible sources is highly technical, the MLA has published a "Deciphering Medspeak" brochure, which you can obtain by sending an e-mail to info@mlahq.org.

1. The American Cancer Society (http://www.cancer.org/) supports education and research in cancer prevention, diagnosis, detection, and treatment. The web pages provide news, information on types of cancer, patient services, treatment options, sections on children with cancer and living with cancer, and cancer statistics. The site is also available in Spanish.

2. The Association of Cancer Online Resources (http://www.acor.org/) has a mission to provide "varied and credible" information to cancer patients and those who care for them through the "creation and maintenance of cancer-related Internet mailing lists and web-based resources." ACOR currently offers access to nearly 100 public e-mail cancer support groups as well as ACOR-supported websites.

3. Cancer Care, Inc. (http://www.cancercare.org/) is a nonprofit organization "whose mission is to provide free professional help to people with all cancers through counseling, education, information and referral, and direct financial assistance." The site maintains links to support, educational, treatment, and information services. Information is also available in Spanish.

4. CancerNet–National Cancer Institute (http://cancer.gov/cancer_information/), produced by the National Cancer Institute of the National Institutes of Health, provides information on types of cancer; treatment options; clinical trials; genetics, causes, risk factors, and prevention; testing; coping, and support resources. It also provides free access to the PDQ and Cancerlit databases. The site is also available in Spanish.

5. Families of Children with Cancer (http://www.fcco.org/resources.html), located in Toronto, Canada, is a support and advocacy group for families living with the effects of childhood cancer. The web page has a wide variety of links to Internet information sources on pediatric cancer, including basic information, treatment and research centers, community organizations, personal web pages, and a chat support line.

6. The Intercultural Cancer Council (http://iccnetwork.org), produced at the Texas Medical Center in Houston, has as its goal the elimination of "the unequal burden of cancer among racial and ethnic minorities and medically underserved populations in the United States." It provides news, press releases, links to cancer information sites, and a calendar of upcoming events.

7. Oncolink (http://oncolink.upenn.edu/) is a collection of Internet resources on the prevention and treatment of cancer maintained by the University of Pennsylvania Cancer Center. The site includes news, book reviews, and disease and patient support links.

8. Women's Cancer Network (http://www.wcn.org/) is the official site of the Gynecologic Cancer Foundation: physicians "dedicated to preventing, detecting and conquering cancer in women." It has information on the organization, the types of cancer that affect women, cancer risks for women, and a search engine to locate gynecologic oncologists. There are also links to related sites, publications, and support groups.

CONCLUDING REMARKS

There is a wealth of available information to assist you in making personal and family health-related decisions (not surprisingly, 80% of all health decisions are made by women). The benefits of being an active consumer exceed the difficulties. People who stay in the health-learning mode fare better clinically, are less depressed by their illness, require less hospitalization, are more comfortable in participating in care, and have financial savings. "A journey of a thousand miles starts with the first step." We optimistically anticipate that this chapter will help to make you a *smart traveler.*

Caveat: As expected, no system is without flaws, and caution and conservatism are highly recommended in decision making. There is no simple solution for the consumer to separate the "good" from the "bad." Nor is it any consolation that even highly trained professionals face a similar situation. Data are never wrong, but interpretations are not always foolproof. General and even health literacy is no guarantee that you will understand the language on a prescription or on a consent form. What if you are faced with a decision related to a new treatment or a new diagnosis? Our advice is to question … question … question! Do not shy from asking your physician, nurse, therapist, and pharmacist about any clinical or financial aspect that you do not understand clearly. Remember, it is far, far better to be embarrassed than to be sorry.

INDEX